Human Lymphoma:
Clinical Implications of the REAL Classification

Springer
London
Berlin
Heidelberg
New York
Barcelona
Hong Kong
Milan
Paris
Santa Clara
Singapore
Tokyo

HUMAN LYMPHOMA:
Clinical Implications of the
REAL Classification

Edited by
David Y Mason and Nancy Lee Harris

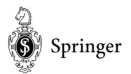
Springer

David Y Mason, Professor of Cellular Pathology, University of Oxford
John Radcliffe Hospital, Oxford, UK

Nancy Lee Harris, Professor of Pathology, Director of Anatomic Pathology
Department of Pathology, Massachusetts General Hospital, Boston, MA., U.S.A.

ISBN 1-85233-129-1 Springer-Verlag London Berlin Heidelberg

British Library Cataloguing in Publication Data
Human lymphoma:clinical implications of the REAL classification
   I. Lymphomas
   I. Mason, David Y. II. Harris, Nancy L.
   616.9´9446
   ISBN 1852331291

Library of Congress Cataloging-in-Publication Data
Human lymphoma: clinical implications of the REAL classification/
   David Y. Mason and Nancy Harris (Eds).
       p.   cm
    Includes bibliographical references and index.
    ISBN 1-85233-129-1 (alk. paper)
    I. Lymphomas—classification—Congresses. I. Mason, D. Y. II. Harris, Nancy L.
    [DNLM: 1. Lymphoma, Non-Hodgkin—classification congresses.
    2. Hodgkin Disease—classification congresses. WH 15 H918 1999]
   RC280.L9H86 1999
   616.99´446´0012—dc21
   DNLM/DLC
   for Library of Congress   98-49714

Typeset by the Medical Informatics Unit
Nuffield Department of Clinical Biochemistry and Cellular Science, University of Oxford, United Kingdom
Printed and bound by Kyodo Printing Company (S'pore) PTE Ltd, Singapore
28/3830-543210 Printed on acid-free paper

Acknowledgment

This book was prepared and typeset in the Nuffield Department of Biochemistry and Cellular Science, University of Oxford by Beata Ozieblowska, Robin Roberts-Gant and Bridget Watson to whom we are indebted for the very extensive work involved.

We would also like to thank Kingsley Micklem and Ellie Parker for recording the contents of the meeting on which this book is based, and all the authors for their contribution to this project.

Foreword

"Nowhere in pathology has a chaos of names so
clouded clear concepts as in the subject of lymphoid
tumors."

Willis R.A.: *Pathology of Tumors*, Mosby 1948

This quotation from one of the most experienced histopathologists of his day indicates the near incomprehensibility of the nomenclature of lymphoid neoplasms half a century ago, and this unsatisfactory state of affairs persisted for many years. This was as much because of the lack of therapeutic options for the treatment of lymphomas – which meant that there was little incentive to categorize them – as because of their morphologic complexity. It was not until Rappaport's classification appeared in the 1960s that some order began to emerge from the chaos. However, no sooner had this scheme achieved widespread acceptance than the Kiel and Lukes/Collins schemes appeared in the mid-1970s, in response to new immunologic data on lymphoid cell differentiation, and these schemes differed not only from the Rappaport scheme but from each other. One reason for these and subsequent discrepancies was disagreement about the preferred "gold standard" for defining different categories. The Rappaport classification was based on growth pattern and cell size, whereas the Kiel and Lukes/Collins schemes related lymphoma types to normal cellular counterparts in the immune system. Yet a third "gold standard" – clinical outcome – was introduced by the Working Formulation. This was a proposal, published in 1982, that aimed to help oncologists deal with discrepancies between classifications.

The limitations of the Working Formulation were soon evident, but more so to pathologists, who faced the problem of using it, than to oncologists, who were often unaware of these practical difficulties. In consequence, the first major development in the understanding of lymphoma following the Working Formulation came from a group of hematopathologists, the International Lymphoma Study Group (ILSG), who published the Revised European American Lymphoma (REAL) classification in 1994. The REAL scheme dispensed with the idea of a single criterion for defining disease entities, and instead used any available data – morphologic, immunologic, genetic and clinical – to define distinct disease entities. The relative importance of individual criteria varied between diseases, and there was no single "gold standard".

Initial reactions were mixed: although the REAL scheme set out very clearly the different categories of lymphoma, the list was nevertheless a substantial one, comprising more than twenty five entities, and also some provisional categories. In consequence, there was some resistance to its use from physicians who recalled the heated debate among pathologists in the past in response to the earlier classification schemes. However, pathologists with experience of lymphoma soon realized that the REAL scheme matched well with their everyday practical experience, and it gained wide acceptance.

It was against this background that a meeting was held with the aim of presenting the REAL scheme to an audience of both pathologists and oncologists, and to consider its impact on the practical management of lymphoma. The meeting was organized by Dr. Nancy Lee Harris of Massachusetts General Hospital, the lead author of the initial description of the REAL classification, together with Dr. Bruce Chabner, Clinical Director of the Massachusetts General Hospital Cancer Center, and it was held in Boston in March 1996. The pathologic features of each disease were presented by members of the ILSG from the US and Europe, and expert oncologists from US and Europe were invited to present clinical features and address problems and new advances in therapy. The audience consisted approximately equally of pathologists and oncologists.

The proceedings of that meeting are presented in this volume. The text is taken directly from the transcript of the meeting, and the numerous figures represent the transparencies shown by the speakers. Unlike many other publications on lymphoma, the chapters include descriptions of both histopathologic and clinical aspects of different disease categories.

An important issue specifically addressed by this meeting was whether the different entities identified in the REAL scheme should be assigned to clinical groupings. The Kiel scheme, which has been widely used in Europe and can be seen as the direct precursor to the REAL classification, grouped non-Hodgkin's lymphoma into two broad categories (low and high grade), but this was based on cell morphology, without data on clinical behavior. The Working Formulation, the scheme widely used in the United States, grouped lymphomas into three grades, but relied on clinical behavior rather than morphologic features. This volume explores the debate on whether the entities in the REAL scheme should also be grouped according to clinical behavior. However, it should be added that since the time of the meeting, there has been a general consensus that such clinical grouping should be avoided, and that each lymphoma category needs to be considered as a unique entity, with a specific clinical pattern of presentation and response to therapy.

One of the presentations (Chapter 3) refers to the "Non-Hodgkin's Lymphoma Classification Project" of Dr. Armitage and his collaborators, that aimed to validate the REAL scheme; the first results have now been published.[1] In this project a group of pathologists, only one of whom had been involved in formulating the REAL scheme, reviewed a large series of lymphoma biopsies from patients on whom there was clinical data. The results demonstrated the reproducibility of the REAL classification and also documented important differences in the clinical behavior of many of the diseases.[2]

This book illustrates the multifaceted nature of lymphoid neoplasia. The meeting raised as many questions as it offered answers. On the clinical side the treatment of mantle cell lymphoma was highlighted as an ongoing challenge, as is an understanding of the optimal approach to the management of MALT lymphomas, where antibiotics, chemotherapy and surgery all have a role to play. Uncertainties also remain on the histopathologic front, despite the great advance represented by the REAL scheme. The diagnostic borderline between Hodgkin's disease and anaplastic large cell lymphoma, for example, represents one area requiring further investigation, as does the controversial category "Burkitt-like" lymphoma.

Thus the REAL scheme provides the setting for a better understanding of lymphoid neoplasms, but it will be many years before all the major current questions have been resolved. The process of lymphoma classification will never end, as long as new data continue to emerge. Since this meeting in Boston, an update of the REAL classification has been in progress under the auspices of the World Health Organisation. This has been a joint project of the two major hematopathology bodies (the American Society and European Association) and, mindful of the initial reactions to the REAL scheme, there has been ongoing interaction between pathologists and clinicians during the development of this updated classification. Such dialog is essential to avoid the confusions of the past, and the contents of this book are very much an embodiment of that spirit.

David Y. Mason   Nancy Lee Harris

REFERENCES

1. The Non-Hodgkin's Lymphoma Classification Project. A clinical evaluation of the International Lymphoma Study Group classification of non-Hodgkin's lymphoma. *Blood* 1997; **89**: 3909-18.

2. Armitage JO, Weisenburger DD. New approach to classifying non-Hodgkin's lymphomas: clinical features of the major histologic subtypes. *J Clin Oncol* 1998; **16**: 2780-95.

Contents

Section 3   High Grade Non-Hodgkin's Lymphoma

Contributors

James O. Armitage, M.D.
Department of Internal Medicine,
University of Nebraska Medical Center,
Omaha, NE,
U.S.A.

Peter M. Banks, M.D.
Carolinas Medical Center,
Charlotte, NC,
U.S.A.

Fernando Cabanillas, M.D.
Dept. of Lymphoma-Myeloma
M.D. Anderson Cancer Center,
The University of Texas,
Houston, TX,
U.S.A.

George P. Canellos, M.D.
Dana-Farber Cancer Institute,
Boston, MA,
U.S.A.

Bertrand Coiffier, M.D.
Service Hématologie,
Centre Hospitalier Lyon-Sud,
Pierre-Bénite,
FRANCE

C. Norman Coleman, M.D.
Joint Center for Radiation Therapy,
Boston, MA,
U.S.A.

Richard I. Fisher, M.D.
Cardinal Bernardin Cancer Center,
Loyola University School of Medicine,
Maywood, IL,
U.S.A.

Arnold S. Freedman, M.D.
Dana-Farber Cancer Institute,
Boston, MA,
U.S.A.

Thomas M. Grogan, M.D.
Department of Pathology,
University of Arizona Health Sciences Center,
Tucson, AZ,
U.S.A.

Nancy Lee Harris, M.D.
Department of Pathology,
Massachusetts General Hospital,
Boston, MA,
U.S.A.

Wolfgang Hiddemann, M.D.
Department of Internal Medicine III,
University Hospital Grosshadern,
Ludwig-Maximilians-University,
Munich,
GERMANY

Sandra J. Horning, M.D.
Division of Oncology,
Stanford University Medical Center,
Palo Alto, CA,
U.S.A.

Peter G. Isaacson, M.D.
Department of Pathology,
University College London Medical School,
London,
UK

Elaine S. Jaffe, M.D.
Laboratory of Pathology,
National Cancer Institute,
Bethesda, MD,
U.S.A.

Marshall E. Kadin, M.D.
Department of Pathology,
Beth Israel Hospital,
Boston, MA,
U.S.A.

Daniel M. Knowles, M.D.
Cornell University Medical College,
New York, NY,
U.S.A.

Peter Koch, M.D.
Westfälische Wilhelms-Universität Münster,
Onkolog.-hämatologische Ambulanz,
Münster,
GERMANY

Peter M. Mauch, M.D.
Department of Radiation Oncology,
Brigham and Women's Hospital,
Dana-Farber Cancer Institute,
Joint Center for Radiation Therapy,
Boston, MA,
U.S.A.

David T. Scadden, M.D.
Massachusetts General Hospital,
Dana-Farber/Partners CancerCare
Boston, MA,
U.S.A.

Margaret A. Shipp, M.D.
Dana-Farber Cancer Institute,
Boston, MA,
U.S.A.

Lawrence N. Shulman, M.D.
Dana-Farber Cancer Institute,
Department of Adult Oncology,
Boston, MA,
U.S.A.

Harald Stein, M.D.
Institut für Pathologie
Universitätsklinikum Benjamin Franklin,
Freie Universität Berlin,
Berlin,
GERMANY

Roger A. Warnke, M.D.
Department of Pathology,
Stanford University Medical Center,
Stanford, CA,
U.S.A.

Howard J. Weinstein, M.D.
Pediatric Hematology/Oncology,
Massachusetts General Hospital,
Boston, MA,
U.S.A.

Wyndham H. Wilson, M.D.
Division of Clinical Sciences,
National Cancer Institute, N.I.H.,
Bethesda, MD,
U.S.A.

Introduction and rationale for the REAL classification

N L Harris

The purpose of this meeting is to introduce pathologists and oncologists, both practising and academic, to the new "REAL" lymphoma classification, and specifically to look at the clinical significance of the lymphoma subtypes that it recognizes.

There have been problems in lymphoma classification for many years [1.1]. These came to a head in the 1970s when six new classifications were proposed, and for a time four classifications were in use in various parts of the world, including those of Rappaport, Lukes and Collins, Kiel and the BNLI. This led to great confusion and difficulty when attempting to interpret the results of clinical studies in different parts of the world.

1.1	**Problems in Lymphoma Classification**

1970's: 4 classifications used
- Rappaport (US)
- Lukes-Collins (US)
- Kiel (Europe)
- BNLI (Britain)

Meetings and NCI-sponsored study: no consensus

1980's: 2 classifications used
- Working Formulation (1982) - US
- Kiel classification (1974, 1988) - Europe

During the 1970s a number of meetings held among pathologists in both the US and Europe failed to arrive at a consensus on classification. This culminated in a study, sponsored by the American National Cancer Institute, of 1,200 patients throughout the world, aimed at reaching at a consensus among pathologists on the best way to classify lymphomas. However, this effort also failed to produce a consensus, and resulted in the Working Formulation, which was designed to translate between existing classifications but which rapidly became a free-standing classification. By the 1980s we had a situation in which two classifi-

cations were widely used, the Working Formulation in the US, and the Kiel classification in many parts of Europe.

The lack of a consensus among pathologists on uniform terminology and definitions caused continuing problems in interpreting clinical trials, and the credibility of pathologists among their clinical colleagues suffered [1.2]. In the US, for instance, many oncologists came to believe that the pathologic classification of lymphomas was largely irrelevant and were only interested in Working Formulation prognostic groups. Adding to the confusion, many new disease identities were described during the 1980s which were not clearly defined in either of the existing classifications. This led to uncertainty among both pathologists and oncologists as to which, if any, of these newly defined entities were real diseases that they should recognize in their daily practice. At the same time, the definition of some of the older disease categories was modified, on the basis of new immunologic or genetic data, and this too led to uncertainty as to which of these criteria were important in defining a disease entity.

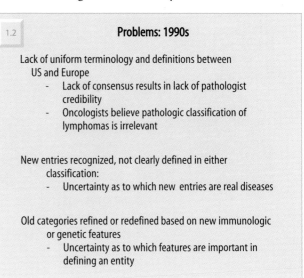

1.2	**Problems: 1990s**

Lack of uniform terminology and definitions between US and Europe
- Lack of consensus results in lack of pathologist credibility
- Oncologists believe pathologic classification of lymphomas is irrelevant

New entries recognized, not clearly defined in either classification:
- Uncertainty as to which new entries are real diseases

Old categories refined or redefined based on new immunologic or genetic features
- Uncertainty as to which features are important in defining an entity

In the early 1990s, it became apparent to many of us at meetings around the world that there was in fact remarkable agreement among experienced hematopathologists about the disease entities that we recognized with available techniques in our daily practice and which appeared to be distinct clinical entities. However, it was clear that a consensus was needed on the definitions and criteria for diagnosis of these diseases, including the relative roles of morphology, immunophenotype, genetic aspects and clinical features. It seemed to us that an appropriate classification for the 1990s could be created by listing the disease entities that pathologists were actually diagnosing in their daily practice; what pathologists actually do, not what they hypothetically should be doing [1.3].

The International Lymphoma Study Group (ILSG) decided to address this problem. The ILSG is an informal group that comprised at the time 19 hematopathologists from the US, Europe, and Asia, which had started meeting annually to discuss problems in lymphoma diagnosis and issues of mutual interest [1.4]. This group gathered in Berlin in 1993 for a three day meeting to see if we could agree on the disease categories to be recognized in a consensus lymphoma classification. At this meeting we found surprisingly little difficulty in reaching agreement and our conclusions were subsequently published as a "Revised European American Classification of Lymphoid Neoplasms" in the fall of 1994. Some of the basic principles of this classification are reviewed in the following pages.

First, we decided to include all lymphoid neoplasms, including non-Hodgkin's lymphomas, lymphoid leukemias and Hodgkin's disease [1.5]. The reasons for this are two-fold: first, lymphomas and lymphoid leukemias are really not distinct diseases. The same tumor may have both a solid and circulating phase, and separating them according to their mode of presentation is artificial and can lead to confusion. Second, it is now recognized that Hodgkin's disease is lymphoid in origin, at least in the vast majority of cases, and that borderline cases can therefore exist between Hodgkin's disease and non-Hodgkin's lymphomas.

1.3   **Lymphoma Classification: Now**

There is a remarkable agreement among hematopathologists about the entities that can be recognized with available techniques, which appear to be distinct clinical entities

Consensus needed on definitions and criteria for diagnosis, including the roles of

     Morphology
     Immunophenotype
     Genetic features
     Clinical features

Classification = List of "REAL" Diseases
What pathologists **do**, not what they **should** do

1.4   **A Revised European-American Classification of Lymphoid Neoplasms**
A Proposal from the International Lymphoma Study Group

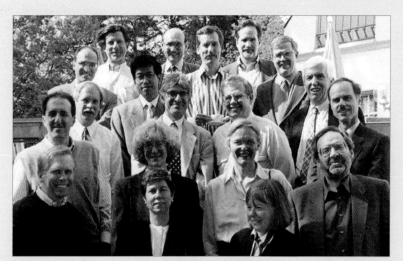

Nancy Harris	-	Boston
Elaine Jaffe	-	Bethesda
Harald Stein	-	Berlin
Peter Banks	-	San Antonio
John Chan	-	Hong Kong
Michael Cleary	-	Stanford
Georges Delsol	-	Toulouse
Chris De Wolf-Peeters	-	Leuven
Brunangelo Falini	-	Perugia
Kevin Gatter	-	Oxford
Thomas Grogan	-	Tucson
Peter Isaacson	-	London
Daniel Knowles	-	Cornell
David Mason	-	Oxford
Konrad Müller-Hermelink	-	Würzburg
Stefano Pileri	-	Bologna
Miguel Piris	-	Toledo
Elizabeth Ralfkiaer	-	Copenhagen
Roger Warnke	-	Stanford

ILSG MEETING - BERLIN 1993

Lymphoma Classification. The Nuffield Department of Clinical Biochemistry and Cellular Science, University of Oxford

Harris *et al.* 1994 [1]

1.5   **Major Categories**

Include all lymphoid neoplasms:

- Non-Hodgkin's lymphomas, lymphoid leukemias
    Hodgkin's disease
- Separation of lymphomas and lymphoid leukemias
    is artificial
- Hodgkin's disease is lymphoid in origin; borderline
    cases exist

Morphology remains the principal basis for this lymphoma classification, and in fact in many cases morphology alone is sufficient for diagnosis. However, immunologic and genetic features play an important role in the definition of many disease entities [1.6]. In fact it was the availability of these relatively objective criteria that finally made a consensus among pathologists in the 1990s that had not been possible in the 1970s, when only subjective morphologic criteria were available.

1.6   **Classification of Lymphoid Neoplasms: Principles**

Morphology
- Principal basis for classification
- Often sufficient for diagnosis

Immunology and genetics
- Important part of the definition of a disease entity
- Not required for diagnosis in every case
- Often useful in differential diagnosis
- Improve reproducibility

Clinical features
- Constellation of clinical features is part of the definition
    of an entity
- Mode of presentation (nodal, extranodal) often
    important in diagnosis

Immunophenotype, and particularly, genetic features are not required for the diagnosis in every case, but they are often useful in the differential diagnosis of difficult cases, and they clearly improve inter-observer reproducibility. An important and novel feature of this approach to classification is recognition that the constellation of clinical features in the patient is an important part of the definition of the disease entity, and that the mode of presentation, for example nodal versus extra-nodal, is also often important for correct diagnosis.

At the 1993 Berlin meeting the issues of "grade" and "aggressiveness" were also discussed [1.7]. The term "grade" has created confusion in recent years because it has been used differently in the Kiel classification and the Working Formulation. In the Kiel scheme it refers to histologic grade, irrespective of clinical behavior, whereas in the Working Formulation it refers to the prognostic group as defined by patient survival. We felt that the term "grade" should be restricted to histologic grade, as it is for other tumor categories (based on cytologic features and features such as the proliferation fraction). The terms "prognostic group" or "clinical aggressiveness" can be used to indicate the known or predicted clinical behavior of the neoplasm, which often, but not always, correlates with histologic grade.

1.7   **Grade and Aggressiveness**

Histologic grade:
- Cytologic features, proliferation

Clinical aggressiveness / prognostic group:
- Known or predicted clinical behavior
- Usually, but not always, correlates with histologic grade

It is important to realize that lymphomas do not constitute a continuous spectrum of disease, with a range of histologic grade and clinical aggressiveness, but in fact represent many different diseases [1.8]. In some instances these are quite unrelated to one another, so it is really not possible or useful to sort these diverse entities according to a spectrum of histologic grade and clinical aggressiveness. In addition, within many of the lymphoma entities, a range of histologic grade and clinical aggressiveness can be found, as we recognize for follicular lymphoma. Therefore, it is impractical simply to sort entities into low, intermediate and high grade categories. Instead we have to get to know each disease entity and to recognize its spectrum of morphology and clinical behavior.

1.8   **Grade and Aggressiveness in Classification**

Lymphomas are not a continuous spectrum of related diseases;
    they are many different diseases

Many distinct lymphoma entities have a range of histologic grade
    and clinical aggressiveness

Impractical to sort entities simply into low, intermediate and high
    grade categories

Must "get to know" each entity and its spectrum of clinical behavior

---

Another issue that the ILSG discussed was the relationship between lymphomas and their normal counterparts [1.9]. This is clearly an important conceptual basis for a lymphoma classification, as it is for any tumor classification, and the normal counterparts for many lymphoma subtypes are known. However, the normal counterpart is not known for some well defined entities, for example hairy cell leukemia, and for this reason we cannot at this time use a scheme of normal counterparts as the sole basis for lymphoma classification. Nevertheless, it is clear that three major categories of lymphoid neoplasms can be distinguished - B cell neoplasms, T and NK cell neoplasms and Hodgkin's disease. In addition, within the B and T cell systems, it is possible to distinguish precursor from peripheral neoplasms, and this is also incorporated into the REAL scheme.

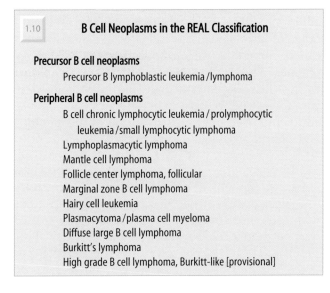

1.9   **Normal Counterparts of Lymphoma Cells**

Important conceptual basis for tumor classification
    Can be postulated for many entities
    Not known for some well-defined entities
    Cannot be sole basis for a classification

Three major categories
    - B cell neoplasms
    - T and NK cell neoplasms
    - Hodgkin's disease

Precursor and peripheral neoplasms

B cell neoplasms recognized in this classification are shown in [1.10]: one precursor neoplasm and nine peripheral neoplasms, ranging from small lymphocytic to large B cell and Burkitt's lymphoma.

1.10   **B Cell Neoplasms in the REAL Classification**

Precursor B cell neoplasms
    Precursor B lymphoblastic leukemia / lymphoma

Peripheral B cell neoplasms
    B cell chronic lymphocytic leukemia / prolymphocytic
       leukemia / small lymphocytic lymphoma
    Lymphoplasmacytic lymphoma
    Mantle cell lymphoma
    Follicle center lymphoma, follicular
    Marginal zone B cell lymphoma
    Hairy cell leukemia
    Plasmacytoma / plasma cell myeloma
    Diffuse large B cell lymphoma
    Burkitt's lymphoma
    High grade B cell lymphoma, Burkitt-like [provisional]

For the T cell system [1.11], we see a similar arrangement, with one precursor neoplasm and then a list of peripheral T and NK cell neoplasms, ranging from T cell CLL to anaplastic large cell lymphoma.

Finally, the REAL scheme deals with Hodgkin's disease [1.12] in a similar fashion to previous classifications, except that we divide it into classical types (which comprise nodular sclerosis, mixed cellularity, lymphocyte depletion and a lymphocyte-rich subtype, which we consider a provisional category). In contrast, "lymphocyte predominance, nodular" is clearly a distinct entity, and, although it is still classified under the general heading of Hodgkin's disease, it should be separated from the classical types.

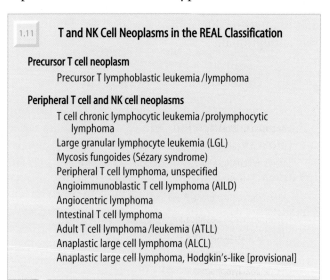

1.11   **T and NK Cell Neoplasms in the REAL Classification**

Precursor T cell neoplasm
    Precursor T lymphoblastic leukemia / lymphoma

Peripheral T cell and NK cell neoplasms
    T cell chronic lymphocytic leukemia / prolymphocytic
       lymphoma
    Large granular lymphocyte leukemia (LGL)
    Mycosis fungoides (Sézary syndrome)
    Peripheral T cell lymphoma, unspecified
    Angioimmunoblastic T cell lymphoma (AILD)
    Angiocentric lymphoma
    Intestinal T cell lymphoma
    Adult T cell lymphoma / leukemia (ATLL)
    Anaplastic large cell lymphoma (ALCL)
    Anaplastic large cell lymphoma, Hodgkin's-like [provisional]

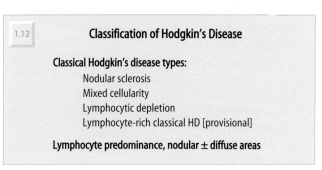

1.12   **Classification of Hodgkin's Disease**

Classical Hodgkin's disease types:
    Nodular sclerosis
    Mixed cellularity
    Lymphocytic depletion
    Lymphocyte-rich classical HD [provisional]

Lymphocyte predominance, nodular ± diffuse areas

If we compare the REAL scheme with the Working Formulation, we see major differences [1.13]. The most important is that it is based on homogeneous disease entities, whereas it was intended that each category in the Working Formulation should be sufficiently broad that all lymphomas could be classified. In addition, the REAL scheme takes advantage of modern immunologic and genetic techniques for the definition and diagnosis of lymphomas. It recognizes important new subtypes of low grade B cell lymphoma and distinctive categories of peripheral T cell lymphomas, none of which were recognized in the Working Formulation.

When we relate the REAL scheme to the Kiel classification [1.13], we see that they are very similar, and that most of the diseases recognized in the Kiel classification are included. However, we have proposed some changes in terminology, largely reflecting the need to compromise between practices in the US and Europe. The most important differences from the Kiel classification are the inclusion of extranodal lymphomas (the Kiel classification being restricted to nodal diseases), and the recognition that peripheral T cell lymphomas are difficult to subclassify reproducibly at this time. In contrast to both the Working Formulation and the Kiel classification, we felt that subclassification of large B cell lymphoma into multiple morphologic subtypes was also poorly reproducible and of questionable clinical significance, and so this was left optional.

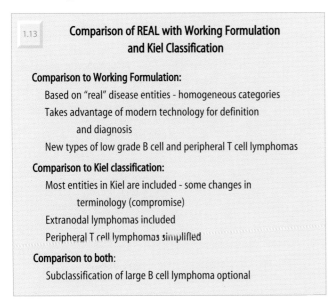

Comparison of REAL with Working Formulation and Kiel Classification

Comparison to Working Formulation:
Based on "real" disease entities - homogeneous categories
Takes advantage of modern technology for definition and diagnosis
New types of low grade B cell and peripheral T cell lymphomas

Comparison to Kiel classification:
Most entities in Kiel are included - some changes in terminology (compromise)
Extranodal lymphomas included
Peripheral T cell lymphomas simplified

Comparison to both:
Subclassification of large B cell lymphoma optional

It is important to realize that this classification contains nothing new, apart from the not inconsiderable fact that it represents a consensus among pathologists. All of the disease entities in the REAL scheme have been well described in the literature, and we have simply compiled a list of the entities found in the existing classifications on which we could all agree. This is the largest group of pathologists ever to agree on a lymphoma classification – or on anything else for that matter! Since it builds on existing European and American classifications we called it the "Revised European-American Lymphoma Classification". As mentioned, most of the entities in the updated Kiel classification are included, and it can certainly also be used together with the Working Formulation, since the latter scheme was designed to translate between different systems. We hope that if these definitions and terminology are adopted by our colleagues it will have the effect of improving international communication.

The clinical relevance of this scheme has already been demonstrated for most of the entities, since they are already well known in their full clinical spectrum to both oncologists and pathologists. However, it is clearly important to evaluate some of the newer entities, both by reviewing cases in existing clinical trials and by prospective studies, to better understand their behavior.

Turning now to the frequency of these entities [1.14], several members of the ILSG applied this classification to their own material and came up with some not very surprising data. The great majority of non-Hodgkin's lymphomas, in both the US and Europe, are of B cell type, comprising 85%. The two most important numerical categories continue to be follicle center (or follicular) lymphoma, and diffuse large B cell lymphoma, which together account for almost 70% of non-Hodgkin's lymphomas. The new categories of low grade B cell lymphomas are relatively uncommon, the most important being mantle cell and small lymphocytic. Within the T cell lymphoma category, the most important are peripheral T cell, anaplastic large cell and angioimmunoblastic lymphomas.

1.14	Nodal Lymphomas: US and Europe	
B cell lymphomas		**85%**
- Follicular lymphoma	35%	
- Diffuse large B cell lymphoma	30%	
- Mantle cell lymphoma	5%	
- B-CLL/SLL	5%	
- Lymphoplasmacytic	1-2%	
- Marginal zone lymphoma	1-2%	
- All others	< 10%	
T cell lymphomas		**15%**
- Peripheral T cell lymphoma	5%	
- Anaplastic large cell lymphoma	5%	
- Angioimmunoblastic lymphoma	2%	

It is important to appreciate the value of recognizing "real" diseases. Lumping diverse entities into broad prognostic groups tends to obscure the distinctive features of the less common entities. For example, a trial of Working Formulation "low grade" lymphomas would be predominantly a trial of follicular lymphoma, contaminated by a small number of mantle cell, MALT type and small lymphocytic lymphomas. Similarly, trials of Working Formulation "intermediate and high-grade" categories are predominately trials of diffuse large B cell lymphoma, but are contaminated by small numbers of less common entities, particularly peripheral T cell lymphomas. We therefore believe that the REAL scheme will allow treatment to be tested on specific entities, which are as homogeneous as it is possible to make them.

Clearly this is not the last word in lymphoma classification. It will need to be updated regularly, for at least as long as there is progress in this field, both to add new disease entities, to delete others that have failed to be substantiated, and to add new defining criteria. A joint project of American and European hematopathology societies is under way, under the auspices of the World Health Organisation, to produce an updated WHO classification. We hope that it will result in a broad consensus on the disease entities in the REAL classification, and will update and expand the list of diseases in that scheme. In the future it may be desirable for hematopathology societies to establish joint classification committees.

Although it is not practical to sort the entities in the REAL scheme rigorously according to clinical features, this meeting is nevertheless organized around clinical groupings. This is because it is to some extent possible to group these diseases in terms of both common clinical presentation and similar survivals. [1.15] shows a scheme proposed by Dr. Longo and his associates. They considered "indolent" neoplasms to be those whose survival, if untreated, would be measured in years; "aggressive" neoplasms those whose survival, if untreated, would be measured in months; and "highly aggressive" neoplasms those whose survival, if treatment were not successful, would be measured in weeks.

> ### Clinical Groupings of Lymphoid Neoplasms
> 1.15
> - **Indolent neoplasms** (survival = years)
> - **Aggressive neoplasms** (survival = months)
> - **Highly aggressive neoplasms** (survival = weeks)

Within the indolent lymphoid neoplasms [1.16] there are actually three major clinical forms of presentation - disseminated, extranodal and nodal.

> ### Indolent Lymphoid Neoplasms
> 1.16
> **Disseminated** (Chronic Leukemias)
> - B-CLL/SLL
> - Lymphoplasmacytic lymphoma/immunocytoma
> - Splenic marginal zone lymphoma (SMZL/SLVL)
> - Hairy cell leukemia
> - Multiple myeloma
> - T/NK LGL
> - T-CLL/PLL
>
> **Nodal**
> - Follicular lymphoma
> - Mantle cell lymphoma
>
> **Extranodal**
> - Marginal zone B cell lymphoma (MALT)
> - Mycosis fungoides/Sézary syndrome

The indolent disseminated lymphoid neoplasms are predominantly those that we know as chronic lymphoid leukemias. The indolent nodal lymphomas are accounted for by just two types of B cell neoplasm - follicular lymphoma and mantle cell lymphoma. And the indolent extranodal lymphomas are marginal zone (MALT) lymphoma and mycosis fungoides.

As for aggressive lymphomas [1.17], the great majority are diffuse large B cell lymphoma, but virtually all peripheral T cell lymphomas also fall into this category. Finally the highly aggressive neoplasms or acute leukemia/lymphomas [1.18] include Burkitt's lymphoma, the precursor B and T neoplasms and adult T cell lymphoma/leukemia.

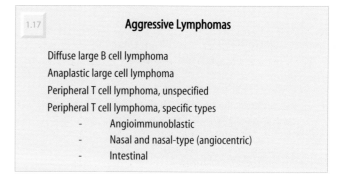

> ### Aggressive Lymphomas
> 1.17
> Diffuse large B cell lymphoma
> Anaplastic large cell lymphoma
> Peripheral T cell lymphoma, unspecified
> Peripheral T cell lymphoma, specific types
> - Angioimmunoblastic
> - Nasal and nasal-type (angiocentric)
> - Intestinal

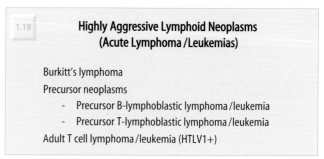

> ### Highly Aggressive Lymphoid Neoplasms
> ### (Acute Lymphoma/Leukemias)
> 1.18
> Burkitt's lymphoma
> Precursor neoplasms
> - Precursor B-lymphoblastic lymphoma/leukemia
> - Precursor T-lymphoblastic lymphoma/leukemia
> Adult T cell lymphoma/leukemia (HTLV1+)

In summary [1.19], lymphomas are a diverse group of neoplasms arising from cells of the immune system, and each disease entity is defined by a combination of morphologic, immunophenotypic and clinical features. Although more than twenty distinct diseases can be recognized, it is important to remember that three or four diseases account for the great majority of patients seen in our clinical practice. We believe that future progress will be facilitated by recognizing homogeneous categories of patients for both pathologic and clinical studies.

> ### Summary: Lymphoma Classification
> 1.19
> - Lymphomas are a diverse group of diseases arising from cells of the immune system
> - A combination of morphologic features, immunophenotype, and clinical features define each entity
> - Although > 20 distinct entities are recognized, 3 or 4 diseases account for the majority of the patients
> - Future progress will be facilitated by recognizing homogeneous categories of patients for studies

Finally, the spirit behind the REAL scheme can be summarized by the following quotation from Albert Einstein: "Everything should be made as simple as possible, but not simpler."

REFERENCES

1. Harris NL, Jaffe ES, Stein H *et al*. A revised European-American classification of lymphoid neoplasms: a proposal from the International Lymphoma Study Group. *Blood* 1994; **84**: 1361-92.

FURTHER READING

Bennett JM, Catovsky D, Daniel MT *et al*. Proposals for the classification of chronic (mature) B and T lymphoid leukemias. French-American-British (FAB) Co-operative Group. *J Clin Pathol* 1989; **42**: 567-84.

Fisher RI, Dahlberg S, Nathwani BN, Banks PM, Miller TP, Grogan TM. A clinical analysis of two indolent lymphoma entities: mantle cell lymphoma and marginal zone lymphoma (including the mucosa-associated lymphoid tissue and monocytoid B-cell subcategories): a Southwest Oncology Group study. *Blood* 1995; **85**: 1075-82.

Harris N. Lymphoma 1987: an interim approach to diagnosis and classification. In: Fechner R, Rosen P, eds. *Pathology Annual*. East Norwalk, CT. Appleton & Lange, 1987; **2**: 1-67.

Hastrup N, Hamilton-Dutoit S, Ralfkiaer E, Pallesen G. Peripheral T-cell lymphomas: an evaluation of reproducibility of the updated Kiel classification. *Histopathology* 1991; **18**: 99-105.

Lennert K, Feller A. *Histopathology of non-Hodgkin's lymphomas*. 2nd edn. New York: Springer-Verlag, 1992.

Lennert K, Mohri N, Stein H, Kaiserling E. The histopathology of malignant lymphoma. *Br J Haematol* 1975; **31** (Suppl): 193-203.

Lennert K. *Malignant lymphomas other than Hodgkin's disease*. New York: Springer-Verlag, 1978.

Longo DL. The REAL classification of lymphoid neoplasms: one clinician's view. In: Rosenberg S, ed. *PPO Updates*. Philadelphia: Lippincott, 1995; **9**: 1-12.

Longo DL, DeVita VT, Jaffe ES, Mauch P, Urba WJ. Lymphocytic Lymphomas. In: De Vita VT, Hellman S, Rosenberg S, eds. *Principles and Practice of Oncology*. Philadelphia: Lippincott, 1993: 1859-1927.

Lukes R, Collins R. Immunologic characterization of human malignant lymphomas. *Cancer* 1974; **34**: 1488-1503.

Nathwani BN, Metter GE, Miller TP *et al*. What should be the morphologic criteria for the subdivision of follicular lymphomas? *Blood* 1986; **68**: 837-45.

Non-Hodgkin's lymphoma pathologic classification project. National Cancer Institute sponsored study of classifications of non-Hodgkin's lymphomas: summary and description of a Working Formulation for clinical usage. *Cancer* 1982; **49**: 2112-135.

Rappaport H. *Tumors of the hematopoietic system*. Armed Forces Institute of Pathology. Washington, DC, 1966.

Sheibani K, Nathwani BN, Swartz WG *et al*. Variability in interpretation of immunohistologic findings in lymphoproliferative disorders by hematopathologists. A comprehensive statistical analysis of interobserver performance. *Cancer* 1988; **62**: 657-64.

Teodorovic I, Pittaluga S, Kluin-Nelemans JC *et al*. Efficacy of four different regimens in 64 mantle-cell lymphoma cases: clinicopathologic comparison with 498 other non-Hodgkin's lymphoma subtypes. European Organization for the Research and Treatment of Cancer Lymphoma Co-operative Group. *Clin Oncol* 1995; **13**: 2819-26.

Lymphocyte differentiation

2

H Stein

Aknowledge of the normal differentiation pathways of the cells of the lymphoid system is an absolute prerequisite for an understanding of lymphomas and their classification. Without this knowledge, it is not possible to understand the morphology, the immunophenotype or even the molecular genetics of lymphomas.

Immunologists subdivide the lymphoid system [2.1] into central and peripheral lymphoid tissue. The peripheral lymphoid tissue is organized in a complex manner. In the lymph node cortex, B cell areas are seen, comprising primary or secondary lymphoid follicles. Other features are the paracortical or T cell zone, the sinuses, the medulla and the interfollicular zone.

2.1	Subdivisions of Lymphoid System	
Central lymphoid tissue:	Bone marrow	
	Thymus	
Peripheral lymphoid tissue:	Spleen	
	Superficial lymph nodes	
	Mucosa associated lymphoid tissue (MALT)	

When a secondary lymphoid follicle is examined in detail [2.2], the germinal center usually contains a dark zone (DZ) and a light zone (LZ). The germinal center is mainly surrounded by the follicle mantle (FM), consisting of small B cells. The cells in the dark zone are rapidly proliferating – as revealed by a marker such as Ki-67 [2.2] – and many of the cells are centroblasts (CB) – large blasts with large nuclei, marginally located nucleoli and sparse basophilic cytoplasm. When these cells move up to the light zone, they differentiate into the other major type of germinal center cell, the centrocyte. These cells have an irregularly shaped nucleus and an inconspicuous cytoplasm, and most are destined to die by apoptosis. In the area between the dark and the light zone, remnants of apoptotic centrocytes, usually phagocytosed by macrophages, can be seen.

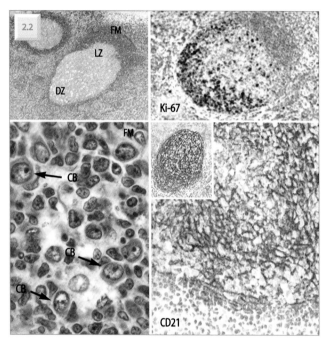

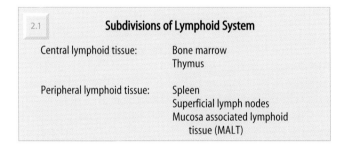

Centroblasts and centrocytes express the aminopeptidase CD10/CALLA [2.3], whereas all other peripheral B cells and T cells are negative, and this is a widely used marker for germinal center cells. Lymphoid follicles also contain a meshwork of follicular dendritic cells (FDC). This cannot be recognized in conventional stains, but is revealed by labeling for CD21 [2.2]. The FDC meshwork is very dense and sharply defined within the germinal center, but extends in a more open and loose arrangement into the mantle zone. The FDC meshwork is responsible for the homing of B cells and is crucial for the germinal center reaction since it captures antigen in the form of antigen-antibody immune complexes. This phenomenon can be visualized by immunostaining for IgM, IgG and complement, which shows immune complexes attached to the FDC processes. Immunostaining shows in addition that the centroblasts, which predominate the dark zone, carry little or no IgM. In contrast, follicle mantle cells express

IgM at a high density. Nearly all germinal center cells are devoid of IgD, whereas the follicle mantle cells stain as strongly for IgD as they do for IgM.

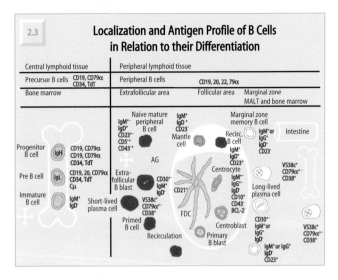

B-CLL and mantle cell lymphomas express both IgD and IgM, as do reactive mantle cells. This supports the notion that the cells of these lymphomas are related to the cells residing in the mantle zone. Both B-CLL and mantle cell lymphomas have in common the expression of CD5. It is therefore of interest to know whether normal mantle cells also express CD5, and immunohistologic studies show that occasionally they do.

There are not only immunophenotypic similarities, but also differences between B-CLL and mantle cell lymphoma. These include expression of CD23 by the former and absence from the latter. In normal lymphoid tissues a large proportion of the cells in the mantle zone and in the blood carry the CD23 molecule. It is tempting to assume that B-CLL is derived from CD23-positive cells, and mantle cell lymphoma cells from CD23-negative cells in the mantle zone.

Many functional and molecular biological studies have addressed the question of the developmental relationship between germinal center and follicular mantle B cells. When an antigen enters the organism for the first time there is a slowly increasing production of IgM antibodies of low affinity. If the antigen is presented to the immune system for a second time, there is an immediate major production of IgG antibodies of high affinity. The higher affinity is caused by a better "fit" of the antigen binding site of the antibodies, resulting from somatic mutations in the V regions of the genes that encode the antibody binding sites. This mutation process is mainly random and can lead to either a better or a poorer binding of antigen by the antibody. B cells expressing poorly binding Ig molecules are eliminated, whereas the others are retained. This process of somatic Ig mutation and negative and positive selection of B cells on the basis of unfavorable or favorable mutations takes place in germinal centers.

Since this mutation process is restricted to germinal centers, B cells with three different patterns of mutations can be distinguished. B cells devoid of somatic mutations have not yet entered a germinal center, and are therefore often called "pre-germinal center" B cells or "mature naive" B cells. In peripheral lymphoid tissue (primary follicles and follicle mantles) and in blood, 90% of B cells are of this type. B cells which have undergone somatic Ig gene mutation may show signs of ongoing mutations, in which case they must derive from the germinal center. Finally, B cells which carry somatic mutations without signs of ongoing mutations represent cells which have left the germinal center, and are termed "post-germinal center" B cells. There are two types – memory B cells and plasma cells. They populate marginal zones, the lamina propria of the intestine and the bone marrow. In the marginal zones the memory B cells predominate.

On the basis of these and other findings, one can construct a differentiation scheme, starting in the bone marrow, where the first recognizable B cells develop [2.4]. These progenitor B cells or pro-B cells become pre-B cells by a differentiation step associated with rearrangement of their Ig heavy chain genes. This is followed by a rearrangement of the Ig light chain genes which results in expression of complete and functional IgM molecules. If they are non-self-reactive the B cells carrying these Ig receptors, designated immature B cells, leave the bone marrow and acquire IgD, whereby they become "naive mature" peripheral B cells. These circulate in the blood and populate primary lymphoid follicles and mantle zones of secondary follicles. As mentioned above, there is some evidence that there are two subsets of these B cells: those which express CD23 and those which do not.

These IgM-positive and IgD-positive mature B cells recirculate continuously until they find antigens recognized by their Ig receptors. They then transform into extrafollicular B-blasts which proliferate and give rise to short-lived plasma cells or primed B cells. The short-lived plasma cells secrete IgM antibodies which form complexes with the antigen responsible for inducing the primary immune response. These Ig complexes bind complement, and the resulting antigen-antibody-complement complexes are captured by FDC. This is probably the signal for the primed B cells to enter the germinal center, and to initiate a germinal center reaction.

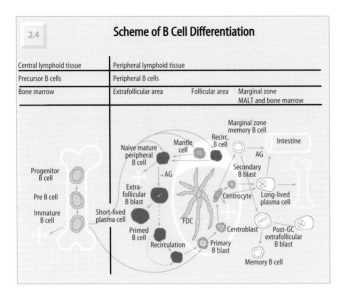

Scheme of B Cell Differentiation

Central lymphoid tissue	Peripheral lymphoid tissue		
Precursor B cells	Peripheral B cells		
Bone marrow	Extrafollicular area	Follicular area	Marginal zone MALT and bone marrow

A comparison of malignant lymphomas with normal lymphoid tissue reveals that low grade B cell lymphomas recapitulate many features of the normal B cell system. For example, follicle center lymphomas arise within a follicle center and subsequently metastasize to other follicles, giving rise to the characteristic follicular growth pattern. It is only late in the disease course that the tumor cells lose their homing properties and manifest a diffuse growth pattern. Another example is mantle cell lymphoma. It starts to develop within a mantle zone and from there other mantle zones are infiltrated. This causes an enlargement of the mantle zones and eventually leads to invasion of the germinal centers and finally of the entire lymph node. A third example is marginal zone lymphoma. The neoplastic cells infiltrate and expand the marginal zone. Germinal centers may secondarily be colonized.

The earliest identifiable germinal centers comprise cells that are smaller than centroblasts and which have been called by some immunologists "primary B blasts" or "pre-centroblasts". They multiply rapidly and differentiate into centroblasts which continue to multiply but simultaneously acquire mutations in their Ig genes and then differentiate into centrocytes. It is at this stage, at which the B cells are selected according to their antigen binding capacity, that the mutation process of the Ig genes gives rise to two populations of centrocytes. Centrocytes that have unfavorable mutations and that bind antigen with low affinity Ig are eliminated by apoptosis. In contrast, centrocytes in which the mutations were favorable and that carry high affinity Ig receive survival signals allowing them to differentiate further, one pathway taking them to the plasma cell stage and one to memory B cells.

Plasma cell differentiation starts in the light zone of the germinal center, although in these cells the nuclei still resemble those of centrocytes even though the cytoplasm has already acquired the feature of plasma cells. Thus B cells start on their differentiation pathway towards plasma cells in the germinal center, from where they emigrate to other tissues, particularly the bone marrow and the intestine.

The other differentiation path that centrocytes follow is towards memory B cells. There is evidence that memory B cells migrate to "marginal zone" areas adjacent to the follicle mantle zones. Well-developed memory or marginal zones are easily seen in the spleen, around the lymphoid follicles and in Peyer's patches, but they are not recognizable in normal superficial lymph nodes. Marginal zone cells are strongly IgM-positive, but, in contrast to mantle cells, are negative or only weakly positive for IgD.

The site of origin and the homing properties of these lymphomas fit well with their pattern of somatic Ig gene mutations. Mantle cell lymphoma is devoid of somatic mutations as are normal mantle cells. Follicle center lymphoma in contrast shows both somatic mutations and signs of on-going mutations. Marginal zone lymphomas of MALT type carry, as expected, mutations. Unexpectedly, some of them also show intraclonal diversity as a sign of ongoing mutations. This suggests a derivation from early marginal zone cells, i.e. centrocytes which have just started to transform into marginal zone cells.

Finally, the T cell system may be briefly referred to. T cell development also starts in the bone marrow. The first cells that can be recognized as T cells in this tissue are progenitor T cells or "pro-T cells" which migrate to the cortex of the thymus and there undergo differentiation, associated with rearrangement of T cell receptor genes. T cells with auto-reactive receptors are eliminated, but non-self-reactive T cells differentiate further into CD4-positive and CD8-positive cells. They emigrate, via the thymus medulla, to the paracortical zones of peripheral lymphoid tissue and become mature naive T cells. If they encounter antigen they undergo transformation to blasts, which are often CD30-positive. Some CD4-positive T cells migrate into germinal centers and promote and modulate the germinal center reaction.

Three different organ-restricted T cell types can be distinguished. Intraepithelial T cells within the glandular epithelium of intestinal mucosa give rise to intestinal T cell lymphoma of enteropathy type. Enteropathy-type T cell lymphoma and intraepithelial T cells have in common the selective expression of mucosal lymphocyte antigen (MLA or CD103). A second cell type is the skin-associated T cell, which gives rise, following malignant transformation, to primary cutaneous T cell lymphomas (i.e. mycosis fungoides and Sézary syndrome). Primary cutaneous T cell lymphomas and skin-associated T cells share (in addition to epidermotropism) expression of CLA, cutaneous lymphocyte antigen. A third organ-restricted type of T cell is the nodal T cell. This cell is devoid of the markers found on cutaneous and intraepithelial T cells, and is the probable cell of origin for most nodal T cell lymphomas. In the last few years it has emerged that T cells and natural killer cells share a common precursor, and it is therefore of no surprise that some T cell lymphomas show features of natural killer cells. The most important examples are large granular lymphocytic leukemia and angiocentric (nasal) lymphoma.

In conclusion, this brief overview of the normal differentiation pathway of the lymphoid system should help to understand better the neoplasms arising in the lymphoid system and the most recent proposal for their classification, the REAL scheme.

Goals of a lymphoma classification for the oncologist

3

J O Armitage

This chapter is a review, from the point of view of someone who sees and cares for lymphoma patients, of what we might reasonably hope to gain from a lymphoma classification.

Obviously the first and most important question is: why do we want to classify lymphomas? The answer is, of course, to help us take better care of patients. So everything that follows is aimed at that particular goal. There are other reasons, and perfectly legitimate ones, to classify lymphomas. For example if this leads to a better understanding of the biology of these diseases and what causes them, it might, in an indirect way, eventually impact on how we take care of patients. However, this chapter focuses specifically on how we can use this information to help us care for the patient.

To address that issue it is helpful to stop and reflect on just how in practice one approaches a patient newly diagnosed as having lymphoma. First of all, we are anxious to confirm that the patient has this disorder and also, if possible, to know its subtype, in order to help us in our task of treating the patient. Here we are obviously concerned about the accuracy of the diagnosis. Then we evaluate the patient, to try to determine those characteristics of the disease that will help us to plan therapy. For example, we are interested in knowing if the disease is localized or disseminated, or if a particularly important organ is involved; and we will be very interested in any hints from the classification system that help us to make these determinations.

Then we treat the patient. We would be interested again in the classification system if it gives us any information as to whether or not the disease can be cured, that is to say information on the relative aggressiveness of this disease and its responsiveness to available therapies, and also whether any particular unique therapy might be appropriate. Finally, since

we will continue to take care of the patients after we initially treat them, we are interested in the natural history of the disease in those who have been apparently successfully treated, so that we can identify patients who are likely to relapse.

Although the approach to the patient is greatly influenced by the pathologists' diagnosis, whatever classification system is used, there are also many other factors that we take into account before we start treatment. For example, the pace of the disease in the individual patient, the particular sites that are involved, whether the patient has symptoms, the patient's age, the risk of the therapy, how well the patient is, and emotional issues - all of these are relevant. A multitude of factors influence treatment decisions, apart from just the classification scheme.

What do we expect from a classification? The answer is that we want it to be clinically relevant, we want it to be reproducible between pathologists, and we want it to be consistent for the individual patient if more than one sample is taken.

One of the things we would like a classification to do is illustrated by [3.1]. This is from the Working Formulation study, although similar illustrations could be shown from the Kiel group or from others. These are the survival curves for different subtypes in the Working Formulation, and one would like, whatever classification system is utilized, to be able to identify in this way different natural histories of the diseases. One would also like the system to be able to do what the REAL classification is aimed at, that is to identify particularly subtypes of lymphoma for which unique therapies are appropriate. For example, gastric MALT lymphomas often seem to respond to the eradication of *Helicobacter pylori* following the administration of antibiotics, and one wants to identify these patients so that this therapy, which would be quite inappropriate for other cases, can be used.

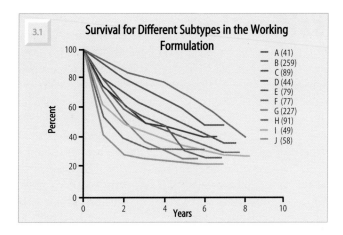

3.1 Survival for Different Subtypes in the Working Formulation

A (41)
B (259)
C (89)
D (44)
E (79)
F (77)
G (227)
H (91)
I (49)
J (58)

The data in [3.4] show that, first of all, pathologists in the UK are no better than Americans at identifying lymphoma subtypes! They also highlight another important issue: in the Working Formulation study, as part of its protocol, the individual pathologists were given the same slides to review again, so it was possible to determine their consistency of diagnosis. It is evident [3.4] that even those pathologists who were considered at the time to be the leading experts, were able to reproduce their own diagnoses on the same slide only 53% to 93% of the time. The point is therefore clearly made that it can be a difficult task to diagnose lymphomas - it is not a precise business.

And of course we would like the diagnosis to be accurate. This is unfortunately an Achilles heel for all lymphoma classification systems, because lymphoma diagnoses have not proved particularly accurate when they have been tested.

Data from three different American study groups [3.2], show, firstly, the accuracy of diagnosis of lymphoma (as opposed to carcinoma or other disorders); secondly, the accuracy of diagnosis of follicularity; and, thirdly, the accuracy of diagnosis of specific sub-types of lymphoma.

3.2 Diagnostic Accuracy in Non-Hodgkin's Lymphoma

Group	Concordance		
	NHL vs other	Nodular vs diffuse	Specific type
SWOG	96%	85%	56%
SECSG	87%	NA	56%
ECOG	96%	NA	NA

The comparison in [3.3] is between institutional hematopathologists and a group of selected experts, the Lymphoma Repository Group.

3.3 Diagnostic Accuracy in Non-Hodgkin's Lymphoma

Group	Concordance		
	DHL	NPDL	DPDL
SWOG	86%	78%	13%
SECSG	71%	81%	46%
ECOG	60%	84%	-

It is evident from these data that the accuracy of lymphoma diagnosis was quite good. The diagnosis of follicularity was also fairly good, but the diagnosis of specific subtypes of lymphoma was not, and in fact was not much better than flipping a coin. This type of study has been carried out on several occasions, and this is fairly consistently the result, a finding which should make clinicians pause and think twice about planning major differences in treatments between closely related lymphoma subgroups.

3.4 Diagnostic Accuracy in Non-Hodgkin's Lymphoma

Group	Concordance	
	Nodular vs diffuse	Specific type
Yorkshire [1]	NA	55%
Working Formulation Panel [2]	90%-95%	53%-93% (ability to reproduce own diagnosis)

From the point of view of the clinician, we are also curious to know how soon we are going to be able to use biologic data to support the histopathologic diagnosis. Physicians concerned with leukemia do this regularly today, being interested in, among other things, genetic information that might alter their treatment decisions.

Some studies have shown genetic differences in DLCL depending on the site of origin [3.5].[3] Little use is made of this approach for lymphoma at present, but there are many hints suggesting that it might be useful. There have been extensive data showing different immunophenotypes within lymphoma categories. One study suggested that, in diffuse large B cell lymphoma, whether or not the neoplasm expressed Class II antigen had a major impact on outcome [3.6].[4]

Several studies [3.7] have measured the ability of tumor cells to proliferate, to see if slowly or rapidly proliferating lymphomas have different natural histories.[5,6] In practice, although some clinical trials are now testing the utility of these factors, at present lymphoma clinicians do not utilize this information. Nevertheless, one could anticipate that these sorts of biologic measurements will some day be used to support the histopathologic diagnosis.

This meeting, organized by Nancy Harris and Bruce Chabner, reflects the fact that lymphoma pathology is not a dead science - its exponents continue to see things that those who preceded them were unable to see. In some cases this is because of new advances in areas such as genetics; in others it is because a clever individual has a new idea; and occasionally it is because clinicians who have made new observations come back to the pathologist and this leads to the identification of new entities. In each instance this leads to the definition of entities. New entities that do not fit into old classifications continue to be observed, and this may well be the natural history of this area. On these grounds, clinicians should be urged to respond, not, as some have done, by saying that the REAL scheme is an attempt by people with a particular interest in lymphomas to keep changing the names so that everyone else stays confused! Instead, this type of evolution can be seen as representing the way things are always going to be - there will continue to be clever pathologists who make new observations. These lead to new proposals about how to classify these disorders, in a way that is clinically useful, and that in turn leads to trials that refute or support the new ideas. We are in this cycle and that is how we will continue to make progress.

A final point to make in the context of this new classification is that a group of us began after the publication of the REAL scheme to perform a field test with the aim of testing its clinical applicability. Individuals from eight sites in Africa, Asia, Europe and N. America were involved. Consecutive cases of lymphoma from each site diagnosed in the late 1980s have all been re-evaluated by an expert group of hematopathologists and classified both by an existing scheme and by the REAL classification. The diagnoses were made before and after immunophenotyping, in an attempt to test the contribution which that makes to clinical decisions. As in the Working Formulation, the pathologists re-reviewed the same slide 20% of the time, to see how accurate this new system is in practice. Consensus diagnoses were made and clinical data were collected. 1,360 cases were studied and this data is now in the process of being analyzed.

The clinical information has been reviewed, trying to answer issues such as the most clinically relevant way to exploit these diagnoses. A number of other interesting things are emerging, including geographic variations in types of lymphoma. The individuals involved are listed in [3.8]. This is a major effort, and five pathologists from the United States and Europe all visited eight different sites to diagnose these cases. Drs. Berard and Harris served as consultants to the project and Dr. Harris attended the first two site visits. The pathologists at the sites that were visited did a lot of work in anticipation of those visits, and the clinicians involved in collecting and analyzing the data are also listed. Saul Rosenberg was one of the important people in giving us advice about how to perform this aspect of the project.

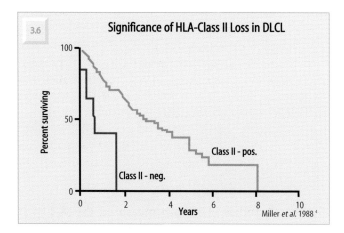

3.5

Genetic Differences in DLCL Depending on Site of Origin (Leiden)

Abnormality	Nodal	Extranodal
BCL-2	40%	< 5%
C-MYC	5%	35%

Raghoebier et al. 1991 [3]

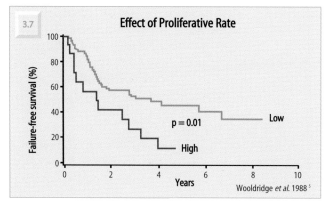

3.6 Significance of HLA-Class II Loss in DLCL

Percent surviving

Class II - pos.

Class II - neg.

Years

Miller et al. 1988 [4]

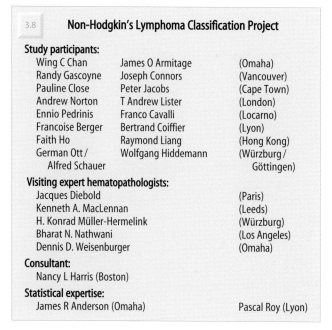

3.7 Effect of Proliferative Rate

Failure-free survival (%)

p = 0.01

Low

High

Years

Wooldridge et al. 1988 [5]

3.8 **Non-Hodgkin's Lymphoma Classification Project**

Study participants:

Wing C Chan	James O Armitage	(Omaha)
Randy Gascoyne	Joseph Connors	(Vancouver)
Pauline Close	Peter Jacobs	(Cape Town)
Andrew Norton	T Andrew Lister	(London)
Ennio Pedrinis	Franco Cavalli	(Locarno)
Francoise Berger	Bertrand Coiffier	(Lyon)
Faith Ho	Raymond Liang	(Hong Kong)
German Ott /	Wolfgang Hiddemann	(Würzburg /
Alfred Schauer		Göttingen)

Visiting expert hematopathologists:

Jacques Diebold	(Paris)
Kenneth A. MacLennan	(Leeds)
H. Konrad Müller-Hermelink	(Würzburg)
Bharat N. Nathwani	(Los Angeles)
Dennis D. Weisenburger	(Omaha)

Consultant:
Nancy L Harris (Boston)

Statistical expertise:

James R Anderson (Omaha)	Pascal Roy (Lyon)

REFERENCES

1. Bird CC, Lauder I, Kellett HS *et al.* Yorkshire Regional Lymphoma Histopathology panel: analysis of five years' experience. *J Pathol* 1984; **143**: 249-58.

2. Classification of non-Hodgkin's lymphomas. Reproducibility of major classification systems. NCI Non-Hodgkin's Classification Project Writing Committee. *Cancer* 1985; **55**: 91-5.

3. Raghoebier S, Kramer MH, van Krieken JH *et al.* Essential differences in oncogene involvement between primary nodal and extranodal large cell lymphoma. *Blood* 1991; **78**: 2680-5.

4. Miller TP, Lippman SM, Spier CM, Slymen DJ, Grogan TM. HLA-DR (Ia) immune phenotype predicts outcome for patients with diffuse large cell lymphoma. *J Clin Invest* 1988; **82**: 370-2.

5. Wooldridge TN, Grierson HL, Weisenburger DD *et al.* Association of DNA content and proliferative activity with clinical outcome in patients with diffuse mixed cell and large cell non-Hodgkin's lymphoma. *Cancer Res* 1988; **48**: 6608-13.

6. Grogan TM, Lippman SM, Spier CM *et al.* Independent prognostic significance of a nuclear proliferation antigen in diffuse large cell lymphomas as determined by the monoclonal antibody Ki-67. *Blood* 1988; **71**: 1157-60.

A multi-institutional evaluation of lymphoma classification

4

T M Grogan

This contribution is made from the position of Chair of the Southwest Oncology Lymphoma Biology Group. The Group has addressed the usefulness of the REAL classification in diagnosing and treating lymphoma patients, and this has been done under the auspices of the SWOG Lymphoma Committee headed by Dr Fisher and Dr. Miller. Our common goal was to find a lymphoma classification that predicts patient outcome and response to therapy, and which suggests biological features that may be of relevance to new therapy. We had worked for almost fifteen years with the Working Formulation and felt comfortable with the fact that morphology equated to outcome. The justification for this was the unique median survival of these patients. We had grown to live with some of the problems, not the least of which is that the original studies on which we have to rely were not based on uniformly staged and treated patients. There had also been difficulties with reproducibility, and of course information on the biological underpinnings of these diseases was frequently lacking.

The almost random way in which different pathologic stages were treated among the patients in the original Working Formulation categorization is revealed in [4.1]. By modern standards, we see too many patients who were not treated with adriamycin-based chemotherapy, who were not uniformly staged, and whom really could hardly be treated as a group. These represent clear limitations to the use of this information.

Equally revealing, from one of the Southwest Oncology Group trials of intensive combination chemotherapy for unfavorable non-Hodgkin's lymphoma (SWOG phase II trials), [4.2] shows how much difficulty there was in reaching agreement on the diagnosis among different third generation treatment protocols. The extent of disagreement and failure to achieve consensus reveals the mythical nature of any belief that we achieve full reproducibility in these studies.

4.2	Expert Pathology Review		
Description	m-BACOD N (%)	Pro-MACE N (%)	MACOP-B N (%)
Registered	140	97	131
Pathology reviewed	107 (100)	71 (100)	67 (100)
Wrong histology	14 (13)	12 (17)	6 (9)
			SWOG 8410. 8503. 8508 (4/87)

The Revised European-American scheme offers the possibility of a fresh approach [4.3] but the problem is that the utility of the scheme is unproven. For this reason, we decided to test these new categories against uniformly staged and treated patients from the Southwest Oncology Group lymphoma protocols.

4.3	Background
Present: Revised European-American (1994) Multiparameter = morphology, phenotype, genotype	
Problems: Utility unproven	
Solution: To test clinical entity of new REAL categories with uniformly staged and treated SWOG lymphoma patients	

Some preliminary observations about the REAL scheme are relevant at this point [4.4]. It adds some new entities and it removes some old ones, and this is relevant to the questions we want to ask. It suggests that follicular large cell and intermediate high grade should be lumped together. It establishes a number

4.1	Working Formulation Clinical Database			
		Pathologic stage (%)		
Treatment	I	II	III	IV
RT	69	61	24	4
RT+CT	16	23	37	28
CT	3	9	34	63
Other	11	5	2	2
None	1	2	3	3

of new categories among the small lymphocytic neoplasms (mantle cell, MALT and monocytoid B marginal zone lymphomas), a new large cell B cell lymphoma category, and a category of peripheral T cell lymphomas. There are consequently questions to ask about the new entities and also some questions about the validity of lumping together old entities.

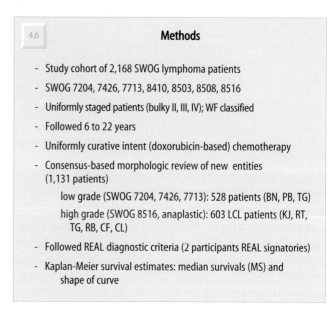

4.4	**The REAL Classification**

Subtracts some old entities
- follicular subsets (WF B, C, D)
- large cell subsets (WF G/H)
- intermediate/high grade subsets (WF F, J)

Adds some new entities
- small lymphocytic
    - mantle cell (MCL), mucosa-associated (MALT)
    - monocytoid B (MCBL)
- large cell: anaplastic (HD-like)

Gives peripheral T cell lymphomas status
- new subgroups e.g. intestinal T

In the study we conducted recently, the overall question was whether the REAL classification was useful [4.5]. Other questions were whether we should lump together all grades of follicular lymphoma, and whether we should unite the diffuse aggressive entities as we know them in the Working Formulation - the diffuse mixed, the large cell immunoblastic and large cell. We also asked whether there are unique clinical behaviors associated with some of these new categories.

4.5	**Questions**

- Is the REAL classification clinically useful?
- As suggested by REAL, should follicular lymphomas be "lumped"?
- As suggested by REAL, should the diffuse aggressive entities (category F, G, H, J) be "lumped"?
- Are there unique clinical behaviors associated with the new REAL categories?
    - small lymphocytic: mantle cell (MCL)
    - mucosa-associated (MALT), monocytoid B
    - large cell types: anaplastic (ALCL)

The strategy adopted was to look at the studies from the early 70s into the mid 80s. These were all patients with bulky Stage II, III or IV disease who had already been assigned to a Working Formulation category, and for whom we had a sizeable amount of follow up data. They were all treated with doxorubicin-based chemotherapy, and the aim was to achieve a consensus-based morphologic review [4.6].

We focused on two major cohorts: a group of 528 patients with WF low grade lymphoma, which was reviewed by three pathologists; and a group of 603

patients with WF high grade lymphoma, reviewed by six pathologists. We followed the diagnostic criteria of the REAL classification, to which two of our senior pathologists were signatories. We looked at the Kaplan-Meier survival estimates, assessing both the median survival and the shape of the curves in these patients.

4.6	**Methods**

- Study cohort of 2,168 SWOG lymphoma patients
- SWOG 7204, 7426, 7713, 8410, 8503, 8508, 8516
- Uniformly staged patients (bulky II, III, IV); WF classified
- Followed 6 to 22 years
- Uniformly curative intent (doxorubicin-based) chemotherapy
- Consensus-based morphologic review of new entities (1,131 patients)
    - low grade (SWOG 7204, 7426, 7713): 528 patients (BN, PB, TG)
    - high grade (SWOG 8516, anaplastic): 603 LCL patients (KJ, RT, TG, RB, CF, CL)
- Followed REAL diagnostic criteria (2 participants REAL signatories)
- Kaplan-Meier survival estimates: median survivals (MS) and shape of curve

Sample survival data from the review of low grade lymphoma is shown in [4.7]. This identifies a new entity, mantle cell lymphoma, lifting it out of familiar Working Formulation categories (A, B, C, D and E). One can see that this new entity – mantle cell lymphoma - had by far the poorest survival curve of any member of this group. Many of the mantle cell lymphomas derive from category E; thus this becomes a shrinking category.

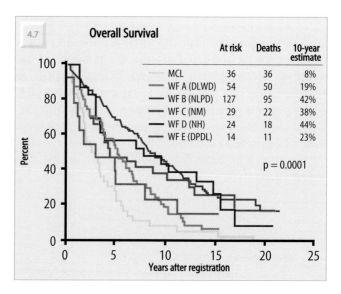

4.7	**Overall Survival**			
		At risk	Deaths	10-year estimate
	MCL	36	36	8%
	WF A (DLWD)	54	50	19%
	WF B (NLPD)	127	95	42%
	WF C (NM)	29	22	38%
	WF D (NH)	24	18	44%
	WF E (DPDL)	14	11	23%

p = 0.0001

Curves B, C and D represent grades of follicular lymphoma. There are some differences in the early five year interval, but over 20 years they overlap, with a very similar outcome [4.8]. There were also similar ten year survivals for the Working Formulation intermediate and high grade categories (diffuse mixed, large cell, immunoblastic and Burkitt-like).

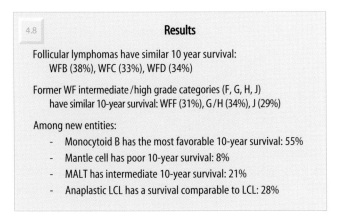

4.8	**Results**

Follicular lymphomas have similar 10 year survival:
  WFB (38%), WFC (33%), WFD (34%)

Former WF intermediate /high grade categories (F, G, H, J) have similar 10-year survival: WFF (31%), G/H (34%), J (29%)

Among new entities:
  - Monocytoid B has the most favorable 10-year survival: 55%
  - Mantle cell has poor 10-year survival: 8%
  - MALT has intermediate 10-year survival: 21%
  - Anaplastic LCL has a survival comparable to LCL: 28%

Among the new entities, the most favorable prognosis is for nodal monocytoid B cell lymphoma, with a survival of 55% at 10 years. The poorest survival was for mantle cell lymphoma, 8% after 10 years. MALT lymphomas had an intermediate survival, but this may reflect the fact that only Stage III or IV patients were included in this study. The survival of anaplastic large cell lymphoma was comparable to that of other large cell lymphomas.

If these data are presented not as simple survival curves but in combination with the therapeutic effect, three histologically distinguishable risk groups emerge [4.9]. There is a low risk group that includes monocytoid B cell lymphoma and follicular lymphoma; an intermediate group that comprises mantle cell lymphoma, Stage III and IV MALT lymphoma, small cell lymphocytic lymphoma and diffuse small cleaved cell lymphoma; and a high risk group comprising anaplastic large cell lymphoma, all large cell lymphomas, diffuse mixed cell lymphoma and Burkitt-like lymphoma. For the low and intermediate cases there is no change in the shape of the curve (no plateau), whereas in the high risk group there is a change in the shape, with the appearance of a plateau, and we can conclude that there are cures among the latter group.

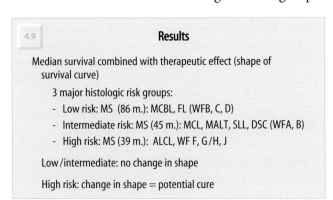

4.9	**Results**

Median survival combined with therapeutic effect (shape of survival curve)

  3 major histologic risk groups:
  - Low risk: MS (86 m.): MCBL, FL (WFB, C, D)
  - Intermediate risk: MS (45 m.): MCL, MALT, SLL, DSC (WFA, B)
  - High risk: MS (39 m.): ALCL, WF F, G/H, J

Low /intermediate: no change in shape

High risk: change in shape = potential cure

The SWOG low histologic risk group is shown in [4.10], comprising the three grades of follicular lymphoma and monocytoid B cell lymphoma. There may be early differences in he follicular grades but over fifteen years they are comparable in outcome. The curve shows a slow steady decline, without a plateau.

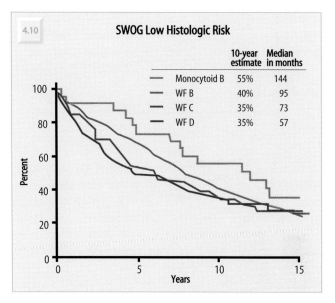

The curves for the (SWOG) intermediate group have a steeper slope, and again there is no plateau [4.11]. Once again, mantle cell lymphoma stands out as a distinct entity. Although originally considered indolent, this clearly has a very poor survival, 8% at 10 years. This intermediate risk group includes small lymphocytic lymphoma and diffuse small cleaved cell lymphoma (non-mantle cell).

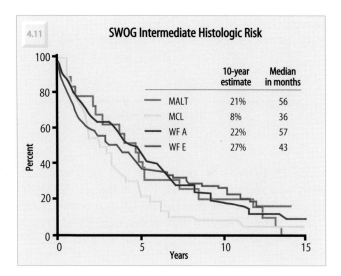

The (SWOG) high histologic risk group [4.12] comprises anaplastic large cell lymphoma, the diffuse mixed category F, large cell lymphoma and immunoblastic lymphoma, without perceptible differences in outcome. The category J cases are largely Burkitt-like lymphomas.

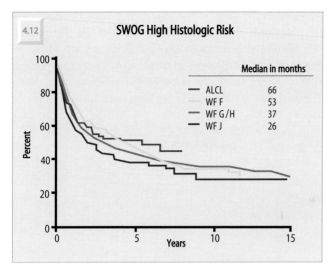

If one compares the low, intermediate and high risk groups, it is the high risk group that stands out with a plateau [4.13]. The low risk group shows no plateau, with a slow but steady decline over time, whereas the intermediate group shows a sharper slope over time again without a plateau.

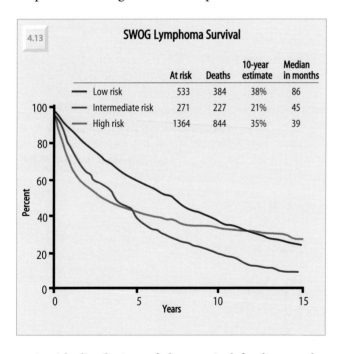

An idealized view of the survival for low grade, intermediate and high risk lymphoma is shown in [4.14]. One can see that the categorization we made comes pretty close to this theoretical ideal, which comprises what we might call the three basic types of lymphoma.

From this we can conclude that the REAL nomenclature is obviously useful in that it identifies distinct clinical entities [4.15]. These entities have predictable outcomes relative to the known Working Formulation categories. We have been able to review the histology of our patients from the 1970s in the

light of the REAL scheme to achieve consensus and then to look at their survival patterns. The REAL categories allows re-grouping of the histologic subsets and gives us a more uniform prognostic scheme.

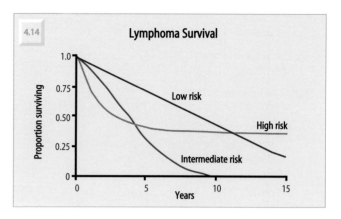

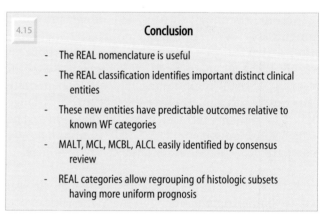

A final point concerns one particular entity and our changing understanding over twenty years. This illustrates that classification is an ongoing process and will continue to evolve in the future. Diffuse, poorly differentiated lymphocytic lymphoma as recognized in 1975 is shown [4.16]. In 1982, in the Working Formulation study, the survival curve for lymphoblastic lymphoma (category I) shows up to the left and the category E, diffuse small cleaved cell lymphoma, moves to the right. Then in 1995, the REAL scheme separated out the mantle cell lymphomas, most of which came from category E, and it is evident that they form another category to the left. Data from 1996, on diffuse small cleaved cell lymphoma cases, reveals that a low proliferative rate allows further stratification of outcome. Thus, with increasing experience and the use of specific markers, our vision of an individual disease evolves progressively and subsets emerge. Those markers are critical in the initial identification of these subsets, but ultimately morphology may find those subsets.

Thus we are witnessing the emergence of discrete homogeneous entities defined by amalgamated data and mantle cell lymphoma is a case in point, with specific phenotypic, genotypic, and clinical features. The SWOG 8819 clinicopathologic definition of mantle cell lymphoma is shown [4.17]. Entities such as mantle cell lymphoma can now be identified with increasing accuracy, and these identifications are clearly useful to clinicians.

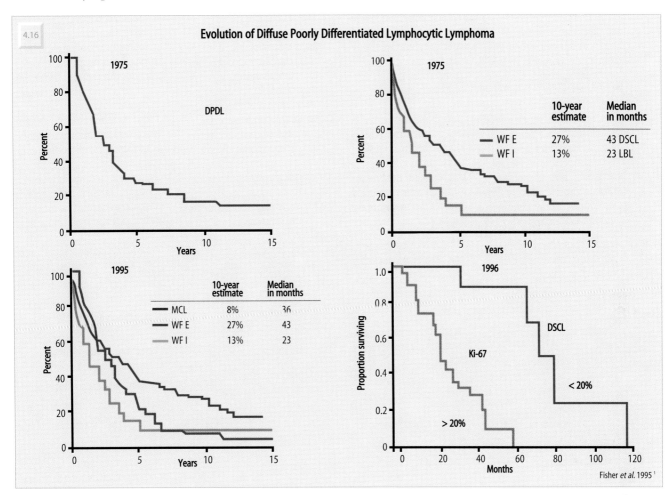

4.16 **Evolution of Diffuse Poorly Differentiated Lymphocytic Lymphoma**

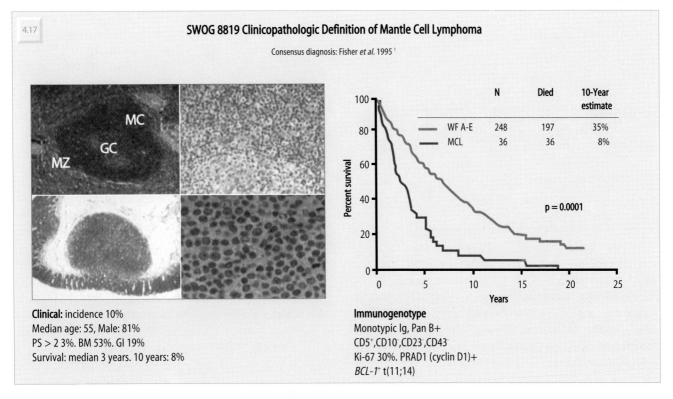

4.17 **SWOG 8819 Clinicopathologic Definition of Mantle Cell Lymphoma**

Consensus diagnosis: Fisher *et al.* 1995 [1]

Clinical: incidence 10%
Median age: 55, Male: 81%
PS > 2 3%. BM 53%. GI 19%
Survival: median 3 years. 10 years: 8%

Immunogenotype
Monotypic Ig, Pan B+
CD5+,CD10-,CD23-,CD43-
Ki-67 30%. PRAD1 (cyclin D1)+
BCL-1+ t(11;14)

REFERENCES

1. Fisher RI, Dahlberg S, Nathwani BN, Banks PM, Miller TP, Grogan TM. A clinical analysis of two indolent lymphoma entities: mantle cell lymphoma and marginal zone lymphoma (including the mucosa-associated lymphoid tissue and monocytoid B-cell subcategories): a Southwest Oncology Group study. *Blood* 1995; **85**: 1075-82.

FURTHER READING

Banks PM, Chan J, Cleary ML *et al.* Mantle cell lymphoma: A proposal for unification of morphologic, immunologic and molecular data. *Am J Sur Pathol* 1992; **16**: 637-40.

Chan JKC, Banks PM, Cleary ML *et al.* A revised European-American classification of lymphoid neoplasms proposed by the International Lymphoma Study Group. A summary version. *Amer J Clin Path* 1995; **103**: 543-60.

Grogan T, Miller T, Dahlberg S *et al.* Morphologic review of 2100 SWOG patients supports the REAL classification of lymphoma as clinically useful. *Lab Invest* 1996; **74**: 650.

Harris NL, Jaffe ES, Stein H *et al.* A revised European-American classification of lymphoid neoplasms: a proposal from the International Lymphoma Study Group. *Blood* 1994; **84**: 1361-92.

Nathwani BN, Metter GE, Miller TP *et al.* What should be the morphologic criteria for the subdivision of follicular lymphomas? *Blood* 1986; **68**: 837-45.

The Non-Hodgkin's Lymphoma Pathologic Classification Project. NCI sponsored study of classifications of non-Hodgkin's lymphoma. Summary and description of a working formulation for clinical usage. *Cancer* 1982; **49**: 2112-35.

POST-SCRIPT

The recently published Nebraska study of the REAL classification[2] adds considerable weight to the above SWOG observations by finding: (1) discrete REAL categories are readily and <u>reproducibly</u> diagnosed in the multi-institutional review; and (2) the distinction of B cell versus T cell lineage in the REAL classification has clinical significance.

REFERENCES

2. The Non-Hodgkin's Lymphoma Classification Project. A clinical evaluation of the International Lymphoma Study Group classification of non-Hodgkin's lymphoma. *Blood* 1997; **89**: 3909-3918.

Morphologic, immunologic and genetic features of B cell CLL/SLL and immunocytoma

R A Warnke

Chronic lymphocytic leukemia (CLL) / small lymphocytic lymphoma (SLL) and lymphoplasmacytic lymphomas (immunocytoma) are two of the four major small B cell categories in the REAL scheme. Together with a couple of T cell disorders, they used to comprise "small lymphocytic" lymphoma in the Working Formulation [5.1].

5.1	"Small Lymphocytic" Lymphoma	
Working Formulation	**REAL Classification**	
	B cell neoplasms	
Small lymphocytic	CLL/PLL/Small lymphocytic	
	Lymphoplasmacytoid	
	Mantle cell	
	Marginal zone	
	Extranodal (MALT type)	
	Monocytoid	
	T cell neoplasms	
	CLL/PLL/small lymphocytic	
	LGL leukemia	

CLL/SLL patients account for about 10% of our adult oncology patients at Stanford, and these disorders are about ten times as common as lymphoplasmacytic lymphoma (immunocytoma), as shown in [5.2]. SLL, which in tissue sections looks indistinguishable from B cell CLL, can be defined as a neoplasm composed of lymphocytes that have the appearance of the unstimulated small B cells seen in primary follicles, or in the mantle zones of secondary follicles [5.3].

At low power, one often sees pseudofollicles, commonly referred to as "proliferation centers" or "growth centers". These are especially common in leukemic cases, so that more than 80% of cases of B cell CLL have these pseudofollicles, compared to about half that number in non-leukemic cases. They are composed of cells which often have prominent central nucleoli, and which comprise both small lymphoid cells, or prolymphocytes, and larger cells, sometimes referred to as paraimmunoblasts or large prolymphocytes. One may also see plasmacytoid lymphocytes and plasma cells, cells with cleaved nuclei, or "centrocyte-like" cells. Dr. Weisenberger and others have shown that if these larger cells and proliferation centers are seen in cases of what used to be called intermediate lymphocytic lymphoma the clinical behavior will be that of CLL or SLL.[1] Generally there is a low mitotic index [5.4].

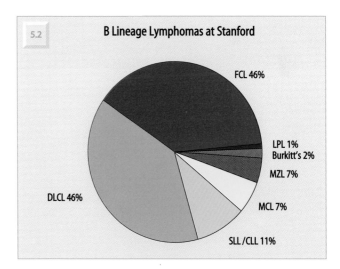

5.2 B Lineage Lymphomas at Stanford

FCL 46%
LPL 1%
Burkitt's 2%
MZL 7%
MCL 7%
SLL/CLL 11%
DLCL 46%

5.3	B-CLL/Small Lymphocytic Lymphoma Definition

Small lymphocytic lymphoma (and B cell CLL which is indistinguishable from SLL in tissue sections), is a neoplasm composed of lymphocytes that have the cytological appearance of the unstimulated lymphocytes normally residing in the primary follicles or the mantle zones of secondary follicles of lymphoid tissue.

5.4	**B-CLL /Small Lymphocytic Lymphoma Morphology**

Pseudofollicles (> 80% in CLL vs 40% in SLL)

Prolymphocytes and paraimmunoblasts

Plasmacytoid lymphocytes and plasma cells

Cleaved cells

Low mitotic index

At low magnification the architecture of the lymph node is typically effaced by sheets of small lymphocytes [5.5], and these are indistinguishable from the normal lymphocytes that occupy the B zones of the lymphoid tissue. Many cases at low magnification contain pale nodular areas [5.6], or pseudofollicles, and these continue to cause problems in diagnosis. For example, a case seen by the author at Stanford was mistakenly diagnosed as a follicular large cell lymphoma, but proved to be a low grade SLL.

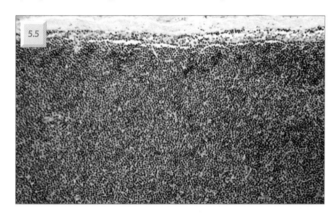

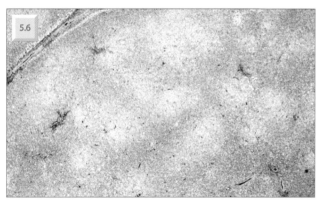

Within these pseudofollicles, there are smaller cells with prominent central nucleoli (prolymphocytes), as well as larger cells also with prominent central nucleoli (paraimmunoblasts). In addition one may see ordinary large lymphoid cells with one or more small nucleoli [5.7].

About 85-90% of cases express IgM and about half of these also express IgD. Typically the amount of immunoglobulin is less than on a normal small lymphocyte, so that staining is weak in tissue sections or by flow cytometry. The great majority of cases express CD5 and this appears to be virtually always present among the CLL cases, but is less common in non-leukemic cases. These neoplasms express CD23, lack CD10, and express a variety of B cell markers. However, about half lack CD22, and most of the remaining cases express CD22 only weakly, another useful immunologic feature [5.8].

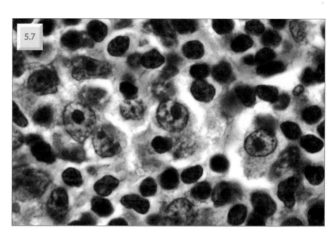

5.8	**B-CLL /Small Lymphocytic Lymphoma**	
Immunology:		**(CLL vs SLL)**
Surface IgM±IgD		+ (weak)
CD5		+ (> 90% vs 50%)
CD10		−
CD19, 20, 79a		+
CD22		±
CD23		+
CD11a/18 (LFA-1)		± (30% vs > 90%)
Mouse RBC rosettes		+ (85% vs 70%)

Dr. Inghirami and others, working with Dr. Knowles,[2] reported that the leukemic cases express the adhesion molecule LFA-1 less frequently than non-leukemic cases, although this has not yet been confirmed. In both types of disease the neoplastic cells may form rosettes with mouse erythrocytes.

Typically most cases have a low proliferative rate, so only a small number of nuclei stained for Ki-67 are seen [5.9 left]. However, there are occasional cases in which a much larger number of cells is labelled [5.9 right].

If one analyzes survival curves, the patients with the low number of proliferating cells have a significantly better outcome than those with a high percentage [5.10].

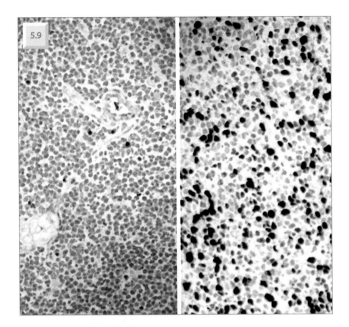

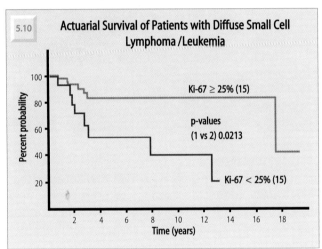

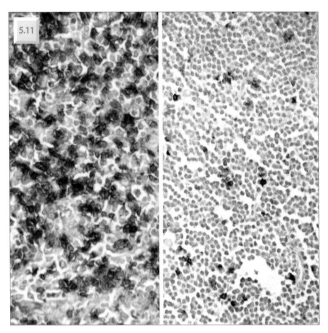

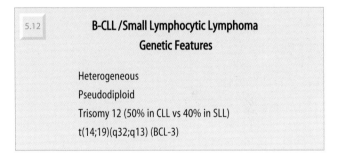

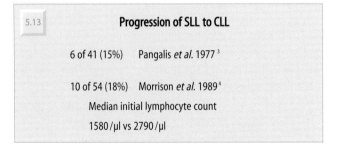

diagnosed as SLL acquired the clinical features of CLL over time. In the more recent study, most of the cases that became leukemic had a higher initial lymphocyte count, in the order of about 3,000/μl.

Most cases contain plentiful reactive host T cells, especially CD4-positive cells [5.11 left]. However, some cases have a very low number of T cells [5.11 right], and the number of CD4-positive cells also correlates with clinical behavior, the survival being better for patients with significant numbers of T cells than for those with few T cells.

The genetic features in this category are heterogeneous [5.12]. Many of the cases are pseudodiploid. Trisomy 12, while not being specific for this category, is seen fairly commonly, and roughly similar numbers are seen whether the cases are leukemic or not. A rare anomaly is the t(14;19) translocation.

It has been suggested that a high percentage of cases of SLL will progress to CLL, and at least two studies have addressed this. One of these was from Rappaport's group in 1977,[3] and the other was reported more recently from Stanford [5.13].[4] The results are virtually identical, in that about 10 to 20% of cases

Lymphoplasmacytic lymphoma (also known as immunocytoma) is a rarer entity [5.14]. This neoplasm is composed of small lymphocytes that show maturation towards plasma cells, but do so without demonstrating features of the other low grade subtypes. This is very important because many B cell lymphomas, including CLL, mantle cell lymphomas, marginal zone lymphomas and even follicular lymphomas, can differentiate towards plasma cells. This feature can be highlighted with a Giemsa stain or methyl green pyronin stain.

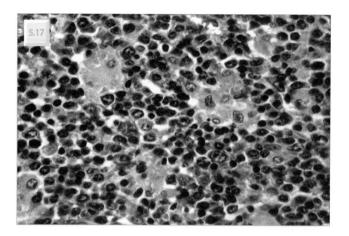

5.14   Lymphoplasmacytic Lymphoma /Immunocytoma Definition

Lymphoplasmacytoid lymphoma (immunocytoma) is a neoplasm composed of small lymphocytes that show maturation toward plasma cells without demonstrating features of other low grade lymphoma subtypes. Many lymphomas occasionally show differentiation to plasma cells including CLL, mantle cell lymphoma, marginal zone B cell lymphoma (monocytoid B cell lymphoma and low grade lymphoma of mucosa-associated lymphoid tissue), and follicular lymphoma.

Immunoglobulin inclusions, Russell bodies or Dutcher bodies, can be revealed with a PAS stain. Mast cells are often frequent and, because many of these patients have an autoimmune hemolytic anemia, prominent hemosiderin deposition may be seen [5.15].

5.15   Lymphoplasmacytic Lymphoma /Immunocytoma Morphology

Giemsa or methyl green pyronin (MGP) stains

Russell bodies or Dutcher bodies (PAS stain)

Mast cells

Hemosiderosis

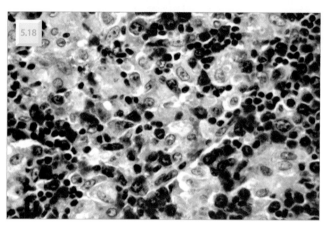

[5.19] illustrates a case with abundant cytoplasmic immunoglobulin inclusions which are PAS-positive. When these indent the nucleus or even appear as if they are intra-nuclear (Dutcher bodies) they can be useful in the diagnosis of this category, although not specific.

The case shown in [5.16] contained numerous epithelioid histiocytes. At higher magnification [5.17], this lymphoma was composed of small lymphocytes, plasmacytoid lymphocytes and plasma cells. Staining for lambda light chain [5.18] confirmed the monotypia, and hence the diagnosis of lymphoma. It also showed that the plasmacytoid cells and plasma cells were part of this lymphoma, and this can be useful in supporting the diagnosis.

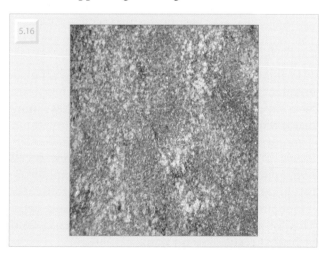

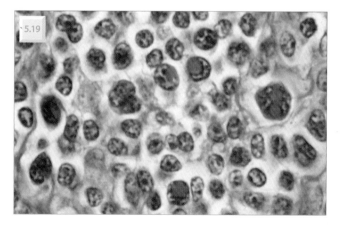

The great majority of these cases express IgM both on the cell surface and in the cytoplasm, and in a number of series there were many more kappa cases than lambda cases. Generally the cases lack CD5 and CD23 and also CD11c and CD10, and express a variety of pan-B markers [5.20]. There are no specific genetic abnormalities in this category but in one small series a (9;14) translocation was identified [5.21].

5.20

Lymphoplasmacytic Lymphoma /Immunocytoma Immunology

Surface and cytoplasmic IgM	+ ($\kappa >> \lambda$)
CD5	-/+
CD11c	-
CD10	-
CD19, 20, 22, 79a	+
CD23	-/+

5.21

Lymphoplasmacytic Lymphoma /Immunocytoma Genetic Features

No specific abnormalities

t(9;14)(q13;q32) in one small series

Some of these cases were in the "diffuse mixed" category in the Working Formulation, because in this disease occasional large lymphoid cells may be seen, just as in marginal zone type lymphomas. Consequently, there is a spectrum of clinical behavior, and cases in which these large cells are very frequent have been termed large cell rich immunocytoma, and have a more aggressive clinical behavior [5.22].

5.22

"Diffuse Mixed Small and Large Cell" Lymphoma

Working Formulation	REAL Classification
	B cell neoplasms
Diffuse mixed small and large cell	Lymphoplasmacytic
	Marginal zone
	Extranodal (MALT type)
	Monocytoid

REFERENCES

1. Weisenburger DD, Duggan MJ, Perry DA, Sanger WG, Armitage JO. Non-Hodgkin's lymphomas of mantle zone origin. *Pathol Annu* 1991; **1**: 139-58.

2. Inghirami G, Wieczorek R, Zhu BY, Silber R, Dalla-Favera R, Knowles DM. Differential expression of LFA-1 molecules in non-Hodgkin's lymphoma and lymphoid leukemia. *Blood* 1988; **72**: 1431-4.

3. Pangalis GA, Nathwani BN, Rappaport H. Malignant lymphoma, well differentiated lymphocytic type. Its relationship with chronic lymphocytic leukemia and macroglobulinemia of Waldenström. *Cancer* 1977; **39**: 999-1010.

4. Morrison WH, Hoppe RT, Weiss LM, Picozzi VJ Jr, Horning SJ. Small lymphocytic lymphoma. *J Clin Oncol* 1989; **7**: 598-606.

FURTHER READING

Aoki H, Takishita M, Kosaka M, Saito S. Frequent somatic mutations in D and/or Jh segments of Ig gene in Waldenström's macroglobulinemia and chronic lymphocytic leukemia (CLL) with Richter's syndrome but not in common CLL. *Blood* 1995; **85**: 1913-9.

BenEzra J, Burke JS, Swartz WG *et al.* Small lymphocytic lymphoma: a clinicopathologic analysis of 268 cases. *Blood* 1989; **73**: 579-87.

Bennett JM, Catovsky D, Daniel MT *et al.* Proposals for the classification of chronic (mature) B and T lymphoid leukemias. French-American-British (FAB) Cooperative Group. *J Clin Pathol* 1989; **42**: 567-84.

Berger F, Felman P, Sonet A *et al.* Nonfollicular small B-cell lymphomas: a heterogeneous group of patients with distinct clinical features and outcome. *Blood* 1994; **83**: 2829-35.

Brittinger G, Bartels H, Common H *et al.* Clinical and prognostic relevance of the Kiel classification of non-Hodgkin lymphomas: results of a prospective multicenter study by the Kiel lymphoma study group. *Hematol Oncol* 1984; **2**: 269-306.

Dighiero G, Travade P, Chevret S, Fenaux P, Chastang C, Binet JL. B-cell chronic lymphocytic leukemia: present status and future directions. *Blood* 1991; **78**: 1901-14.

Dimopoulos MA, Alexanian R. Waldenström's macroglobulinemia. *Blood* 1994; **83**: 1452-9.

Engelhard M, Brittinger G, Heinz R *et al.* Chronic lymphocytic leukemia (B-CLL) and immunocytoma (LP-IC): clinical and prognostic relevance of this distinction. *Leukemia Lymphoma* 1991; Supplement: 161-73.

Gehan EA. A generalized two-sample Wilcoxon test for doubly censored data. *Biometrika* 1965; **52**: 650-3.

Juliusson G, Oscier D, Fitchett M *et al.* Prognostic subgroups in B-cell chronic lymphocytic leukemia defined by specific chromosomal abnormalities. *N Engl J Med* 1990; **323**: 720-4.

Küppers R, Gause A, Rajewsky K. B cells of chronic lymphatic leukemia express V genes in unmutated form. *Leuk Res* 1991; **15**: 487-96.

Lennert K, Tamm I, Wacker HH. Histopathology and immunocytochemistry of lymph node biopsies in chronic lymphocytic leukemia and immunocytoma. *Leukemia Lymphoma* 1991; Supplement: 157-60.

Medeiros LJ, Picker LJ, Gelb AB *et al.* Numbers of host "helper" T cells and proliferating cells predict survival in diffuse small-cell lymphomas. *J Clin Oncol* 1989; **7**: 1009-17.

Patsouris E, Noel H, Lennert K. Lymphoplasmacytic/ lymphoplasmacytoid immunocytoma with a high content of epithelioid cells: histologic and immunohistochemical findings. *Am J Surg Pathol* 1990; **14**: 660-70.

Pozzato G, Mazzaro C, Crovatto M *et al.* Low-grade malignant lymphoma, hepatitis C virus infection, and mixed cryoglobulinemia. *Blood* 1994; **84**: 3047-53.

Wagner SD, Martinelli V, Luzzatto L. Similar patterns of Vκ gene usage but different degrees of somatic mutation in hairy cell leukemia, prolymphocytic leukemia, Waldenström's macroglobulinemia, and myeloma. *Blood* 1994; **83**: 3647-53.

Zukerberg L, Medeiros L, Ferry J, Harris N. Diffuse low-grade B-cell lymphomas: four clinically distinct subtypes defined by a combination of morphologic and immunophenotypic features. *Am J Clin Pathol* 1993; **100**: 373-85.

POST-SCRIPT

Small lymphocytic lymphoma and chronic lymphocytic leukemia are regarded as the same disease with differences in the clinical manifestations. Nevertheless, a lower incidence of pseudofollicles and CD5 expression has been reported for small lymphocytic lymphoma. These differences may be real or may have resulted from inclusion of marginal zone lymphomas in the category of small lymphocytic lymphoma in older studies.

Recent studies have addressed the molecular features of the immunoglobulin gene loci in small lymphocytic lymphoma/chronic lymphocytic leukemia and lymphoplasmacytic lymphoma (Waldenström's macroglobulinemia). In contrast to the B cells of CLL which express V genes in unmutated form, progression of CLL (Richter's transformation) and Waldenströms macroglobulinemia show frequent mutations in the D and/or JH segments of the immunoglobulin heavy chain gene.[5-7]

REFERENCES

5. Aoki H, Takishita M, Kosaka M, Saito S. Frequent somatic mutations in D and/or Jh segments of Ig gene in Waldenström's macroglobulinemia and chronic lymphocytic leukemia (CLL) with Richter's syndrome but not in common CLL. *Blood* 1995; **85**: 1913-9.

6. Küppers R, Gause A, Rajewsky K. B cells of chronic lymphatic leukemia express V genes in unmutated form. *Leuk Res* 1991; **15**: 487-96.

7. Wagner SD, Martinelli V, Luzzatto L. Similar patterns of Vκ gene usage but different degrees of somatic mutation in hairy cell leukemia, prolymphocytic leukemia, Waldenström's macroglobulinemia, and myeloma. *Blood* 1994; **83**: 3647-53.

Clinical aspects and treatment options of B cell CLL/SLL and immunocytoma

B Coiffier

One of the merits of the REAL classification is that it emphasizes different entities and particularly small lymphocytic and lymphoplasmacytic lymphomas. As noted in a preceding chapter, small lymphocytic lymphoma is found in the Working Formulation in category A and also among the diffuse small cell and diffuse mixed cell lymphomas [6.1]. There appears to be a continuum between CLL/small lymphocytic lymphoma, small cell lymphoplasmacytic lymphoma, and large cell rich immunocytoma. It is sometimes difficult to separate these, so that in this chapter all of these categories are considered together.

6.1	Small Lymphocytic and Lymphoplasmacytic Lymphoma	
Working Formulation		**REALity**
Low grade		**Small lymphocytic**
Small lymphocytic		**lymphoma/CLL**
Follicular, small cleaved cell		**Marginal zone lymphoma**
Follicular mixed		MALT lymphoma
Intermediate grade		Monocytoid B cell
Follicular large cell		Splenic lymphoma
Diffuse small cleaved cell		**Mantle cell lymphoma**
Diffuse mixed		**Immunocytoma**
Diffuse large cell		CLL-like
High grade		LCRI
Immunoblastic		Others
Lymphoblastic		**T small cell lymphomas**
Small non-cleaved cell		

Lymphoplasmacytic and small lymphocytic lymphomas are quite frequent in our center, accounting for slightly more than 10% of lymphoma patients [6.2]. They are therefore commoner than mantle cell or marginal zone lymphoma. There are very few studies in the literature that focus on this category because they were mixed in the Kiel classification with CLL patients, and in the Working Formulation with low grade lymphoma, principally follicular lymphoma. In the pie chart showing data from the NCI Surveillance, Epidemiology and End Results

(SEER) program on more than 30,000 patients [6.3], one sees again that the percentage is about 10% of all lymphoma patients.

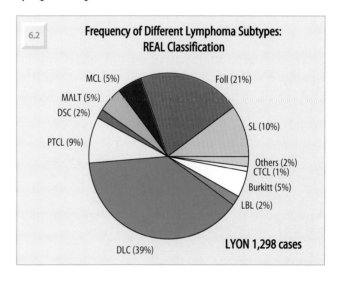

Frequency of Different Lymphoma Subtypes: REAL Classification

MCL (5%), MALT (5%), DSC (2%), PTCL (9%), DLC (39%), Foll (21%), SL (10%), Others (2%), CTCL (1%), Burkitt (5%), LBL (2%)

LYON 1,298 cases

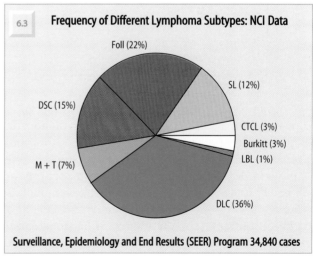

Frequency of Different Lymphoma Subtypes: NCI Data

Foll (22%), DSC (15%), M + T (7%), DLC (36%), SL (12%), CTCL (3%), Burkitt (3%), LBL (1%)

Surveillance, Epidemiology and End Results (SEER) Program 34,840 cases

The survival of all patients attending our center are summarized in [6.4]. The features are similar to those detailed elsewhere by Dr. Grogan. The marginal zone lymphomas include MALT lymphomas, which are mostly localized, and this explains their better prognosis. Follicular lymphoma is also shown, as is the survival for the small lymphocytic lymphomas. One sees clearly that small lymphocytic/ lymphoplasmacytic lymphoma has a worse outcome than follicular lymphoma.

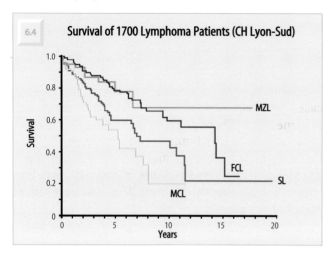

There is little information on this subject in the literature, but [6.5] shows survival data, published some years ago by Dr. Lister. He also observed a poor outcome and no cures for small lymphocytic and lymphoplasmacytic lymphoma.

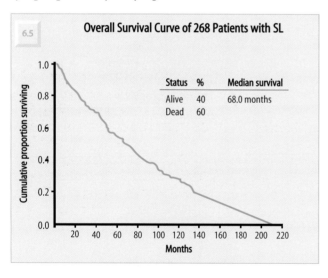

The results shown in [6.6] are from Dr. Fisher, and probably correspond to the data of Dr. Grogan. One can again see clearly that lymphoplasmacytic lymphoma has a worse outcome than follicular lymphoma.

These patients should therefore be considered separately because they also differ from CLL patients. CLL patients mostly have blood and bone marrow involvement and sometimes lymph node and spleen involvement whereas usually small lymphocytic/ lymphoplasmacytic lymphoma cases have lymph node involvement, as well as sometimes blood involvement.

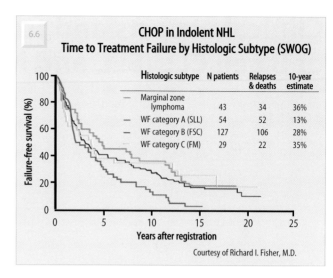

To diagnose classical B CLL [6.7], one needs to see at least four or five of the following features: weak surface immunoglobulin, expression of CD5 and CD23; absence of FMC7; and a weak or negative reaction for CD22. Most of the lymphoplasmacytic lymphomas have only one of two of these markers; they are usually FMC7-positive and CD23-negative, with strong immunoglobulin and CD22 positivity.

6.7	Immunophenotyping	
	LPL	**CLL/SLL**
Surface Ig	Weak	Moderate/strong
CD5	Positive	Negative
CD23	Positive	Negative
FMC7	Negative	Positive
CD22	Weak/negative	Moderate/strong

Matutes *et al.* 1994 [1]

Cytologic features may also be of value in making the diagnosis. Figure [6.8] is from a patient who was referred to our center with an initial diagnosis of CLL. However, the appearance of the cells in cytologic smears was different from that of classical CLL in that they were large, with atypical features, such as abundant cytoplasm and clearly visible nucleoli.

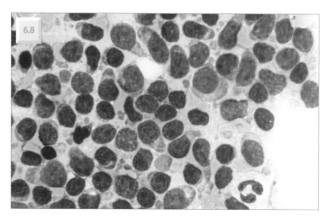

Chromosomal abnormalities are frequently found in lymphoplasmacytic lymphoma. The karyotype shown in [6.9] is characteristic of a new entity we have observed in our center, characterized by a deletion in the long arm of chromosome 11 at 11q13, which may be recognized in the future as a recurrent anomaly.

6.9 Karyotyping of Lymphoplasmacytic Lymphoma

Summarized in [6.10] are the differences between CLL, lymphoplasmacytic lymphoma, and other lymphoma categories. CLL and LPL can be distinguished by the pattern of expression of LFA-1, which is mostly negative in CLL patients and usually positive in lymphoplasmacytic lymphoma. The same is true for CD54 and this can be of help in diagnosis. Currently, CLL and SLL cells have the same phenotype and cannot be distinguished.

6.10 Expression of Adhesion Molecules in Lymphoproliferative Disorders				
	CD44	LECAM-1	LFA-1 (CD11a/CD18)	CD54 (ICAM-1)
CLL	+	+/-	-/+	-
LPL	+	-/+	+/-	+/-
MCL	+	-	-	-
FCL	+	-	+/-	+/-
DLCL	+	-	-/+	+/-
B L / LAL	-	-	-	-

As far as the clinical picture is concerned [6.11], there are differences between lymphoplasmacytic lymphoma and large cell rich immunocytoma and marginal zone lymphoma. The patients typically have a good performance status, except for the small group of patients with large cell rich immunocytoma. Most patients have bone marrow involvement. Between 10% and 30% have blood involvement, but usually only at a low level, i.e. usually with less than 5,000/ml neoplastic cells. There is spleen involvement in at least 30-40% of patients.

6.11 Diffuse Small Cell Lymphoma Patients Treated in CH Lyon-Sud (%)				
	Poor PS	BM+	Blood+	Spleen+
LPL	12	79	30	39
WD	21	90	8	21
LCRI	31	71	18	42
MZL	8	70	18	65

When the disease stage is reviewed [6.12], most cases have blood or bone marrow involvement, but in some 10 to 20% of patients the disease is localized to only one or two lymph nodes. If one includes blood and bone marrow, most of the patients have involvement of more than one extranodal site, but otherwise the figure is less than 20%. Few have bulky tumors at diagnosis.

6.12 Diffuse Small Cell Lymphoma Patients Treated in CH Lyon-Sud (%)				
	Localized stage	No extranodal site	1 extranodal site	> 1 extranodal site	Bulky tumor
LPL	13	12	30	58	21
WD	19	-	69	31	4
LCRI	14	17	34	49	29
MZL	19	11	27	62	32

A serum M component is always, by definition, present in Waldenström's disease, but it is also found in 20-30% of the other diseases. Very few have high LDH levels, except the patients with large cell rich immunocytoma, who also tend to have low serum albumin levels. High β_2-microglobulin levels are frequent in all categories, and particularly so in large cell rich immunocytoma. Large cell rich immunocytoma patients therefore present with worse features than those in other categories [6.13].

6.13 Diffuse Small Cell Lymphoma Patients Treated in CH Lyon-Sud (%)				
	M comp	High LDH	Low S alb	High β_2-m
LPL	20	33	13	49
WD	100	13	20	61
LCRI	32	53	39	70
MZL	25	35	20	43

We have treated approximately 120 of these patients in our center. The results shown in [6.14] represent not a randomized trial but a retrospective study based on different treatments. One sees that the complete remission rate is low, although it is slightly higher in large cell rich immunocytoma. This is probably because the latter cases represent a more aggressive disease, but is not statistically significant. Most of these patients responded to treatment in that they achieved partial remission, but nearly all of them relapsed at some time after initial treatment.

Details from the study in which we compared survival and freedom from progression for these patients are shown in [6.14] and [6.15]. LPL patients had an intermediate outcome, worse than MZL patients but better than LCRI patients.

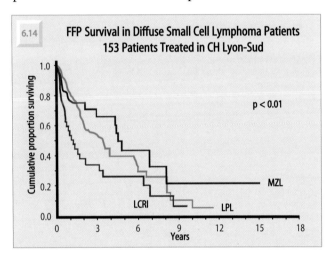

If one looks at the time to progression in all patients [6.15], lymphoplasmacytic lymphoma was intermediate between mantle zone lymphoma and large cell rich immunocytoma. However, survival is not good, and all patients showed disease progression at some time. If survival is reviewed, marginal zone lymphoma has a good prognosis - they progress but have good survival. The survival for large cell rich immunocytomas is slightly worse than for lymphoplasmacytic lymphoma.

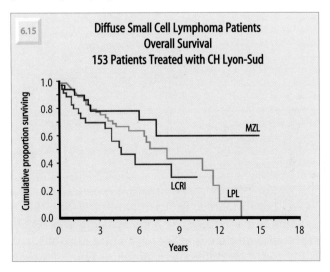

Clearly there is no cure for these patients, and better treatment strategies are needed [6.16]. Very few trials have analyzed only small lymphocytic lymphoma or lymphoplasmacytic lymphoma, since these patients are usually mixed with follicular lymphoma or other so called low grade lymphomas. No curative treatment has been described for these patients. Our current recommendation is not to treat patients older than 65 years, but to wait until clinical manifestations appear. For young patients, without adverse parameters, single agent chemotherapy is probably best. In the past this meant chlorambucil or cyclophosphamide, but today we would consider fludarabine. For patients with adverse prognostic parameters, more aggressive treatment is needed – for example, fludarabine and CHOP – followed, if there is a good response, by bone marrow transplantation.

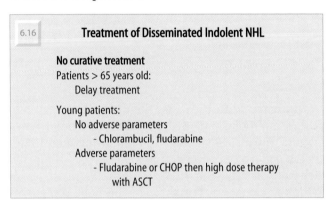

Shown in [6.17], are the results of a trial in which we treated 150 patients with fludarabine at different stages of the disease. The response rate to fludarabine was very low, and only a small percentage of patients achieved complete remission. The same was true for lymphoplasmacytic lymphoma. However, most patients, at least 50-70%, responded. If the results of fludarabine treatment are reviewed, the curve in blue is for patients where it was first line treatment, the red curve is for patients in whom it was used as second line therapy, and the yellow curve is for other patients. There was clearly a good response and a good survival in lymphoplasmacytic lymphoma patients treated in this way.

6.17	**Fludarabine in Indolent Lymphomas and CLL Patients** **Response According to Types of Lymphoma**		
	CR	% CR	% Response
CLL	3	7	59
LPL	5	18	79
Waldenström	1	9	55
MZL	3	60	80
FCL	19	44	72
MCL	1	6	17
CTCL	0	0	0

Finally, large cell rich immunocytoma represents a problem which appears not to have been recognized in the past, because these patients were included in the diffuse mixed cell lymphoma category and often treated as large cell lymphoma [6.18]. These patients present with aggressive disease and many adverse prognostic factors. They are refractory to standard treatment, and we see no complete responses, and a very low response rate. CHOP gave better results, but overall the response was disappointing and no patients were cured. Clearly, we have to find new treatment strategies for these patients.

6.18	**Large Cell Rich Immunocytoma Patients**
	Aggressive disease
	Stage IV, bone marrow and blood
	High LDH and β_2-microglobulin levels
	Refractory to standard treatments
	No CR, PR in 60%, SD in 20% and PD in 20%
	Better results with CHOP
	To be tested:
	High dose therapy with ASCT in first response
	Monoclonal antibodies

REFERENCES

1. Matutes E, Owusu-Ankomah K, Morilla R *et al*. The immunological profile of B-cell disorders and proposal of a scoring system for the diagnosis of CLL. *Leukemia* 1994; **8**: 1640-5.

FURTHER READING

Baldini L, Guffanti A, Cro L, *et al*. Poor prognosis in non-villous splenic marginal zone cell lymphoma is associated with p53 mutations. *Brit J Haematol* 1997; **99**: 375-8.

Brynes RK, Almaguer PD, Leathery KE, *et al*. Numerical cytogenetic abnormalities of chromosomes 3, 7, and 12 in marginal zone B-cell lymphomas. *Mod Pathol* 1996; **9**: 995-1000.

Fisher RI, Dahlberg S, Nathwani BN, Banks PM, Miller TP, Grogan TM. A clinical analysis of two indolent lymphoma entities: Mantle cell lymphoma and marginal zone lymphoma (including the mucosa-associated lymphoid tissue and monocytoid B-cell subcategories). A Southwest Oncology Group study. *Blood* 1995; **85**: 1075-82.

de Wolf-Peeters C, Pittaluga S, Dierlamm J, Wlodarska I, van den Berghe H. Marginal zone B-cell lymphomas including mucosa-associated lymphoid tissue type lymphoma (MALT), monocytoid B-cell lymphoma and splenic marginal zone cell lymphoma and their relation to the reactive marginal zone. *Leuk Lymphoma* 1997; **26**: 467-78.

POST-SCRIPT

Since the meeting at which this presentation was made, the discussions concerning the WHO proposal for lymphoma classification, which will be an update of the REAL classification, have separated marginal zone lymphoma (MZL) as a specific entity, encompassing MALT lymphoma, splenic lymphoma, and nodal MZL. Most of the cases we described previously as LPL or LCRI are now recognized as MZL with or without a large cell component. These cases are defined by the specific pattern of infiltration, the particular composition of cells (frequently showing lymphoplasmacytic differentiation), the CD5/CD23/CD10-negative phenotype, and the same karyotypic abnormalities as those described in MALT lymphoma.

We currently recognize three clinical subtypes of non-MALT marginal zone lymphomas: splenic lymphomas with or without villous lymphocytes, nodal MZL with or without monocytoid B cells, and disseminated cases. Bone marrow infiltration is observed in nearly all splenic and disseminated cases but in only 30% of nodal cases. A high component of large cells is frequent in disseminated cases, less common in nodal cases, and rare in splenic cases.

Median time-to-progression and median survival are longer in splenic MZL compared to nodal or disseminated MZL, with figures of 7 and 9 years compared to 1 and 6 years, respectively. However, the presence of a high component of large cells is not associated with a worse outcome (data unpublished).

Splenic marginal zone B cell lymphoma

P G Isaacson

The entity of splenic marginal zone lymphoma was listed originally in the REAL classification as a provisional entity but it is rapidly gaining full membership of the club. The histologic features which define it are listed [7.1].

| 7.1 | **Splenic Marginal Zone Lymphoma Histologic Features** |

Perifollicular (white pulp) involvement
  - +/– preservation of reactive follicle centres
  - mantle zone not preserved
  - biphasic cytology: central small lymphocytes, peripheral (marginal) zone of cells with more abundant pale cytoplasm and scattered transformed blasts

Red pulp
  - diffuse infiltrate of small cells and micronodular aggregates of larger cells
  - invasion of sinuses

Splenic hilar (and peripheral) lymph nodes
  - sinuses preserved and dilated
  - folliculocentric infiltrate without "marginal" zone

Bone marrow
  - interstitial (non-paratrabecular) nodules

In summary, a nodular infiltrate of the white pulp of the spleen is seen, centred on pre-existing follicles, and there is sometimes preservation of reactive follicle centers. An important point is that the mantle zone is not preserved. The cytology of these cells is "biphasic", with a central area of small lymphocytes, and a peripheral, or marginal, zone of cells with more abundant pale cytoplasm, mixed with scattered transformed blasts. The red pulp of the spleen is also involved, with diffuse infiltrates of small cells and micronodular aggregates of larger cells, and there is invasion of sinuses. The splenic hilar lymph nodes are almost always involved, and occasionally peripheral lymph nodes are also involved. These nodes are distinguished by preservation and dilatation of the sinuses, and an infiltrate centred, as in the spleen, on the follicles. However, there is no marginal zone pattern. The infiltration in the bone marrow is also characteristic - it is interstitial, again nodular, and non-paratrabecular.

The low power view of the spleen in [7.2] shows the nodules with the marginal zone pattern which gives the entity its name. It is evident that there is infiltration of the red pulp.

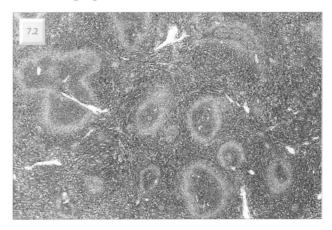

In a white pulp nodule [7.3 left] the follicle center is preserved. The biphasic nature of this infiltrate is evident, with a central darker zone (which sometimes infiltrates into the follicle center) and a paler marginal zone. In another nodule [7.3 right], which is perhaps more typical, the follicle center has been totally effaced.

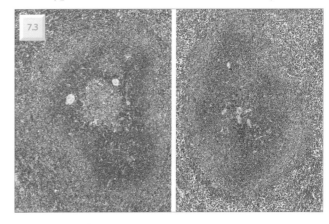

At higher power [7.4], the gradual transition from the central darker zone outwards to the marginal zone appearance is seen, within which there are transformed blasts.

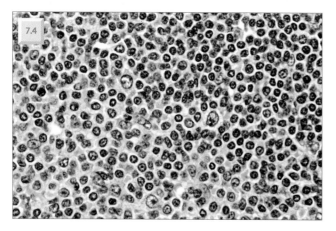

In the red pulp [7.5], nodules of the larger cells which comprise the marginal zone area, and diffuse infiltrates of the smaller cells, with prominent sinus invasion, are seen.

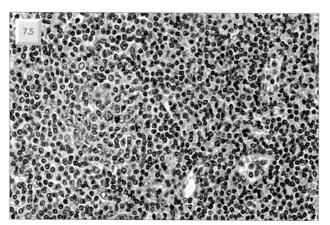

The pattern of involvement in the lymph node [7.6] is unique, in that there is a nodular pattern and these nodules are all based on pre-existing follicles. There are also prominent dilated sinuses.

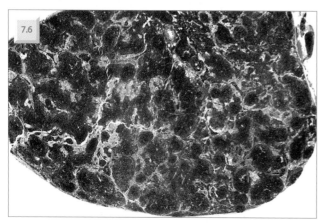

Within the nodule shown in [7.7], a very small residual follicle center can be identified, and an infiltrate within and around it. At higher power

occasional transformed blasts are seen, accompanied by smaller lymphocytes. It is of note that there is no marginal zone appearance in the lymph node.

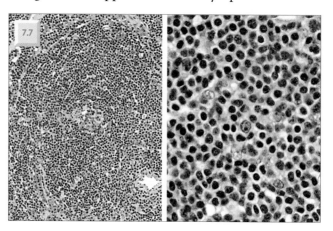

The infiltrate in the bone marrow [7.8] has a non-paratrabecular interstitial pattern, and the nodules that comprise the infiltrate are similar to those seen in the lymph nodes. Small reactive follicle centers are often present (although not seen in [7.8]).

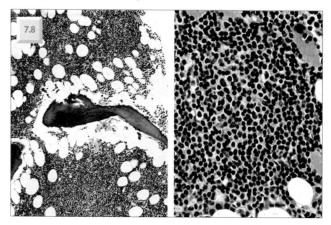

This disease can occur as a primary lymphoma of the spleen without peripheral blood involvement, but when neoplastic cells are seen in the circulation they often have polar villi, and the term "splenic lymphoma with villous lymphocytes" is used by hematologists. However, circulating neoplastic cells which lack these distinctive villi are sometimes found. Furthermore, the bone marrow may be involved, even when the peripheral blood is not [7.9].

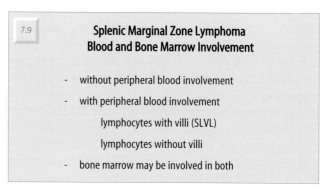

7.9 **Splenic Marginal Zone Lymphoma
Blood and Bone Marrow Involvement**

- without peripheral blood involvement
- with peripheral blood involvement
    lymphocytes with villi (SLVL)
    lymphocytes without villi
- bone marrow may be involved in both

Shown in [7.10] is the typical appearance seen in the peripheral blood. The two cells seen here have fine polar villi which are quite different in appearance from those of hairy cells.

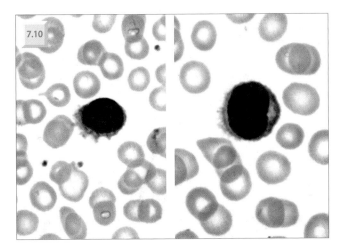

The neoplastic cells typically express IgM and in most, but not all, cases IgD [7.11]. They express mature B cell antigens, and two antigens which are typical of marginal zone B cells (CD21, CD35) are variably expressed. In contrast to many other B cell lymphomas, the author has yet to see a case in which CD43 has been expressed.

7.11	Splenic Marginal Zone Lymphoma Immunophenotype	
Ig	M+, D+(−)
CD20	+
CD10	−
CD5	−
CD23	−
CD21	+/−
CD35	+/−
CD43	−
Cyclin D1	−

Shown in [7.12] is a nodule containing a reactive follicle center in the spleen. The neoplastic cells express both IgM and also IgD. The follicle center is negative, as one expects, for IgD, but no residual strongly IgD-positive mantle zone cells are present.

In a second case [7.13] the tumor is IgM-positive but IgD-negative. If these cells were truly in the marginal zone, a residual IgD-positive mantle zone should be present, but again this is not seen.

These tumors are frequently very rich in T cells [7.14]. The tumor cells in this sample are negative for CD43, as is probably true for all cases.

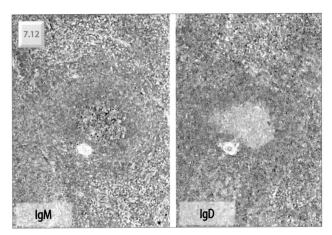

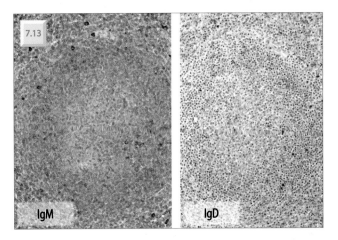

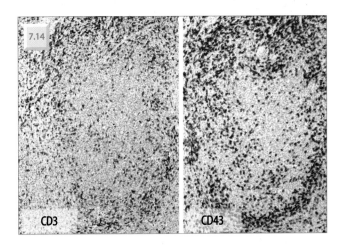

BCL-2 immunostaining can be of value when it highlights the reactive germinal centers seen in at least some of the splenic nodules [7.15]. Ki-67 is also a valuable immunostain which can now be detected in paraffin sections. This reveals a high proliferation fraction in the marginal zone area, and a very low proliferation fraction in the area of small dark cells. A target-like appearance is frequently seen, representing a tiny area of proliferating residual reactive follicle cells at the center, and can be a useful diagnostic aid.

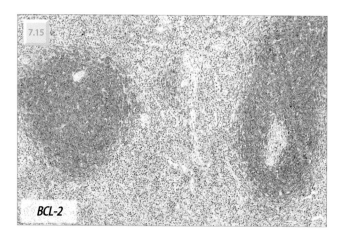

BCL-2

The genotypic features of this condition [7.16] remain to be fully documented. Immunoglobulin genes are rearranged, and they are also somatically mutated. One study, based on peripheral blood samples, has reported no ongoing mutations, but in the author's own study ongoing mutations and evidence of antigen selection were found. Cytogenetic studies have been performed by the Catovsky group, mainly on peripheral blood samples. They found a number of abnormalities, including the (11;14) translocation in a number of cases, but these may in reality have been true mantle cell lymphomas, and not splenic marginal zone lymphomas. In a study from Holland, trisomy 3 was found in half of the cases, but the numbers were small.

Splenic Marginal Zone Lymphoma
Genotype

Immunoglobulin genes
Monoclonal rearrangement
Mutated
No ongoing mutations (SLVL)
                          Zhu *et al.* 1995 [1]
Ongoing mutations, antigen selected (SMZL)
                          Dunn-Walters *et al.* 1998 [2]
Cytogenetics
    31 patients (all SLVL): t(11;14) in 5;7q del /trans in 7;
        iso 17q in 4; 2p11 trans in 4
                          Oscier *et al.* 1993 [3]
    7 patients (SLVL in 3): +3 in 3; various others
                          Dierlamm *et al.* 1996 [4]

What is the normal cell counterpart [7.17]? Our group was responsible for suggesting that this is a marginal zone B cell lymphoma, because it arises as a primary splenic lymphoma, and has a marginal zone pattern. The cytology of the cells, at least at the periphery of the infiltrate, also approximates to that of splenic marginal zone B cells, as does the immunophenotype. However, there is now a considerable array of evidence against this. First of all, the mantle zone is not preserved, as it is in other marginal zone lymphomas. Furthermore, the cells are not

confined to marginal zones, and they have an unusual biphasic cytology, which is not seen in normal marginal zones. Moreover, the marginal zone pattern is seen only in the spleen and not in the lymph nodes. Another point is that the histology and immunophenotype are slightly different from that of normal marginal zone cells, and of other marginal zone cell lymphomas when they involve the spleen. Finally, a number of other low grade lymphomas can adopt a marginal zone pattern when they infiltrate the spleen.

Splenic Marginal Zone Lymphoma
Normal Cell Counterpart

In favor of the marginal zone B-cell
- a primary splenic lymphoma
- a marginal zone pattern
- cytology at periphery +/−=marginal zone cells
- immunophenotype +/−=marginal zone cells

Against the marginal zone B-cell
- mantle zone not preserved
- cells not confined to marginal zone
- biphasic cytology; "marginal zone" cells only at periphery of nodules and only in spleen
- histology and phenotype are dissimilar from other marginal zone lymphomas when they involve spleen or lymph nodes
- other LG lymphomas adopt a marginal zone pattern in spleen

When the immunophenotype of splenic marginal zone lymphoma is compared to that of the normal marginal zone and of other marginal zone lymphomas, including MALT lymphoma [7.18], distinct differences emerge. There is a high frequency of IgD expression, and variable expression of the two markers of splenic marginal zone cells (CD21 and CD35). Furthermore, there is almost complete absence of CD43, which is frequently expressed, not by normal splenic marginal zone cells, but by other marginal zone lymphomas.

Immunophenotype of SMZL, Marginal Zone B Cells and Marginal Zone Lymphoma

	SMZL	Mar Z	Mar ZL
Ig	M$^+$, D$^+$	M$^+$, D$^-$	M$^+$, D$^-$
CD20	+	+	+
CD10	−	−	−
CD5	−	−	−
CD23	−	−	−
CD21	+/−	+	+
CD35	+/−	+	+
CD43	−	−	+/−
Cyclin D1	−	−	−

[7.19] shows that when the spleen is involved by a true marginal zone lymphoma, an IgM-positive MALT lymphoma, the IgD-positive mantle zone and the reactive follicle center are preserved. The neoplasm clearly occupies the marginal zone of the spleen, which is delineated from the follicle center by the mantle zone, and this pattern is not seen in splenic marginal zone lymphoma.

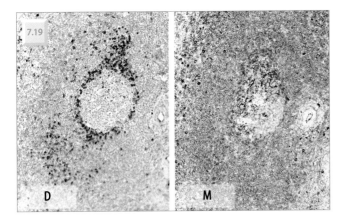

Follicular lymphoma involving the spleen can be a major diagnostic trap [7.20]. The lymphoma frequently adopts a marginal zone-like pattern, surrounding the dense central area of follicle center cells.

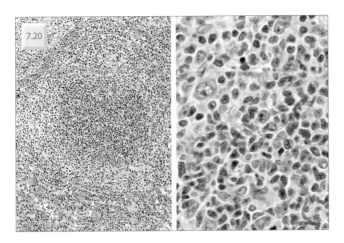

Mantle cell lymphoma involving the spleen [7.21] is also easily mistaken for a marginal zone lymphoma. Fortunately, cyclin D1 is now well established as a marker of mantle cell lymphoma [7.22].

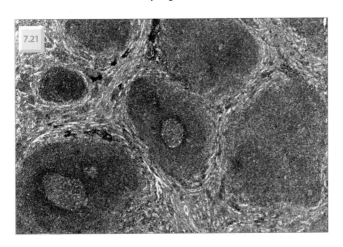

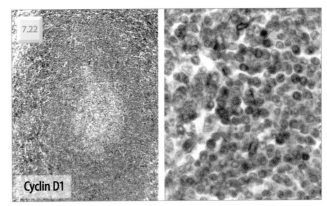

Cyclin D1

What are the clinical features of this disease [7.23]? Most of the cases are over 50. It is difficult to give an accurate estimate of its frequency but in our experience it is not a rare lymphoma. The sex incidence is equal. Patients present with splenomegaly, often with peripheral blood involvement; bone marrow involvement is also common. The liver is also often found to be involved if biopsied at the time of splenectomy. Patients may present with signs of hypersplenism, autoimmune hemolytic anemia or thrombocytopenia.

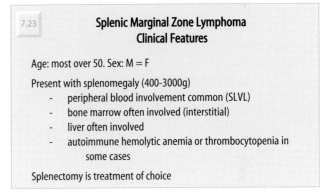

**Splenic Marginal Zone Lymphoma
Clinical Features**

Age: most over 50. Sex: M = F

Present with splenomegaly (400-3000g)
- peripheral blood involvement common (SLVL)
- bone marrow often involved (interstitial)
- liver often involved
- autoimmune hemolytic anemia or thrombocytopenia in some cases

Splenectomy is treatment of choice

Their response to chemotherapy is poor, and splenectomy is the treatment of choice for this disease. The survival curve shown in [7.24] is from Dr. Piris of Toledo, who has collected more than 100 cases of this disorder. This shows that these patients have a very favourable outcome after splenectomy.

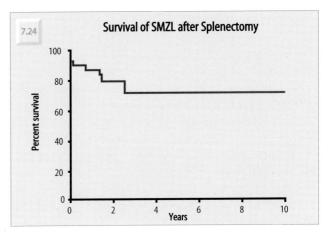

Survival of SMZL after Splenectomy

REFERENCES

1. Zhu D, Oscier DG, Stevenson FK. Splenic lymphoma with villous lymphocytes involves B cells with extensively mutated Ig heavy chain variable region genes. *Blood* 1995; **85:** 1603-7.

2. Dunn-Walters DK, Boursier L, Spencer J, Isaacson PG. Analysis of immunoglobulin genes in splenic marginal zone lymphoma suggests ongoing mutation. *Hum Pathol* 1998; **29:** 585-93.

3. Oscier DG, Matutes E, Gardiner A *et al.* Cytogenetic studies in splenic lymphoma with villous lymphocytes. *Br J Haematol* 1993, **85:** 487-91.

4. Dierlamm J, Pittaluga S, Wlodarska I *et al.* Marginal zone B-cell lymphomas of different sites share similar cytogenetic and morphologic features. *Blood* 1996; **87:** 299-307.

FURTHER READING

Catovsky D. Splenic B cell lymphoma with circulating villous lymphocytes: Differential diagnosis of B cell leukemias with large spleens. *J Clin Pathol* 1987; **40:** 642-51.

Isaacson PG, Matutes E, Burke M, Catovsky D. The histopathology of splenic lymphoma with villous lymphocytes. *Blood* 1994; **84:** 3828-34.

Neiman RS, Sullivan AL, Jaffe R. Malignant lymphoma simulating leukemic reticuloendotheliosis. A clinicopathologic study of 10 cases. *Cancer* 1979; **43:** 329-42.

Mollejo M, Menarguez J, Lloret E *et al.* Splenic marginal zone lymphoma: a distinctive type of low-grade B-cell lymphoma. A clinicopathological study of 13 cases. *Am J Surg Pathol* 1995; **19:** 1146-57.

Mulligan SP, Matutes E, Dearden C, Catovsky D. Splenic lymphoma with villous lymphocytes: Natural history and response to therapy in 50 cases. *Br J Haematol* 1991; **78:** 206-9.

Schmid C, Kirkham N, Diss TC, Isaacson PG. Splenic marginal zone cell lymphoma. *Am J Surg Pathol* 1982; **16:** 455-66.

T cell CLL /prolymphocytic leukemia and T /NK cell large granular lymphocyte leukemia 8

P M Banks

This chapter summarizes the features of two rare disorders: chronic lymphocytic leukemia (CLL) of T cell phenotype (sometimes referred to as T cell prolymphocytic leukemia), and large granular lymphocytosis [8.1].

8.1	T Cell Chronic Lymphocytic Leukemia (T-CLL) and T Cell Prolymphocytic Leukemia	
Morphology:	Many cases feature some degree of prolymphocytic appearance	
Immunophenotype:	A relatively complete CD4+ T cell phenotype, with CD7 expression.	
Genetic features:	Clonal TCR gene rearrangements; inv 14(q11;q32) in 75%; also trisomy 8q.	
Clinical features:	More aggressive than B cell CLL	
Postulated normal cell counterpart:	Circulating peripheral CD4+ T cell	

T cell CLL often has the same morphologic features as typical B cell CLL, including the presence of so called "smudge" cells, representing fragile neoplastic cells which are ruptured during blood smear preparation. These cases often show a range of neoplastic cell types. Typical small lymphocytes, with heterochromatin, are seen, but Catovsky's group has emphasized that most cases have a "prolymphocytic" appearance. However, some cases are microscopically indistinguishable from typical B cell CLL, with uniform clumped nuclear chromatin and scant cytoplasm [8.2].

The question is therefore raised as to whether immunophenotyping, and in particular flow cytometry, should be routinely used in the diagnosis of CLL, in order to detect rare cases of T cell type. The disease is difficult to distinguish in tissue sections by conventional microscopy alone from B cell small lymphocytic lymphoma. However, one does not find proliferation centers, so that if the typical appearance of small lymphocytic lymphoma is seen, but proliferation centers are absent, T cell CLL is a possible diagnosis. Furthermore, epithelioid venules are often conspicuous [8.3].

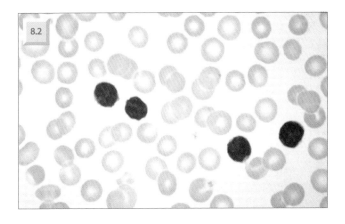

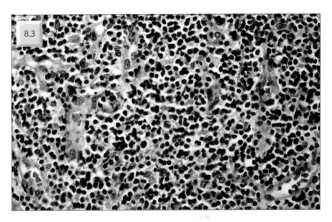

Shown in [8.4] are two-color flow cytometry profiles, which identify the process as a T cell neoplasm, expressing common T cell markers such as CD2, CD3, and CD5. It is exclusively of helper CD4 phenotype, not of CD8 type, and it does not co-express B cell antigens such as CD19.

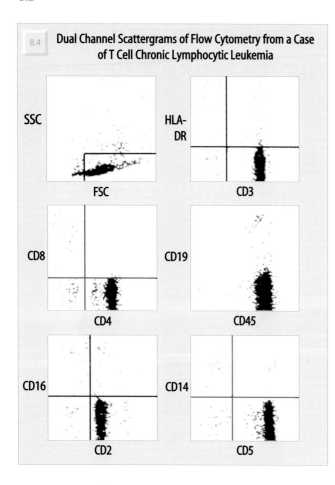

8.4 Dual Channel Scattergrams of Flow Cytometry from a Case of T Cell Chronic Lymphocytic Leukemia

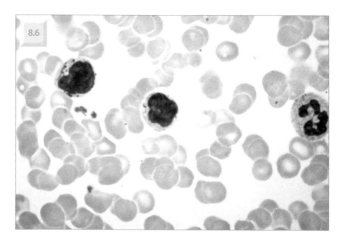

A phenotypically similar but distinct disorder, with an entirely different clinical behavior, is large granular lymphocyte leukemia, which can manifest either a T cell or a natural killer cell phenotype [8.5]. One often suspects this process on conventional microscopy when large granular lymphocytes, with round or slightly irregular nuclei, relatively abundant, usually pale cytoplasm, and azurophilic large granules are seen [8.6].

There is a morphologic spectrum in this disease, in terms of both size and the degree of granularity, and this should be taken into account. Furthermore, the disease is difficult or impossible to recognize in conventional paraffin sections, as in the spleen section shown in [8.7].

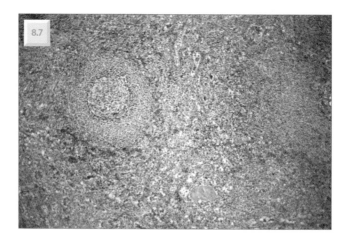

Residual lymphoid tissue may be present [8.7] and in the red pulp there is a subtle diffuse infiltration of small lymphoid elements [8.8], which is indistinguishable from low grade B cell chronic lymphocytic leukemia or small lymphocytic lymphoma.

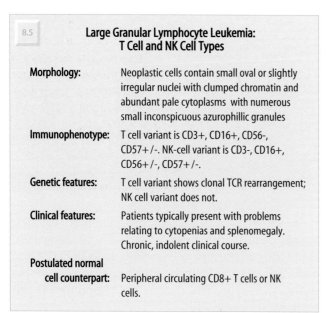

8.5	**Large Granular Lymphocyte Leukemia: T Cell and NK Cell Types**
Morphology:	Neoplastic cells contain small oval or slightly irregular nuclei with clumped chromatin and abundant pale cytoplasms with numerous small inconspicuous azurophillic granules
Immunophenotype:	T cell variant is CD3+, CD16+, CD56-, CD57+ /-. NK-cell variant is CD3-, CD16+, CD56+ /-, CD57+ /-.
Genetic features:	T cell variant shows clonal TCR rearrangement; NK cell variant does not.
Clinical features:	Patients typically present with problems relating to cytopenias and splenomegaly. Chronic, indolent clinical course.
Postulated normal cell counterpart:	Peripheral circulating CD8+ T cells or NK cells.

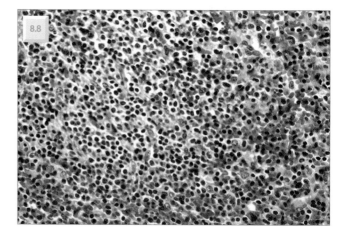

[8.9] shows a different case, with a natural killer immunophenotype, in which the same red pulp distribution is seen. The changes are again extremely subtle, and it would be difficult to diagnose this morphologically as anything other than a low grade B cell process. However, if one makes imprint preparations from tissue samples (right), one can, on careful examination recognize relatively abundant pale cytoplasm containing, at least in this case, a few azurophilic granules [8.10].

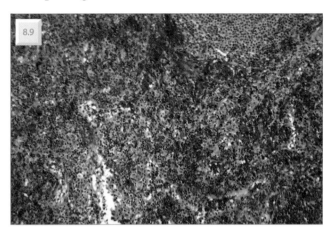

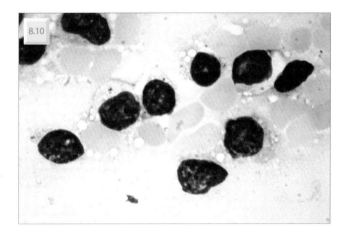

On phenotyping [8.11], a T cell phenotype, without B cell markers is again seen. However, in this case CD8 and not CD4 is expressed, and T cell markers are co-expressed with CD16.

The importance of the disease distribution and clinical manifestations in distinguishing between T cell CLL and large granular lymphocytosis should be emphasized. Even though they may be very difficult or impossible to distinguish from typical small lymphocytic lymphoma/chronic lymphocytic leukemia of B cell type by conventional microscopic appearance, they are clinically quite distinct.

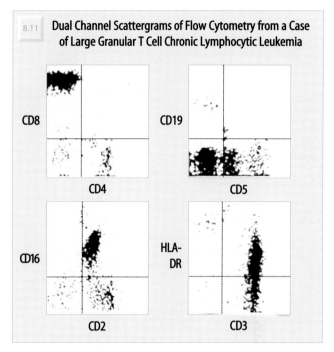

8.11 Dual Channel Scattergrams of Flow Cytometry from a Case of Large Granular T Cell Chronic Lymphocytic Leukemia

Chronic lymphocytic leukemia of T helper type is a relatively aggressive disorder, usually presenting with a high white count. If one has the ability to do molecular or cytogenetic studies, T cell receptor gene arrangement can be detected, and typically an inversion of chromosome 14 can be found. In contrast, patients with large granular lymphocytosis, whether of T cell or natural killer phenotype, are relatively asymptomatic, but usually have cytopenias and splenomegaly. A significant minority of these patients have manifestations of rheumatoid arthritis and can therefore be categorized as having Felty's syndrome.

Large granular lymphocytosis, when it presents as a leukemic or systemic process without constitutional symptoms, is entirely different clinically and prognostically from the very aggressive T cell and natural killer cell neoplasms, otherwise known as angiocentric nasal T cell and natural killer cell lymphomas. Those neoplasms present as tumors, often in the upper airway, or occasionally in the skin and other sites. They are Epstein-Barr virus-positive, whereas the disorders discussed above are Epstein-Barr virus-negative, and very different in their clinical manifestations.

FURTHER READING

Agnarsson BA, Loughran TP Jr, Starkebaum G, Kadin ME. The pathology of large granular lymphocyte leukemia. *Hum Pathol* 1989; **20**: 643-51.

Catovsky D, Matutes E. Leukemias of mature T cells. In: Knowles DM, ed. *Neoplastic Hematopathology.* Baltimore: Williams & Wilkins, 1992; 1267-79.

Hoyer JD, Ross CW, Li CY *et al.* True T-cell chronic lymphocytic leukemia: a morphologic and immunophenotypic study of 25 cases. *Blood* 1995; **86**: 1163-9.

Loughran TP, Kadin ME. Large granular lymphocyte leukemia. In: Beutler E, Lichtman MA *et al*, eds. *Williams Hematology,* fifth edition. New York: McGraw-Hill, 1995; 1047-9.

Matutes E, Brito-Babapulle V, Swansbury J *et al.* Clinical and laboratory features of 78 cases of T-prolymphocytic leukemia. *Blood* 1991; **78**: 3269-74.

Nakamura S, Suchi T, Koshikawa T *et al.* Clinicopathologic study of CD56 (NCAM)-positive angiocentric lymphoma occurring in sites other than the upper and lower respiratory tract. *Am J Surg Pathol* 1995; **19**: 284-96.

Pelicci PG, Allavena P, Subar M *et al.* T-cell receptor (alpha, beta, gamma) gene rearrangements and expression in normal and leukemic large granular lymphocytes/natural killer cells. *Blood* 1987; **70**: 1500-8.

Suchi T, Lennert K, Tu LY *et al.* Histopathology and immunohistochemistry of peripheral T cell lymphomas: a proposal for their classification. *J Clin Pathol* 1987; **40**: 995-1015.

Morphologic, immunologic and genetic features of mantle cell lymphoma

N L Harris

Mantle cell lymphoma was surrounded by controversy for about fifteen years, but quite abruptly became a clearly defined entity, and now presents no great diagnostic difficulty for pathologists [9.1].

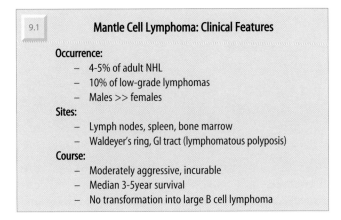

9.1 Mantle Cell Lymphoma: Clinical Features

Occurrence:
- 4-5% of adult NHL
- 10% of low-grade lymphomas
- Males >> females

Sites:
- Lymph nodes, spleen, bone marrow
- Waldeyer's ring, GI tract (lymphomatous polyposis)

Course:
- Moderately aggressive, incurable
- Median 3-5 year survival
- No transformation into large B cell lymphoma

The problem that it poses has now become principally a clinical one because, although it is easy to diagnose, it is very difficult to treat.

Mantle cell lymphoma is defined morphologically as a neoplasm of monomorphic medium-sized B lymphoid cells, with irregular nuclei. The growth pattern may be diffuse, but it is more commonly vaguely nodular, and may have a mantle zone pattern. Large transformed basophilic blast cells and pseudofollicles are absent. Typically it involves both lymph nodes and extranodal sites, particularly the gastrointestinal tract and the bone marrow [9.2].

The important immunophenotypic features are expression of CD5 and lack of CD10 or CD23. The tumor shows rearrangement of the *BCL-1* (or PRAD-1) oncogene caused by the (11;14) translocation, and this results in over-expression of cyclin D1 protein.

Mantle cell lymphoma corresponds virtually exactly to the entity that was known for many years as centrocytic lymphoma in the Kiel classification [9.3].

The term "mantle cell" was chosen because it is now believed that this tumor does not arise from germinal center centrocytes. As Professor Stein has found from Ig gene mutation studies, it probably corresponds to a pre-germinal center naive B cell found in the normal follicle mantle. We believe that some examples of what has been called "centroblastic lymphoma of centrocytoid type" in the Kiel classification represent an aggressive variant of mantle cell lymphoma.

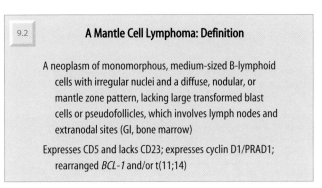

9.2 A Mantle Cell Lymphoma: Definition

A neoplasm of monomorphous, medium-sized B-lymphoid cells with irregular nuclei and a diffuse, nodular, or mantle zone pattern, lacking large transformed blast cells or pseudofollicles, which involves lymph nodes and extranodal sites (GI, bone marrow)

Expresses CD5 and lacks CD23; expresses cyclin D1/PRAD1; rearranged *BCL-1* and/or t(11;14)

Cases of centrocytic lymphoma were included in the Working Formulation study [9.3], and the majority of cases fell into the "diffuse small cleaved cell" category. However, others, made up of rather small cells, were categorized as small lymphocytic lymphoma, and a few cases can be found in the diffuse mixed and diffuse large cleaved cell categories.

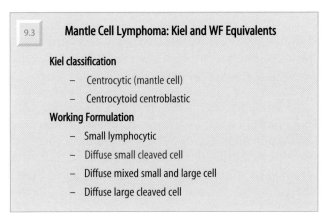

9.3 Mantle Cell Lymphoma: Kiel and WF Equivalents

Kiel classification
- Centrocytic (mantle cell)
- Centrocytoid centroblastic

Working Formulation
- Small lymphocytic
- Diffuse small cleaved cell
- Diffuse mixed small and large cell
- Diffuse large cleaved cell

In an individual case, the cells are usually quite monotonous. However there is variation from case to case. Most cases are composed of medium-sized cells with irregular "cleaved" nuclei, but some are composed of small round lymphocyte-like cells. A "blastoid" variant also exists, in which the tumor cells have dispersed chromatin and a high proliferation index [9.4]. These latter cases often resemble lymphoblastic lymphoma. There are also rare cases containing large pleomorphic cleaved cells, which might be confused with diffuse large B cell lymphoma.

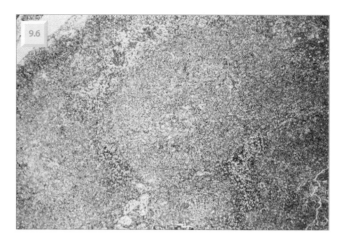

9.4   **Mantle Cell Lymphoma: Morphology**

Pattern: diffuse, nodular, mantle zone

Cytology: small to medium sized cells, irregular nuclei, inconspicuous nucleoli, scant cytoplasm, no blasts or pseudofollicles

Variants/grades:
– lymphocyte-like or round cells
– blastoid (dispersed chromatin and high proliferation index)
– large, pleomorphic cleaved cells
– ? centroblastoid

Most cases have a predominantly diffuse pattern, but on closer examination areas of nodularity are often evident. Frequently, there is a suggestion of a "starry sky" pattern, created by the presence of scattered epithelioid histiocytes [9.5].

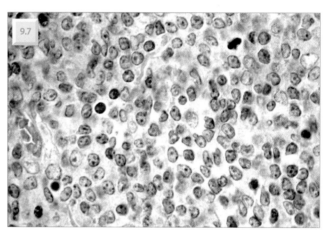

In the blastoid variant, the chromatin is more dispersed and nucleoli are more prominent. However, in contrast to true lymphoblastic lymphoma, the cytoplasm is not basophilic, even in a Giemsa stained section [9.8].

When the tumor has a mantle zone pattern, reactive germinal centers are surrounded by broad mantle zones of atypical lymphoid cells [9.6].

At higher magnification [9.7] one sees very monomorphous small lymphoid cells with dispersed chromatin, slightly irregular nuclei and inconspicuous cytoplasm. Large transformed basophilic cells are absent. The scattered epithelioid histiocytes are quite characteristic, and can be very helpful in diagnosing this entity in routine sections.

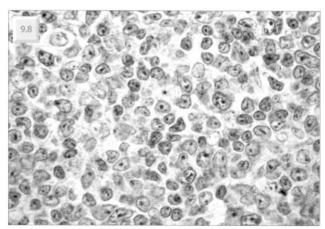

The rare "large pleomorphic" cases might be categorized in the Kiel classification as anaplastic centrocytic lymphoma. This change is usually found focally in lymph nodes that elsewhere contain typical mantle cell lymphoma, but it may also be encountered as a form of cytologic transformation in relapsing cases [9.9].

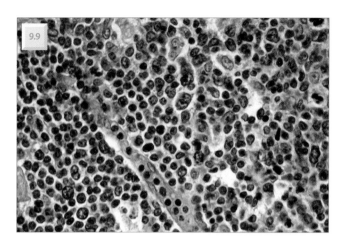

The pattern of antigen expression in mantle cell lymphoma is characteristic, although immuno-phenotyping may not be necessary in a histologically typical case [9.10]. In distinction from B cell CLL, CD23 is absent, and in distinction from follicular lymphoma, CD5 is present. The normal counterpart is thought to be the CD5-positive, CD23-negative B cell of the follicle mantle. The availability of anti-bodies to the cyclin D1 protein allows this specific and useful marker for this disorder to be detected in routine sections [9.11].

9.10	Phenotype /Genetics

Immunophenotype:
- SIg M+ D+ Pan B+ CD5+ CD10- CD23- CD43+
- Loose FDC clusters
- Cyclin D1 protein+

Genetics:
- IgH and IgL genes rearranged
- t(11;14) BCL-1 rearranged (cyclin D1/PRAD1+)

Normal counterpart:
CD5+ CD23- B cell of follicle mantle

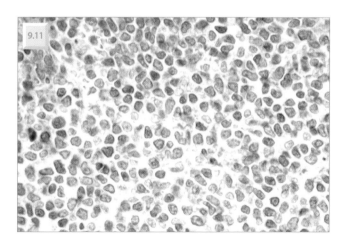

A number of questions remain about mantle cell lymphoma [9.12], most of which will be addressed in subsequent chapters. We have addressed the diagnostic specificity of immunophenotypic and genetic features

in mantle cell lymphoma. In a large number of low grade B cell neoplasms stained with a polyclonal antibody to cyclin D1 [9.13], only one case of mantle cell lymphoma lacked detectable cyclin D1, although, when using paraffin sections, there are inevitably occasional cases in which problems with fixation or other technical factors will prevent satisfactory staining. Three of the positive cases, which were morphologically typical of mantle cell lymphoma, were CD5-negative, indicating that cyclin D1 may be a more consistent marker than CD5.

9.12	Mantle Cell Lymphoma Questions

- Diagnostic specificity of immunophenotypic and genotypic features
  CD5- cases
  CD23+ cases
  BCL-1 rearrangement, Cyclin D1 expression
- Clinical relevance of pattern
  mantle zone, nodular, diffuse
- Clinical relevance of variant morphologies
- Optimal treatment

9.13	Cyclin D1 Protein in Low Grade B Cell Neoplasms	
Lymphoma	N cases	CCND1
MCL (3 CD5-)*	36	35
B-CLL/SLL	25	1**
CB/CC	20	0
MALT (2 CD5+)	15	0
SMZL	21	0
Splenic ML unclass.	2	2**
HCL	17	2
Plasmacytoma	22	1
Total	**149**	**41**

* includes 2 cases originally classified as B-CLL
** unusual morphology and aggressive course

Among 25 cases of B cell small lymphocytic lymphoma, most of which were associated with a leukemic blood picture, we have found only one cyclin D1-positive case. The morphology in this case was very atypical, with increased prolymphocytes and paraimmunoblasts, and the patient had an extremely aggressive clinical course. This was one of the earliest cases of B cell CLL studied and there have been no other positive cases. In consequence, cyclin D1 expression appears to be rare in B cell CLL, and, when present, possibly indicates a more aggressive disease.

We have not found staining for cyclin D1 in a large number of follicular lymphomas and MALT type lymphomas, including two cases of MALT lymphoma that were CD5-positive. Among 21 examples of splenic marginal zone lymphoma, some cases of which are said to contain the (11;14) translocation and to over-express cyclin D1, we did not find a typical case that was cyclin D1-positive. However, we have found two splenic lymphomas, one from our own material and one from Dr. Piris' group in Toledo, which had unusual morphology and were cyclin D1-positive. One of these had a very aggressive clinical course. These cases warrant further study, but it does appear that cyclin D1 can be used to distinguish typical splenic marginal zone lymphoma from mantle cell lymphoma.

Finally, many cases of hairy cell leukemia and some plasmacytomas express cyclin D1; in multiple myeloma, there have been cases reported with the t(11;14). However, taking these data together, it seems that cyclin D1, although not absolutely specific for mantle cell lymphoma, is a very useful marker for this disease in most clinically important situations.

Diffuse large B cell lymphoma can sometimes enter into the differential diagnosis of a mantle cell lymphoma. In 35 cases, including five CD5-positive large B cell lymphomas, we found none that expressed cyclin D1. Together with the Stanford group, we have studied precursor B lymphoblastic lymphomas, since this is relevant to the differential diagnosis of the blastoid variant, and found none that expressed cyclin D1 [9.14].

9.14	**Cyclin D1 Protein in High Grade Lymphomas**		
Lymphoma		N cases	CCND1
Large BCL(5 CD5+)		35	0
	13 LN, 9 bone,		
	6 WR, 7 other		
BT/BL		9	0
	3 LN, 6 other		
T-LBL (LN)		4	0
B-LBL		8	0
ATL/L (Bone)		1	0
Total		57	0

In conclusion, it is clear from these studies that the cyclin D1 protein is of diagnostic value in mantle cell lymphoma. The other immunophenotypic characteristics, such as CD5, are also valuable, but it does appear that there are occasional CD5-negative cases.

FURTHER READING

Banks PM, Chan J, Cleary ML *et al*. Mantle cell lymphoma. A proposal for unification of morphologic, immunologic, and molecular data. *Am J Surg Pathol* 1992; **16**: 637-40.

Berger F, Felman P, Sonet A *et al*. Nonfollicular small B-cell lymphomas: a heterogeneous group of patients with distinct clinical features and outcome. *Blood* 1994; **83**: 2829-35.

Fisher RI, Dahlberg S, Nathwani BN, Banks PM, Miller TP, Grogan TM. A clinical analysis of two indolent lymphoma entities: mantle cell lymphoma and marginal zone lymphoma (including the mucosa-associated lymphoid tissue and monocytoid B-cell subcategories): a Southwest Oncology Group study. *Blood* 1995; **85**: 1075-82.

Harris N, Nadler L, Bhan A. Immunohistologic characterization of two malignant lymphomas of germinal center type (centroblastic/centrocytic and centrocytic) with monoclonal antibodies: follicular and diffuse lymphomas of small cleaved cell types are related but distinct entities. *Am J Pathol* 1984; **117**: 262-72.

Hummel M, Tamaru J, Kalvelage B, Stein H. Mantle cell (previously centrocytic) lymphomas express VH genes with no or very little somatic mutations like the physiologic cells of the follicle mantle. *Blood* 1994; **84**: 403-7.

Inghirami G, Foitl D, Sabichi A, Zhu B, Knowles D. Autoantibody-associated cross reactive idiotype bearing human B lymphocytes: distribution and characterization, including IgVH gene and CD5 antigen expression. *Blood* 1991; **78**: 1503-15.

Isaacson P, MacLennan K, Subbuswamy S. Multiple lymphomatous polyposis of the gastrointestinal tract. *Histopathology* 1984; **8**: 641-56.

Lardelli P, Bookman M, Sundeen J, Longo D, Jaffe E. Lymphocytic lymphoma of intermediate differentiation. Morphologic and immunophenotypic spectrum and clinical correlations. *Am J Surg Pathol* 1990; **14**: 752-63.

Lennert K. *Malignant lymphomas other than Hodgkin's disease*. New York: Springer Verlag, 1978.

Meusers P, Engelhard M, Bartels H *et al*. Multicentre randomized therapeutic trial for advanced centrocytic lymphoma: anthracycline does not improve the prognosis. *Hematol Oncol* 1989; **7**: 365-80.

Norton AJ, Matthews J, Pappa V *et al*. Mantle cell lymphoma: natural history defined in a serially biopsied population over a 20-year period. *Ann Oncol* 1995; **6**: 249-56.

Ott MM, Ott G, Kuse R *et al*. The anaplastic variant of centrocytic lymphoma is marked by frequent rearrangements of the bcl-1 gene and high proliferation indices. *Histopathology* 1994; **24**: 329-34.

Rosenberg CL, Wong E, Petty EM *et al*. PRAD1, a candidate BCL1 oncogene: mapping and expression in centrocytic lymphoma. *Proc Natl Acad Sci USA* 1991; **88**: 9638-42.

Stein H, Lennert K, Feller A, Mason DY. Immunohistological analysis of human lymphoma correlation of histological and immunological categories. *Adv Cancer Res* 1984; **42**: 67-147.

Vandenberghe E, De Wolf-Peters C, van den Oord J *et al*. Translocation (11;14): a cytogenetic anomaly associated with B-cell lymphomas of non-follicle centre cell lineage. *J Pathol* 1991; **163**: 13-8.

Yang WI, Zukerberg LR, Mokotura I, Arnold A, Harris NL. Cyclin D1 (Bcl-1, PRAD1) protein expression in low-grade B-cell lymphomas and reactive hyperplasia. *Am J Pathol* 1994; **145**: 86-96.

Zukerberg LR, Medeiros LJ, Ferry JA, Harris NL. Diffuse low-grade B-cell lymphomas. Four clinically distinct subtypes defined by a combination of morphologic and immunophenotypic features. *Am J Clin Pathol* 1993; **100**: 373-85.

Zukerberg LR, Yang WI, Arnold A, Harris NL. Cyclin D1 expression in non-Hodgkin's lymphomas. Detection by immunohistochemistry. *Am J Clin Pathol* 1995; **103**: 756-60.

Clinical features and response to current treatment modalities in mantle cell lymphoma

R I Fisher

This chapter addresses the important question of whether mantle cell lymphoma should be excluded from the indolent or low grade lymphomas, and presents strong evidence that it should be [10.1].

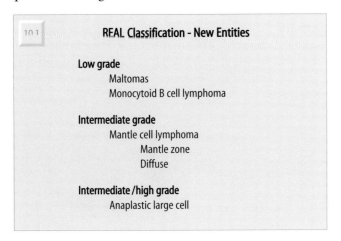

RFAL Classification - New Entities

Low grade
Maltomas
Monocytoid B cell lymphoma

Intermediate grade
Mantle cell lymphoma
Mantle zone
Diffuse

Intermediate /high grade
Anaplastic large cell

This disease has a long history. European pathologists and oncologists are well aware of the term "centrocytic", and Dr. Berard included such cases in his "intermediate" cell category, as did Dr. Weisenburger in his "mantle zone" variant [10.2]. As discussed below, the importance of a mantle zone growth pattern remains a challenge for pathologists. Failure to classify reproducibly this latter category leaves open the question of whether there is a subset of patients with a mantle zone pattern who may have a more indolent behavior than others.

Previous Descriptions of Mantle Cell Lymphoma

1. Centrocytic lymphoma (Lennert-Kiel)
2. Intermediate cell lymphoma (Berard)
3. Lymphocytic lymphoma of intermediate differentiation
4. Mantle zone lymphoma (Weisenburger)

Shown in [10.3] is a schematic of the structure of a normal lymph node, as a reminder of the location of the mantle zone.

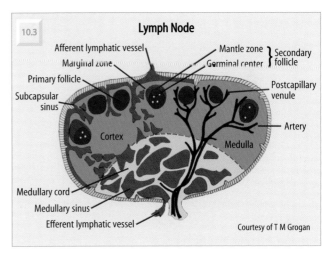

Lymph Node

Courtesy of T M Grogan

Immunophenotyping (and the importance of CD5 expression) and the value of the (11;14) translocation in differentiating mantle cell lymphoma from other entities is detailed elsewhere [10.4].

Comparative Immunophenotype of Mantle Cell Lymphomas

Surface marker	Mantle cell lymphoma	Follicular lymphoma	Small lymphocytic lymphoma
CD5	++	-	++
Surface Immunoglobulin	++	+++	+
CD19	++	++	++
CD20	+++	++	+
CD10	-	80%+	-
CD23	-	±	+

The key feature, from a pathophysiologic point of view, is that mantle cell lymphoma is a very different disease from follicular lymphoma and other indolent lymphomas. There are good reasons to believe that this reflects the consequences of the expression of the *BCL-1* gene [10.5] which encodes cyclin D1, a protein that moves cells rapidly through the cell cycle. Overproduction of *BCL-1* is therefore suspected to cause an abnormally high rate of cell proliferation [10.6], and this stands in great contrast to the rest of the indolent lymphomas.

10.5 | **Comparative Morphologic and Immunophenotypic Features of Indolent NHLs**

Entity	Characteristic morphology	Phenotypic /genotypic features
Small lymphocytic lymphoma (SLL)	Small round lymphocytes; proliferation centres	Faint Ig, CD19>CD20, CD5⁺, CD10⁻, CD23⁺; BCL-3⁺, t(14;19)
Follicular small cleaved lymphoma (FSCL)	Small cleaved lymphocytes in nodules	Strong Ig, Pan B⁺, CD5⁻, CD10⁺, BCL-2⁺, t(14;18)
Follicular mixed lymphoma (FML)	Small cleaved cells and large cells in nodules	Strong Ig, Pan B⁺, CD5-, CD10⁺; BCL-2⁺, t(14;18)

10.6 | ***BCL-1* Oncogene**

Involved in the t(11;14)(q13;q32) translocation associated with intermediate lymphocytic, or mantle cell, lymphoma

Identical to *PRAD1* gene in benign parathyroid tumors

Also implicated in breast, squamous cell, and esophageal cancers

Encodes cyclin D1, a protein that acts to propel cells through the cell cycle

Overproduction of BCL-1 protein is suspected to cause an abnormally high rate of cell proliferation

---

To gain some insight into the clinical behavior of this neoplasm, we have reviewed cases from a study performed by the South West Oncology Group [10.7].[1] This project was started in 1972, so that more than 20 years of follow-up data are available on all these patients. Furthermore, these were not early stage patients - they were previously untreated patients with advanced disease. We looked through all the classic low grade indolent lymphomas, and analyzed Working Formulation categories D and E. These patients all initially received full dose CHOP, and this creates a unique perspective, since in studies published in the *New England Journal of Medicine* we had shown that CHOP is equivalent to any of the other third generation regimes for the treatment of aggressive lymphoma.[2] In consequence, we found that we had, more or less by chance, 20 years ago chosen what we would today consider state-of-the-art therapy.

10.7 | **Eligibility Requirements**

SWOG 7204, 7426, or 7713
Stage III or IV
No prior therapy
Working Formulation A, B, C, D, or E
Received initial full dose CHOP

Fisher et al. 1995[1]

Three pathologists - Dr. Grogan, Dr. Banks and Dr. Nathwani - re-reviewed all of the patients in the trial [10.8]. They identified 36 cases of mantle cell lymphoma, which represented 10% of this group of relatively indolent lymphomas. The cases tended to be found within the old category of "PDL diffuse", or Working Formulation Category E, and this is important because 20 years ago, when these studies began, PDL was a very poor prognosis category. We now know that the reason for this is that they represent a heterogeneous group. Lymphoblastic lymphomas could be removed from it, and mantle cell lymphomas can now also be identified. What remains, the small cell type of follicular lymphoma, has a much better prognosis.

10.8 | **Consensus Pathologic Review of SWOG Lymphoma Cases**

Original diagnosis	Total	Mantle cell (MCL)
WF A (SL) /DLWD	70	6
WF B (FSC) /NLPD	171	9
WF C (FM) /NM	40	0
WF D (FL) /NH	29	0
WF E (DSC) /DLPD	66	21
Total reviewed	**376**	**36 (10%)**

Fisher et al. 1995[1]

Subtypes of mantle cell have been described - diffuse, mantle zone, lymphoblastoid, and nodular [10.9]. In our study, the three pathologists identified about a third of the cases as nodular, a third as diffuse and a third as lymphoblastoid [10.10]. They did not identify cases with the classic mantle zone pattern of the sort that are now being described by Dr. Weisenburger and by Drs. Cabanillas and Pugh, as having a better prognosis.

10.9 | **Mantle Cell Lymphoma Histologic Patterns**

1. Diffuse
2. Mantle zone (vaguely nodular)
3. Lymphoblastoid ("blastoid")
4. (Nodular)

10.10	Subclassification of REAL Categories	
		Number of patients
Mantle cell lymphoma (MCL)	36	
Nodular		14 (39%)
Diffuse		10 (28%)
Blastic		12 (33%)
Marginal zone lymphoma (MZL)	43	
Maltoma		19 (44%)
Monocytoid B		21 (49%)
Not classifiable		(7%)

What were the clinical characteristics of these mantle cell cases? There was a striking male predominance, which is seen throughout the world, and there was a higher incidence of gastrointestinal involvement than in follicular lymphomas. Those stand out as the two major clinical presenting features [10.11].

10.11	Patient Characteristics		
	WF A-E (N = 248)	Mantle cell (N = 36)	Marginal zone (N = 43)
Median age in years (range)	55 (18-81)	55 (18-76)	51 (23-76)
% Male (95% CI)	54 (48-61)	81 (64-92)	51 (35-67)
% PS > 2	8	3	5
% Bone marrow	46	53	49
% GI disease (95% CI)	4 (2-7)	19 (8-36)	23 (12-39)

Fisher *et al.* 1995 [1]

Shown in [10.12] is a summary of the clinical outcome. When the 36 mantle cell lymphomas were compared to the other indolent lymphomas, it is clear that all have relapsed due to treatment failure, or died. The estimated 10 year survival is only 6%, and the median survival is very short, at about 2 - 3 years. Furthermore, we see that of all categories of relatively indolent lymphoma, mantle cell lymphoma clearly has the worst prognosis. It is true that in our experience the Working Formulation Category A also has a relatively poor prognosis compared to follicular lymphomas, but it is necessary to realize the type of patients in the study who fall into that category. They were not examples of CLL diagnosed on a blood count from an asymptomatic patient. All suffered from advanced stage lymphocytic lymphomas and were entered on a protocol because they needed treatment. In this context, it is worth making the point that if one reviews cases of CLL who require therapy, the prognosis is likely to be poor. This is evident from Dr. Coiffier's series, and from many others, that these patients are in a poor prognosis

group, and the disease they suffer from should not to be confused with the "lag phase" in CLL, when many of the patients are asymptomatic.

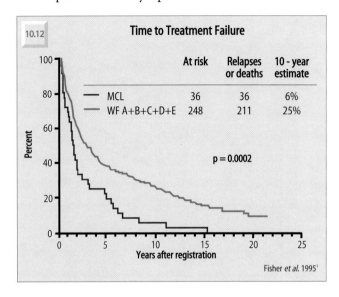

Fisher *et al.* 1995 [1]

When overall survival was reviewed, the curve was again poor, and only 8% of the patients were alive at 10 years. In effect, this disease represents the worst of all possible situations. When the diseases in the REAL scheme are reviewed in terms of survival patterns, three categories emerge. Follicular lymphoma typifies a relatively indolent lymphoma; although it has a median survival of about 7 - 10 years, the year-on-year mortality risk remains the same. The curve for aggressive lymphoma shows an initial fall but then flattens to create a "hockey stick" curve, ending with a survival of 30 - 35%. The worst situation is a survival curve which falls rapidly and keeps on falling, and mantle cell lymphoma provides the best example of this pattern.

When the histologic subtypes were reviewed – blastic, diffuse and nodular [10.13] – there was some difference in survival, the nodular group faring a little better early on, but ultimately they all died. Thus, mantle cell lymphoma clearly carries a very poor prognosis. The only unresolved question is whether there is a subset among mantle cell lymphomas that is of better prognosis. Larger numbers are needed to establish this, but it is difficult to be optimistic about the existence of such a group.

Dr. Press and the author have reviewed the world literature on mantle cell lymphoma,[3] and [10.14] represents a compilation of 13 published series. The clinical characteristics are those which are now well recognized - a clear male predominance, a high median age, frequent adenopathy, bone marrow involvement and splenomegaly. Hepatomegaly is seen in about a third, gastrointestinal involvement in about 20%, and B symptoms and elevated LDH in about a third. High β2-microglobulin levels are common. It may be pointed out that these characteristics are obviously associated in essentially all lymphomas with a relatively poor prognosis.

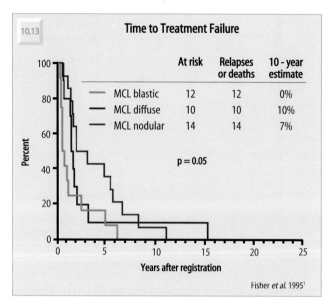

10.13

Time to Treatment Failure

	At risk	Relapses or deaths	10 - year estimate
MCL blastic	12	12	0%
MCL diffuse	10	10	10%
MCL nodular	14	14	7%

p = 0.05

Percent / Years after registration

Fisher *et al.* 1995[1]

10.14   Clinical Presentation of Mantle Cell Lymphoma

Male predominance	2/1
Median age	58
Generalized adenopathy	71-90%
Bone marrow positivity	53-93%
Splenomegaly	35-81%
Hepatomegaly	18-35%
Gastrointestinal involvement	15-28%
Lymphocytosis	10-69%
B symptoms	35-55%
LDH elevated	30-50%
β2-microglobulin elevation	54%

See references: [1, 3-14]

As already noted, no cases in our own series were classified as being of mantle zone type, but the EORTC study identified about 3% of their cases as being mantle cell lymphomas, and the number is

higher in the MD Anderson series. The numbers are still small, but it would be of obvious interest to see if this group has a better prognosis.

All of the published series show a very similar progression-free survival at under twenty months. In those 500 published patients, there was an average 45% complete remission rate, and the overall survival only 3 years. These results are essentially superimposable with the data from our own institution.

All cases in our series were treated with CHOP, so it appears that standard aggressive lymphoma therapy does not work, and this raises a very commonly voiced question: what therapeutic approach should we take to these patients? Unfortunately there is no clear answer. Small numbers treated by bone marrow transplantation have been published in a preliminary communication, but the results certainly do not provide evidence that we can change the natural history by curing these patients. Currently in the South West Oncology Group we are entering these patients in a dose intensified category, using dose-escalated or double dose CHOP or ProMACE cytaBOM. However, nobody in the clinical field has shown that this can achieve a good outcome for the majority of patients.

What other conclusions can we draw [10.15]? Firstly, it is clear that this is a discrete clinical pathologic entity; that it has a short survival and therefore is not indolent; and that it is not curable with any standard therapy. The management of these patients is therefore going to remain a major challenge for the oncologist for some years to come.

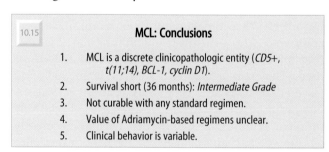

10.15   MCL: Conclusions

1. MCL is a discrete clinicopathologic entity (*CD5+, t(11;14), BCL-1, cyclin D1*).
2. Survival short (36 months): *Intermediate Grade*
3. Not curable with any standard regimen.
4. Value of Adriamycin-based regimens unclear.
5. Clinical behavior is variable.

ACKNOWLEDGEMENTS

Figures [10.12] and [10.13] are reproduced from *Blood* 1995, **85:** 1075-82 with copyright permission from W.B. Saunders Company.

REFERENCES

1. Fisher RI, Dahlberg S, Nathwani BN, Banks PM, Miller TP, Grogan TM. A clinical analysis of two indolent lymphoma entities: mantle cell lymphoma and marginal zone lymphoma (including the mucosa-associated lymphoid tissue and monocytoid B-cell subcategories): a Southwest Oncology Group study. *Blood* 1995; **85**: 1075-82.

2. Fisher RI, Gaynor ER, Dahlberg S *et al.* Comparison of a standard regimen (CHOP) with three intensive chemotherapy regimens for advanced non-Hodgkin's lymphoma. *N Engl J Med* 1993; **328**: 1002-6.

3. Teodorovic I, Pittaluga S, Kluin-Nelemans JC *et al.* Efficacy of four different regimens in 64 mantle-cell lymphoma cases. clinicopathologic comparison with 498 other non-Hodgkin's lymphoma subtypes. European Organization for the Research and Treatment of Cancer Lymphoma Cooperative Group. *J Clin Oncol* 1995; **13**: 2819-26.

4. Weisenburger DD, Nathwani BN, Diamond LW, Winberg CD, Rappaport H. Malignant lymphoma, intermediate lymphocytic type: a clinicopathologic study of 42 cases. *Cancer* 1981; **48**: 1415-25.

5. Norton AJ, Matthews J, Pappa V *et al.* Mantle cell lymphoma: natural history defined in a serially biopsied population over a 20-year period. *Ann Oncol* 1995; **6**: 249-56.

6. Duggan MJ, Weisenburger DD, Ye YL *et al.* Mantle zone lymphoma. A clinicopathologic study of 22 cases. *Cancer* 1990; **66**: 522-9.

7. Meusers P, Engelhard M, Bartels H *et al.* Multicentre randomized therapeutic trial for advanced centrocytic lymphoma: anthracycline does not improve the prognosis. *Hematol Oncol* 1989; **7**: 365-80.

8. Zucca E, Roggero E, Pinotti G *et al.* Patterns of survival in mantle cell lymphoma. *Ann Oncol* 1995; **6**: 257-62.

9. Narang S, Wolf BC, Neiman RS. Malignant lymphoma presenting with prominent splenomegaly. A clinicopathologic study with special reference to intermediate cell lymphoma. *Cancer* 1985; **55**: 1948-57.

10. Pittaluga S, Wlodarska I, Stul MS *et al.* Mantle cell lymphoma: a clinicopathological study of 55 cases. *Histopathology* 1995; **26**: 17-24.

11. Berger F, Felman P, Sonet A *et al.* Nonfollicular small B-cell lymphomas: a heterogeneous group of patients with distinct clinical features and outcome. *Blood* 1994; **83**: 2829-35.

12. Zucca E, Fontana S, Roggero E, Pedrinis E, Pampallona S, Cavalli F. Treatment and prognosis of centrocytic (mantle cell) lymphoma: a retrospective analysis of twenty-six patients treated in one institution. *Leuk Lymphoma* 1994; **13**: 105-10.

13. Coiffier B, Hiddemann W, Stein H. Mantle cell lymphoma: a therapeutic dilemma. *Ann Oncol* 1995; **6**: 208-10.

14. Stewart DA, Vose JM, Weisenburger DD *et al.* The role of high-dose therapy and autologous hematopoietic stem cell transplantation for mantle cell lymphoma. *Ann Oncol* 1995; **6**: 263-6.

FURTHER READING

Banks PM, Chan J, Cleary ML *et al.* Mantle cell lymphoma. A proposal for unification of morphologic, immunologic, and molecular data. *Am J Surg Pathol* 1992; **16**: 637-40.

New treatment options in mantle cell lymphoma

W Hiddemann

Mantle cell lymphoma has only recently been generally accepted as a distinct lymphoma entity. Hence, available clinical information is hampered by the lack of a uniformly accepted pathologic classification [11.1]. Furthermore, all series published so far are small, and mostly based on retrospective evaluations.

11.1	Mantle Cell Lymphoma - Clinical Characteristics Problems and Limitations
-	No uniformly accepted patho-histologic classification until recently
-	Small series of patients
-	Mostly retrospective clinical evaluations
-	Very few prospective clinical studies with standardized therapy

As discussed elsewhere, this disease is however not new, in that it has long been recognized as "centrocytic lymphoma" in the Kiel classification. In an overview published by Dr. Brittinger more than ten years ago [11.2], centrocytic lymphoma accounted for as many as 7% of cases in a series of more than 1,000 patients. The Kiel group also reported already that these lymphomas had a very poor outcome, and that, compared to follicular lymphomas and high grade lymphomas, they had a very specific clinical behavior. However, it was only after the detection of the (11;14) translocation and the description of the immunophenotype that it became possible to identify this new entity reproducibly.

The importance of making the right diagnosis emerges from a survey performed of 573 patients from nine participating institutions in Europe that was carried out by the European Lymphoma Task Force. Each case was reviewed and the participating pathologist had to confirm that the features defined in the REAL classification were present and that the updated Annecy criteria were fulfilled. Following this assessment, 392 of the 573 patients were confirmed as mantle cell lymphomas, 15 did not fulfil the criteria, and in the remaining cases no material was available for pathologic review.

11.2	Frequency of Non-Hodgkin's Lymphomas within the Kiel Lymphoma Study Group		
Low grade lymphomas		782	69%
	Lymphocytic (incl. CLL)	28	25%
	Lymphoplasmacytic-cytoid	213	19%
	Centrocytic	87	7%
	Centroblastic-centrocytic	157	14%
	Unclassifiable	45	4%
High grade lymphomas		341	30%
	Centroblastic	157	14%
	Immunoblastic	83	7%
	Lymphoblastic	60	5%
	Unclassifiable	41	3%
Unclassifiable grade lymphomas		4	1%

Brittinger *et al.* 1984 [1]

The clinical features of the confirmed MCL cases at presentation [11.3] include a male predominance, and in most patients, bone marrow involvement and extranodal disease. Furthermore, many patients had B symptoms.

11.3	Mantle Cell Lymphoma. A European Survey Patient characteristics	
Age		63 years (20-89 years)
Sex	male	73%
	female	27%
Stage	I/II	11%
	III/IV	89%
Bone marrow involvement		67%
Extranodal involvement		87%
B symptoms		35%

An important point to emerge is that making the right diagnosis has major prognostic implications. Patients initially classified as mantle cell lymphoma, but found on review to have another disease, had a comparatively good prognosis. For the other 392 patients the prognosis was poor, and the pattern of survival was very similar at the different participating institutions [11.4].

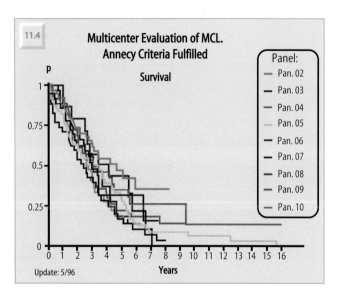

What are the options for therapy? [11.5] summarizes several published reports and shows that most of the regimes investigated have really not solved the problem, and that the overall survival of these patients has not improved.

11.5	Therapy of Mantle Cell Lymphomas with Conventional Chemotherapy Regimens				
Author	N Cases	CR (%)	CR + PR (%)	Failure-free survival (months)	Overall survival (months)
Fisher [2]	36	53	86	20	36
Wagner/Press [3]	51	30	90	11	30
Berger [4]	52	31	56	14	52
Zucca # 1 [5]	26	50	NA	19	33
Weisenburger [6]	42	41	NA	NA	31
Meusers (COP group) [7]	37	41	84	10	32
Meusers (CHOP group) [7]	26	58	88	7	37
Norton [8]	66	9	71	10	36
Pittaluga [9]	55	NA	NA	NA	32
Stewart [10]	14	29	NA	18	32
Zucca # 2 [11]	65	51	86	NA	42
Narang [12]	19	NA	NA	NA	34
Duggan * [13]	22	50	NA	NA	88
Total	511	41	86	12.5	32.5

*Patients in this series all apparently had the "mantle zone" variant

This problem has also been addressed by the Kiel Lymphoma Study Group in Germany in a study which investigated the impact of anthracyclines in mantle cell lymphoma by carrying out a prospective randomized comparison between COP and CHOP. [11.6] and [11.7] show that the complete remission rate was increased by the addition of anthracyclines, but that the overall survival was not improved.

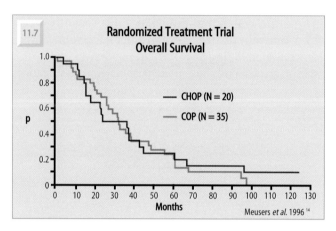

11.6	Mantle Cell Lymphomas: Impact of Anthracyclines	
	COP	CHOP
CR	43%	60%
PR	46%	40%
Failure	11%	-

Meusers *et al.* 1996 [14]

Randomized Treatment Trial
Overall Survival

Meusers *et al.* 1996 [14]

There has been some indication from the EORTC lymphoma study group that more intensive drug combinations might improve the disease-free and overall survival, but these data are based on small numbers of patients only, and are preliminary. It does not appear that any currently available drug combination can change the overall survival pattern dramatically, and the question remains - what can we do?

In our prospective randomized trial in Germany of follicle cell lymphomas and mantle cell lymphomas, we asked two questions. One related to the efficacy of initial cytoreductive chemotherapy, with either COP or prednimustine, mitoxantrone (PM). The other assessed, for patients who responded to chemotherapy, whether alpha interferon had any impact on disease-free survival.

It emerged that there was very little difference between mantle cell lymphoma and follicle center cell lymphoma in terms of response to chemotherapy [11.8]. There may be a 15% lower complete and partial remission rate in the mantle cell lymphomas, but overall the response to initial chemotherapy is reasonable.

The real question is therefore not how to induce remissions, but how to prolong remission once it has been achieved. For that purpose we included mantle cell lymphoma in a prospective randomized comparison of alpha interferon versus observation. At the last evaluation we found a highly significant difference in the event-free interval in favor of the interferon group for the total study population. When we broke this down for the follicular lymphomas and for the mantle cell lymphomas, we could see that in both subtypes there was an advantage in favor of alpha interferon maintenance [11.9]. The numbers are still small but there is at least some indication that alpha interferon may be as effective in patients with mantle cell lymphomas as it is for patients with follicle center cell lymphomas.

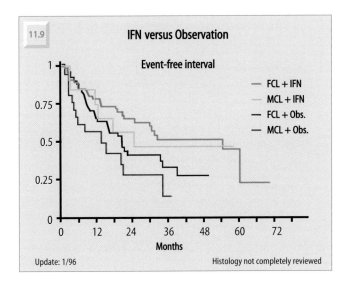

The same suggestion is found in the EORTC study by Teodorovic et al.[15] That paper did not show a curve for the disease-free interval, but a comparison of CVP with CVP plus interferon was given in a table which indicated that interferon may prolong disease-free survival [11.10].

Interferon therefore represents an interesting new approach to therapy, but it is certainly not curative. The question remains – can we achieve a better outcome for patients when we apply myeloablative radio-chemotherapy with subsequent blood stem cell

transplantation? [11.11] shows survival data published by Dr. Armitage's group (Stewart et al.).[10] The results may appear disappointing, but one has to take into account that all of these patients had advanced disease, and had relapsed previously.

11.10	Mantle Cell Lymphoma (EORTC Study)	
	CVP	CVP + IFN
Progression free survival	20	27
Median survival	45	median not reached

Teodorovic et al. 1995 [15]

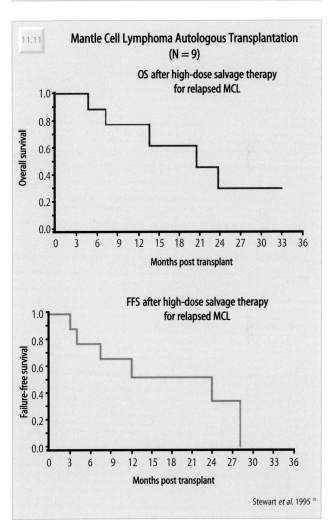

When [11.11] is compared to the results of a trial carried out in Germany, the curves look very different [11.12]. The main difference between these two groups is that most patients in the German study were treated in first remission. Although the numbers are small, there are some patients who have now survived for more than three years without relapse, and are in continuing first remission after myelo-ablative radio-chemotherapy, followed by stem cell transplantation.

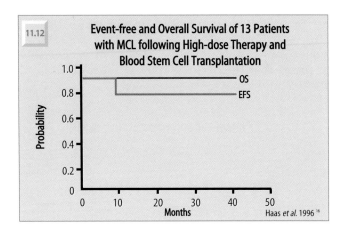

Event-free and Overall Survival of 13 Patients with MCL following High-dose Therapy and Blood Stem Cell Transplantation

Haas *et al.* 1996 [16]

In summary, conventional cytotoxic agents, including the anthracyclines and the purine analogues, do not offer much hope for mantle cell lymphoma. There is some evidence from Dr. Cavalli's group that epipodophyllotoxins might be of some benefit, but this is certainly not a striking effect. There is some hope, which has to be investigated in the future, that alpha interferon may offer a new approach. There is also strong evidence that high dose radio-chemotherapy with stem cell transplantation might be the best treatment option at the current time. However, this needs to be confirmed by prospective studies.

REFERENCES

1. Brittinger G, Bartels H, Common H *et al.* Clinical and prognostic relevance of the Kiel classification of non-Hodgkin lymphomas results of a prospective multicenter study by the Kiel Lymphoma Study Group. *Hematol Oncol* 1984; **2**: 269-306.

2. Fisher RI, Dahlberg S, Nathwani BN, Banks PM, Miller TP, Grogan TM. A clinical analysis of two indolent lymphoma entities: mantle cell lymphoma and marginal zone lymphoma (including the mucosa-associated lymphoid tissue and monocytoid B-cell subcategories): a Southwest Oncology Group study. *Blood* 1995; **85**:1075-82.

3. Wagner R, Press OW. Educational Booklet. *Am Soc Hematol* 1995: 36-44.

4. Berger F, Felman P, Sonet A *et al.* Nonfollicular small B-cell lymphomas: a heterogeneous group of patients with distinct clinical features and outcome. *Blood* 1994; **83**: 2829-35.

5. Zucca E, Fontana S, Roggero E, Pedrinis E, Pampallona S, Cavalli F. Treatment and prognosis of centrocytic (mantle cell) lymphoma: a retrospective analysis of twenty-six patients treated in one institution. *Leuk Lymphoma* 1994; **13**: 105-10.

6. Weisenburger DD, Nathwani BN, Diamond LW, Winberg CD, Rappaport H. Malignant lymphoma, intermediate lymphocytic type: a clinicopathologic study of 42 cases. *Cancer* 1981; **48**: 1415-25.

7. Meusers P, Engelhard M, Bartels H *et al.* Multicentre randomized therapeutic trial for advanced centrocytic lymphoma: anthracycline does not improve the prognosis. *Hematol Oncol* 1989; **7**: 365-80.

8. Norton AJ, Matthews J, Pappa V *et al.* Mantle cell lymphoma: natural history defined in a serially biopsied population over a 20-year period. *Ann Oncol* 1995; **6**: 249-56.

9. Pittaluga S, Wlodarska I, Stul MS *et al.* Mantle cell lymphoma: a clinicopathological study of 55 cases. *Histopathology* 1995; **26**: 17-24.

10. Stewart DA, Vose JM, Weisenburger DD *et al.* The role of high-dose therapy and autologous hematopoietic stem cell transplantation for mantle cell lymphoma. *Ann Oncol* 1995; **6**: 263-6.

11. Zucca E, Roggero E, Pinotti G *et al.* Patterns of survival in mantle cell lymphoma. *Ann Oncol* 1995; **6**: 257-62.

12. Narang S, Wolf BC, Neiman RS. Malignant lymphoma presenting with prominent splenomegaly. A clinicopathologic study with special reference to intermediate cell lymphoma. *Cancer* 1985; **55**: 1948-57.

13. Duggan MJ, Weisenburger DD, Ye YL *et al.* Mantle zone lymphoma. A clinicopathologic study of 22 cases. *Cancer* 1990; **66**: 522-9.

14. Meusers P, Engelhard M, Bartels H *et al.* Mantle cell (centrocytic) lymphoma: long-term survival with advanced disease is possible. *Blood* 1996; **86** (Suppl 1): 53a.

15. Teodorovic I, Pittaluga S, Kluin-Nelemans JC *et al.* Efficacy of four different regimens in 64 mantle-cell lymphoma cases: clinicopathologic comparison with 498 other non-Hodgkin's lymphoma subtypes. European Organization for the Research and Treatment of Cancer Lymphoma Cooperative Group. *J Clin Oncol* 1995; **13**: 2819-26.

16. Haas R, Brittinger G, Meusers P *et al.* Myeloablative therapy with blood stem cell transplantation is effective in mantle cell lymphoma. *Leukemia* 1996; **10**: 1975-9.

Morphologic, immunologic and genetic features of follicular lymphoma, and the problem of grading

N L Harris

Follicular lymphoma is the commonest category of lymphoma in Western countries. It is referred to in the REAL classification as follicle center lymphoma, because it is composed of cells normally found in germinal centers, that is to say, both centrocytes and centroblasts. Also we require for the diagnosis a growth pattern which is (at least partially) follicular.

The immunophenotype is characteristic [12.1] but not absolutely specific, in that the cells lack CD5, and are usually also CD43-negative. Often, but by no means always, they express CD10. The great majority, at least of the low grade cases, have the (14;18) translocation and rearrangement of the *BCL-2* gene. This results in overexpression of BCL-2 protein, contrasting with reactive germinal centers, which are BCL-2-negative.

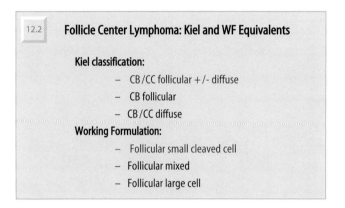

12.1   Follicle Center Lymphoma: Definition

A neoplasm composed of cells normally found in germinal

centers (centrocytes and centroblasts), with at least a partially

follicular growth pattern

Typically lacks CD5 and CD43; expresses CD10; overexpresses

BCL-2; t(14;18) and rearranged *BCL-2*

In the Kiel classification, follicle center lymphoma would usually be categorized as centroblastic centrocytic lymphoma [12.2]. However, the ILSG felt that any lymphoma with a purely follicular pattern, even if composed entirely of centroblasts, should be considered to be of follicle center origin, and therefore follicular centroblastic lymphoma is included in the category of follicle center lymphoma [12.2].

12.2   Follicle Center Lymphoma: Kiel and WF Equivalents

Kiel classification:
– CB/CC follicular +/- diffuse
– CB follicular
– CB/CC diffuse

Working Formulation:
– Follicular small cleaved cell
– Follicular mixed
– Follicular large cell

The REAL scheme includes a provisional category of "diffuse follicle center lymphoma", which would correspond to the Kiel entity of diffuse centroblastic-centrocytic lymphoma. In the Working Formulation study, the majority of cases in all three of the follicular lymphoma categories would have corresponded to the REAL definition of follicle center lymphoma, although one should recognize that some cases in that study, since they were classified without immunophenotyping, may have been mantle cell or MALT type lymphomas.

A typical case [12.3] shows uniform follicles replacing the lymph node architecture and presents no problem in diagnosis. At higher magnification [12.4] we see a reactive germinal center on the left, showing the two characteristic types of cells. The centroblast is a large non-cleaved cell with vesicular chromatin, usually with peripherally located small nucleoli, and a narrow rim of basophilic cytoplasm. The centrocyte, or cleaved cell, has an elongated, irregular nucleus with more dispersed chromatin, inconspicuous nucleoli, and usually no evident cytoplasm, even on Giemsa staining. The follicle center lymphoma seen on the right contains the same two cell types, although typically there are many more centrocytes than are seen in normal germinal centers.

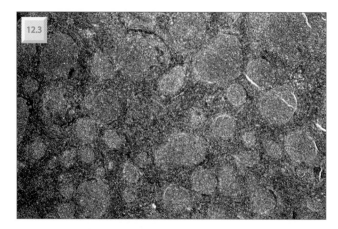

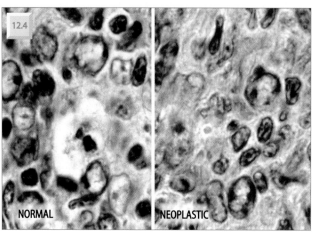

NORMAL   NEOPLASTIC

The *BCL-2* gene, which protects cells against apoptosis, is switched off in normal follicle center cells. This permits the elimination by negative selection of B cell clones with immunoglobulin gene mutations that have resulted in a poorly fitting or low affinity antibody. The (14;18) translocation is thought to occur at a pre-B cell stage, and cells with *BCL-2* rearrangement can be detected in normal adult lymphoid tissues, suggesting that in some people populations of cells may arise that have undergone this translocation in the process of rearranging their immunoglobulin genes. One can imagine that if some of these cells encountered antigen and became stimulated, they would not be able to undergo apoptosis, and this would result in the accumulation of long-lived B cells, the typical picture of follicular lymphoma. In terms of the "two hit" hypothesis of tumorogenesis, the first event would be the rearrangement of *BCL-2* in an early B cell, and the second might be something as simple as antigen stimulation. This raises the intriguing question of whether or not antigen stimulation may be involved in follicular lymphoma proliferation, similar to the mechanism proposed in MALT lymphomas.

In the Working Formulation and the Rappaport classification, follicle center lymphoma is subdivided according to grade, and this is generally felt to have clinical significance. This grading process has been referred to as subclassification, but it is important to recognize that it describes histologic grades of a single disease rather than different diseases.

There is no consensus among pathologists about the optimal way of grading follicle center lymphoma, and there are no objective criteria that permit one to do this reproducibly. The technique of Mann and Berard, which involves counting the number of centroblasts in a certain number of high power fields, has been widely used [12.5]. This gives three grades of follicle center lymphoma: grade I, corresponding to small cleaved cell lymphoma; grade II, corresponding to mixed lymphoma; and grade III, corresponding to large cell lymphoma.

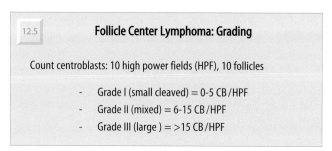

Follicle Center Lymphoma: Grading

Count centroblasts: 10 high power fields (HPF), 10 follicles

- Grade I (small cleaved) = 0-5 CB/HPF
- Grade II (mixed) = 6-15 CB/HPF
- Grade III (large) = >15 CB/HPF

Shown in [12.6] is a typical grade I follicle center lymphoma, with a predominance of small centrocytes and only rare centroblasts. [12.7] would be categorized as grade II, with much more numerous centroblasts, again with a background of centrocytes. [12.8] would be an example of the rare grade III, which consists predominantly of large centroblasts.

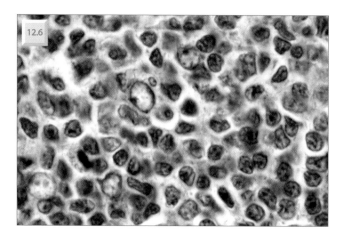

An important question for both pathologists and clinicians concerns the optimum method for grading and its clinical relevance. Another question relates to follicular large cell lymphoma or grade III follicle cell lymphoma, a tumor referred to as "centroblastic, follicular" in the Kiel classification. Should this be included in the spectrum of follicle center lymphoma or should it be treated for clinical purposes as a variant of large B cell lymphoma? Finally, we would like to know the clinical relevance of diffuse areas, and whether there is such a thing as a purely diffuse follicle center lymphoma. If so, how can it be recognized and what are its clinical features?

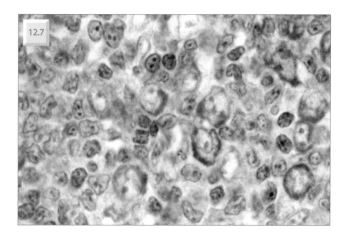

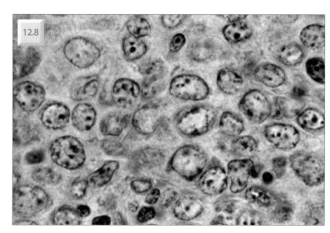

There are two major approaches to grading of follicular lymphoma. We can estimate the percentage of large cells, or we can use the cell counting method of Berard [12.9]. A number of studies have showed that estimating the proportion of large cells was not repro-ducible, whereas several studies in the early 1980s purported to show that the cell counting method was more reproducible. However, anyone who has ever sat down and counted cells will know that it is extremely tedious. It is also probably not accurate, because different microscopes have different sized high power fields, and this can significantly affect grading.

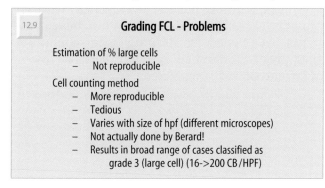

12.9   **Grading FCL - Problems**

Estimation of % large cells
  – Not reproducible
Cell counting method
  – More reproducible
  – Tedious
  – Varies with size of hpf (different microscopes)
  – Not actually done by Berard!
  – Results in broad range of cases classified as
      grade 3 (large cell) (16->200 CB/HPF)

Finally, if one uses the published method of Mann and Berard, it may result in a very large number of cases that are classified as large cell. This category would range from cases with 16 large cells per high power field to those with solid sheets of large cells, or more than 200 centroblasts per high power field. It is hard to believe that all cases in this broad range should be lumped together for clinical purposes.

Follicle center lymphoma is defined differently in the Kiel Classification and Working Formulation [12.10]. In the Working Formulation (and the Rappaport classification) the definition is based on pattern, so that a follicular lymphoma is a lymphoma with any follicular area. This criterion is in fact the one which most pathologists use, except for the large cell type. It is unlikely that many pathologists would make a diagnosis of follicular large cell lymphoma if they found a single follicle in a case of diffuse large cell lymphoma, although, if one adheres strictly to the Working Formulation, that is what should be done. As indicated, these classifications also ask the pathologist to grade the lymphoma according to the number of large cells.

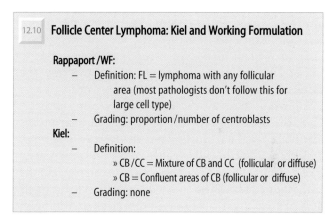

12.10   **Follicle Center Lymphoma: Kiel and Working Formulation**

Rappaport/WF:
  – Definition: FL = lymphoma with any follicular
      area (most pathologists don't follow this for
      large cell type)
  – Grading: proportion/number of centroblasts
Kiel:
  – Definition:
      » CB/CC = Mixture of CB and CC (follicular or diffuse)
      » CB = Confluent areas of CB (follicular or diffuse)
  – Grading: none

The Kiel classification, in contrast, defines the tumors according to cytology, and only secondarily according to pattern. Thus, centroblastic-centrocytic lymphoma is defined as containing a mixture of centro-blasts and centrocytes, with centrocytes predominating. The growth pattern may be either follicular or diffuse. In contrast, in any case that has confluent areas of centroblasts, a diagnosis of centroblastic lymphoma is made. Within each category the tumor may also be follicular or diffuse, but this is considered to be of secondary importance. No histologic grading of centroblastic-centrocytic lymphoma is attempted.

This difference in approach is schematically summarized in [12.11]. In the Working Formulation, the pathologist looks predominantly for the pattern, and if there is any follicular area, even if there is a predominance of centroblasts, makes a diagnosis of follicular lymphoma. Only when it is entirely diffuse, is it called diffuse large cell lymphoma. In contrast, in the Kiel classification, if there are solid sheets of centroblasts, even if the pattern is follicular, the neoplasm is called centroblastic.

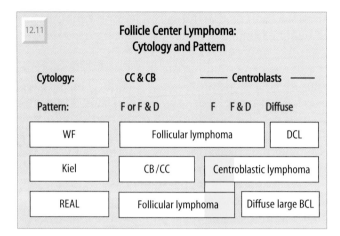

In the REAL classification, we tried a compromise approach, which is to define follicle center lymphoma as either being comprised of a mixture of centroblasts and centrocytes, or, in a case with a predominance of centroblasts, as having a purely follicular pattern. If there is any diffuse component in a case with a predominance of centroblasts, we would make a diagnosis of diffuse large B cell lymphoma. But we recognize that this is an area of controversy that needs to be resolved.

A few observations can be made that bear on this issue [12.12]. First, the impetus to grade follicle center lymphoma is clinical, because of its presumed prognostic importance. There is a paradox in the fact that although grading was started by pathologists in the Rappaport classification, in practice pathologists find it difficult to perform reproducibly. The second observation is that the clinical relevance of separating grades 1 and 2, that is the "small cleaved" and "mixed" categories, is still debated by oncologists. A third point is that pathologists can usually recognize confluent areas of centroblasts within follicles, and are better at doing this than estimating the percentage or number of these cells. And the last observation is that many follicular large cell lymphomas behave more like aggressive lymphomas, similar to diffuse large B cell lymphoma. Based on these observations and problems, a proposal can be put forward for discussion [12.13].

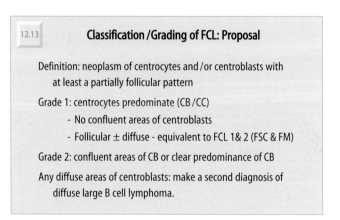

a proposal can be put forward for discussion [12.13].

Since many studies have shown that most pathologists can reproducibly agree on pattern, at least a partially follicular pattern should be required for the diagnosis; thus, the name, follicular lymphoma can be used. In contrast to the Working Formulation, other lymphomas with a nodular or follicular pattern (such as mantle cell) are excluded. We should consider a scheme with only two grades: a low-grade lesion (Grade 1), in which centrocytes predominate, corresponding to WF small cleaved and mixed or Kiel CB/CC, and a high grade lesion (Grade 2), in which centroblasts clearly predominate, corresponding to WF follicular large cell and Kiel centroblastic, follicular. This approach would require pathologists to do only what we know they are capable of doing (recognize a follicular pattern and sheets of large cells), and should provide the most important clinical information, a distinction between indolent and aggressive behavior. This approach should, however, not be adopted until it has been tested for its prognostic significance. Until then, a published approach such as that of Mann and Berard is suggested.

FURTHER READING

Anderson JR, Vose JM, Bierman PJ *et al*. Clinical features and prognosis of follicular large-cell lymphoma: a report from the Nebraska Lymphoma Study Group. *J Clin Oncol* 1993; **11**: 218-24.

Anderson T, Bender R, Fisher R *et al*. Combination chemotherapy in non-Hodgkin's lymphoma results of long-term follow-up. *Cancer Treat Rep* 1977; **61**: 1057-66.

Bartlett NL, Rizeq M, Dorfman RF, Halpern J, Horning SJ. Follicular large-cell lymphoma intermediate or low grade? *J Clin Oncol* 1994; **12**: 1349-57.

Brittinger G, Bartels H, Common H *et al*. Clinical and prognostic relevance of the Kiel classification of non-Hodgkin lymphomas: results of a prospective multicenter study by the Kiel lymphoma study group. *Hematol Oncol* 1984; **2**: 269-306.

Cleary M, Mecker T, Levy S *et al*. Clustering of extensive somatic mutations in the variable region of an immunoglobulin heavy chain gene from a human B cell lymphoma. *Cell* 1986; **44**: 97-106.

de Jong D, Voetdujk B, Baverstock G, van Ommen G, Willemze R, Kluin P. Activation of the c-myc oncogene in a precursor B-cell blast crisis of follicular lymphoma, presenting as composite lymphoma. *N Engl J Med* 1988; **318**: 1373-8.

Ezdinli E, Costello W, Kucuk O, Berard C. Effect of the degree of nodularity on the survival of patients with nodular lymphomas. *J Clin Oncol* 1987; **5**: 413-8.

Fisher RI, Dahlberg S, Nathwani BN, Banks PM, Miller TP, Grogan TM. A clinical analysis of two indolent lymphoma entities: mantle cell lymphoma and marginal zone lymphoma (including the mucosa-associated lymphoid tissue and monocytoid B-cell subcategories): a Southwest Oncology Group study. *Blood* 1995; **85**: 1075-82.

Glick J, Barnes J, Ezdinli E, Berard C, Orlow E, Bennett J. Nodular mixed lymphoma results of a randomized trial failing to confirm prolonged disease-free survival with COPP chemotherapy. *Blood* 1981; **58**: 920-5.

Glick J, McFadden E, Costello W, Ezdinli E, Berard C, Bennett J. Nodular histiocytic lymphoma factors influencing prognosis and implications for aggressive chemotherapy. *Cancer* 1982; **49**: 840-5.

Harris NL, Nadler LM, Bhan AK. Immunohistologic characterization of two malignant lymphomas of germinal center type (centroblastic/centrocytic and centrocytic) with monoclonal antibodies. Follicular and diffuse lymphomas of small cleaved cell types are related but distinct entities. *Am J Pathol* 1984; **117**: 262-72.

Hockenbery D, Zutter M, Hickey W, Nahm M, Korsmeyer S. BCL-2 protein is topographically restricted in tissues characterized by apoptotic cell death. *Proc Natl Acad Sci USA* 1991; **88**: 6961-5.

Hu E, Weiss L, Hoppe R, Horning S. Follicular and diffuse mixed small cleaved and large cell lymphoma a clinicopathologic study. *J Clin Oncol* 1985; **3**: 1183-7.

Hummel M, Tamaru J, Kalvelage B, Stein H. Mantle cell (previously centrocytic) lymphomas express VH genes with no or very little somatic mutations like the physiologic cells of the follicle mantle. *Blood* 1994; **84**: 403-7.

Lee JT, Innes DJ Jr, Williams ME. Sequential *bcl-2* and *c-myc* oncogene rearrangements associated with the clinical transformation of non-Hodgkin's lymphoma. *J Clin Invest* 1989; **84**: 1454-9.

Lennert K. *Malignant lymphomas other than Hodgkin's disease.* New York: Springer-Verlag, 1978.

Limpens J, de Jong D, van Krieken J *et al*. Bcl-2 in benign lymphoid tissue with follicular hyperplasia. *Oncogene* 1991; **6**: 2271-6.

Mann R, Berard C. Criteria for the cytologic subclassification of follicular lymphomas: a proposed alternative method. *Haematol Oncol* 1982; **1**: 187-92.

Martin AR, Weisenburger DD, Chan WC *et al*. Prognostic value of cellular proliferation and histologic grade in follicular lymphoma. *Blood* 1995; **85**: 3671-8.

McDonnell T, Deane N, Platt F *et al*. Bcl-2 immunoglobulin transgenic mice demonstrate extended B cell survival and follicular lymphoproliferation. *Cell* 1989; **57**: 79-88.

Metter G, Nathwani B, Burke J *et al*. Morphological subclassification of follicular lymphoma: variability of diagnosis among hematopathologists, a collaborative study between the Repository Center and Pathology Panel for Lymphoma Clinical Studies. *J Clin Oncol* 1985; **3**: 25-38.

Nathwani B, Metter G, Miller T *et al*. What should be the morphologic criteria for the subdivision of follicular lymphomas? *Blood* 1986; **68**: 837-45.

Non-Hodgkin's lymphoma pathologic classification project. National Cancer Institute sponsored study of classifications of non-Hodgkin's lymphomas: summary and description of a Working Formulation for clinical usage. *Cancer* 1982; **49**: 2112-35.

Paryani SB, Hoppe RT, Cox RS, Colby T, Rosenberg S, Kaplan H. Analysis of non Hodgkin's lymphomas with nodular and favorable histologies, stages I and II. *Cancer* 1983; **52**: 2300-7.

Sander CA, Yano T, Clark HM *et al*. p53 mutation is associated with progression in follicular lymphomas. *Blood* 1993, **82**: 1994-2004.

Stein H, Lennert K, Feller A, Mason DY. Immunohistological analysis of human lymphoma correlation of histological and immunological categories. *Adv Cancer Res* 1984; **42**: 67-147.

Tsujimoto T, Cossman J, Jaffe E, Croce C. Involvement of the bcl-2 gene in human follicular lymphoma. *Science* 1985; **288**: 1440-3.

Warnke R, Kim H, Fuks Z, Dorfman R. The co-existence of nodular and diffuse patterns in nodular non-Hodgkin's lymphomas. *Cancer* 1977; **40**: 1229-33.

Yano T, Jaffe ES, Longo DL, Raffeld M. MYC rearrangements in histologically progressed follicular lymphomas. *Blood* 1992; **80**: 758-67.

Yuen AR, Kamel OW, Halpern J, Horning SJ. Long-term survival after histologic transformation of low-grade follicular lymphoma. *J Clin Oncol* 1995; **13**: 1726-33.

Clinical aspects of follicular lymphoma and the relevance of grading

13

J O Armitage

This section is concerned with some of the clinical aspects of follicular lymphomas, and with how a clinician approaches the issue of grading. Follicular lymphoma [13.1] is one of the commonest types of lymphomas, and one might hope that as a consequence, we could do better than we do in treating these patients. In practice, the ultimately poor clinical outcome makes this one of the most frustrating classes of lymphomas for clinicians.

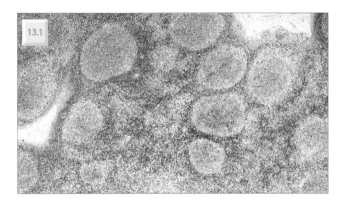

There are a number of ways in which one can divide up follicular lymphomas; for example, one is based on the degree of follicularity. The proposal described elsewhere by Dr Harris is a very practical one in that, when large cells predominate, follicularity is probably less of an issue. Clinicians will, however, continue to be interested in knowing how pathologists separate follicle center lymphomas, and whether they are applying the older rule that any follicularity makes the tumor a follicular lymphoma.

Follicular lymphomas raise several problems for clinicians, but this chapter will focus upon just two of them [13.2]. First of all, are any patients with follicular lymphoma curable? If they are, it is clearly very important to identify them so that we do not fail to treat them. Secondly, can follicular lymphomas be usefully subdivided – or "graded" – in a way that will improve our management?

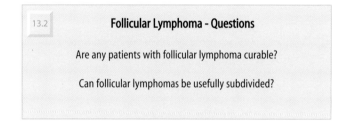

The issue of curability has been an exceedingly contentious issue over the years among clinicians. Many people take the position that follicular lymphomas cannot be cured, and argue strongly that this is true. At the opposite extreme, there have been repeated claims made that certain subtypes of follicular lymphomas can be cured. Almost 20 years ago, there was much debate as to whether or not follicular lymphoma of mixed cell type, "nodular mixed" lymphoma as it was known then, was a curable disease. Some very striking evidence that it was a curable disease was published, but at the same time other publications reported that it was quite incurable. This led to many interesting discussions at American Society of Clinical Oncology meetings. Similar debates have been heard over follicular large cell lymphoma. However, as Dr. Harris has pointed out, it is difficult to distinguish different subtypes of follicular lymphoma reproducibly, and this of course further confuses these issues.

Dr. Horning, together with Dr. Rosenberg and other colleagues at Stanford, have argued that follicular lymphoma is not a curable disease [13.3]. However, the data from Stanford [13.4] also show that if patients with follicular small cleaved and follicular mixed lymphoma) achieve a complete remission, 25% will still be in complete remission after ten years. This flat part of the survival curve is short, and one might or might not choose to call it a plateau. However, at least a significant proportion of patients stay well for very long periods if a complete remission is achieved, even among the more indolent subgroups of follicular lymphoma. If one also takes into account the fact that most lymphomas occur in older people, patients who go into remission and survive for many years and then die without having a relapse have achieved what in practice one can call a cure, whatever the future would have held.

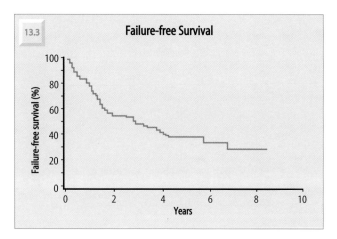

As discussed elsewhere, there are certain subgroups of patients for whom most oncologists believe a cure is possible. One group comprises patients with localized follicular lymphoma, in whom radiotherapy is often used. Data from Nebraska [13.5] indicate that these patients do very well, and that a high proportion of them survive for extended periods of time, especially if they are young.

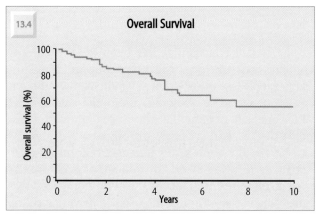

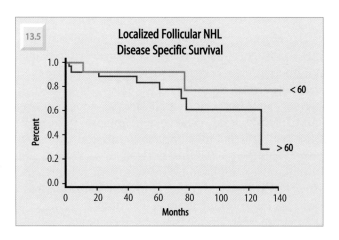

A number of studies have shown that follicular lymphomas can be subdivided clinically on the basis of certain characteristics. For example, data from the Working Formulation study [13.6], which analyzed follicular small cleaved, follicular mixed and follicular large cell lymphomas showed that there are differences in the chances of having disseminated disease, or localized disease, and that patients with fewer large cells are more likely to be bone marrow-positive and to show a different median survival. Findings such as these clearly hint at the possibility of distinctive prognostic groups.

13.6	Clinical Comparison of Follicular Lymphoma (WF Study)		
Characteristic	FSC	FM	FLC
Stage I/II	18%	27%	27%
BM pos.	51%	30%	34%
Median survival	7.2 years	5.1 years	3.0 years

One point to consider in relation to attempts to subdivide, or to grade, follicular lymphomas is that the number of large cells correlates with their proliferative capacity. The proliferative index (PI), i.e. the number of cells undergoing DNA synthesis, varies, and a higher index is seen in cases containing more large cells [13.7].

13.7	Association of PI With Histologic Subtypes of FL		
Classification	N	Mean	p-value
Berard (NLSG) method			
FSC + FM	42	32.1	< 0.0001
FLC	64	43.4	< 0.0001
Rappaport/Jaffe methods			
FSC + FM	85	36.6	0.0002
FLC	21	48.3	0.0002
Lukes-Collins method			
FSC	64	35.3	0.0005
FLC	42	44.3	0.0005

Survival in follicular lymphomas can also be related to Stage, as data from London show [13.8]. The newly described International Index is very predictive, not only in large cell lymphomas, but also in follicular lymphomas. These tumors are therefore not uniform in their clinical manifestation. They can be divided on the basis of characteristics at diagnosis, and this may be associated with different outcomes.

A second issue of importance from the clinical point of view concerns subdivision based on the number of large cells. A study was carried out at our Institution by Drs. Martin, Weisenburger, Chan *et al* which used the methods of Berard, of Rappaport, of Lukes and Collins, and of Jaffe to divide up cases according to the number of large cells.[1] These were consecutive patients treated in the 1980s on whom data was available for analysis. The series included only patients who received what were felt to be comparable therapies – if the disease was localized, patients were treated with radiotherapy, but if the disease was disseminated, they were all treated with adriamycin or anthrocyclin-based combination chemotherapy.

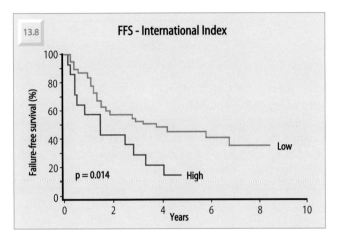

A total of 106 patients were studied [13.9], and they had a median age of just under 60. The great majority of patients were asymptomatic. As is usually the case with follicular lymphoma, most patients were in the low risk category, based on the International Index. Two thirds achieved complete remission following treatment, and a quarter showed partial or no response. The failure-free survival for these patients, showed a median time to treatment failure of about 3 years. Overall this is fairly typical of follicular lymphoma, as compared to the literature. The ten year overall survival was somewhat better than 50%.

If we look at overall survival, and then at failure-free survival, we see that if we take the proliferative index we can divide these tumors into two clinically distinct groups. They are divided on the basis of the number of large cells, using the criteria described by Lukes and Collins [13.10] or by Rappaport [13.11], or the Berard counting method [13.12], or the Jaffe modification of Berard's method [13.13]. The pathologist was able to separate these cases into two groups, comprising cases containing mostly large cells versus other cases. This identified two groups of patients who showed a clear difference in overall survival. However, if we look at failure-free survival, the results are less encouraging, and with three of the techniques no significant difference was seen. Perhaps the counting method identified a group of large cell lymphoma patients who fared better, but that is probably an optimistic interpretation.

13.9	Clinical Characteristics of 106 Patients with FL	
Characteristic		**N**
Age (years)		
	< 60	51 (48)
	≥ 60	55 (52)
Sex		
	Male	50 (47)
	Female	56 (53)
Stage		
	I	27 (26)
	II	13 (12)
	III	23 (22)
	IV	43 (40)
Symptoms		
	A	85 (80)
	B	21 (20)
International Index		
	Low risk	88 (86)
	High risk	14 (14)
Response to treatment		
	Complete	66 (62)
	Partial /none	25 (24)
	Not evaluable	15 (14)

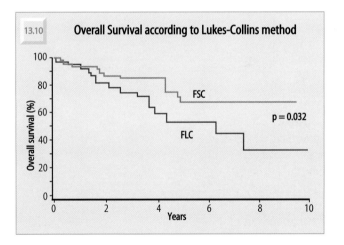

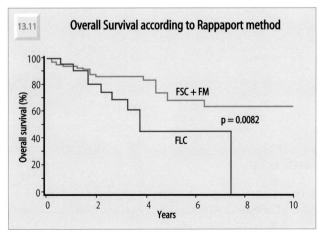

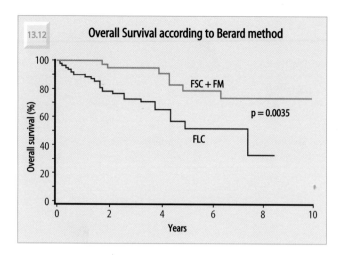

13.12 **Overall Survival according to Berard method**

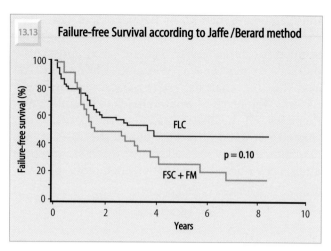

13.13 **Failure-free Survival according to Jaffe /Berard method**

In conclusion, follicular lymphoma is an indolent malignancy, which combines a high level of responsiveness to chemotherapy with a good number of complete remissions. However, in seeming violation of one of the rules of oncology, complete remissions are not difficult to obtain but it is still far from certain that any more than a very small minority of patients are cured. Although we can divide them clinically into prognostically distinct groups and thereby make informed treatment decisions, it is still unclear if histopathologic methods can identify subgroups who should be treated in a particular way, or whom more effective therapies might cure.

REFERENCES

1. Martin AR, Weisenburger DD, Chan WC *et al.* Prognostic value of cellular proliferation and histologic grade in follicular lymphoma. *Blood* 1995; **85**: 3671-8.

When to treat early stage follicular lymphoma

S J Horning

In the curves shown elsewhere in this volume (see Chapter 15) for Stanford advanced stage follicular lymphoma patients, there is a small plateau at about 25%. However, with time this has decreased to less than 10%, and in fact the author saw one of these patients recently with a recurrence after 33 years. As physicians and medical oncologists, we focus on cure and freedom from relapse, but it is important to keep in mind that survival is really the most important parameter.

This chapter is concerned with limited stage low-grade lymphoma. Shown in [14.1] from the original Working Formulation paper[1] is data for the small cleaved cell subset of follicular lymphomas and it makes the point that limited stage disease is in fact rather uncommon. More than twenty years ago Dr. Chabner at the NCI and Dr. Goffinet at our institution showed that the proportion of patients with limited stage disease falls if a lymphangiogram is performed. That is also true for its modern replacement, CT scanning. It will also fall after bone marrow biopsy, and in that context it can be argued that this is one of the situations where bilateral bone marrow samples are indicated. It also falls following staging laparotomy.

A further point to make is shown in [14.2]. In a copy of *Clinical Oncology Alert* sent out ten years ago it was claimed that early stage patients are curable. This chapter considers whether this statement is true – and, if so, at what price?

Early reports of the outcome of radiation therapy for Stage I, II and even Stage III low grade lymphomas were published by Dr. Paryani, who was then a radiation oncology resident at Stanford, together with Dr. Hoppe and the late Dr. Kaplan.[2] More recently, Dr. MacManus, a visiting scholar at Stanford, has updated these results and some of the following illustrations are from his work [14.3].[3]

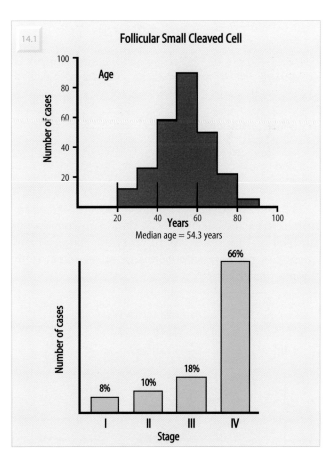

14.1 **Follicular Small Cleaved Cell**

Number of cases vs Years (Age). Median age = 54.3 years

Number of cases vs Stage:
I = 8%, II = 10%, III = 18%, IV = 66%

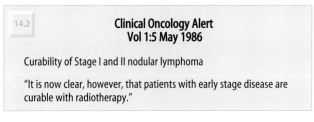

14.2 **Clinical Oncology Alert**
Vol 1:5 May 1986

Curability of Stage I and II nodular lymphoma

"It is now clear, however, that patients with early stage disease are curable with radiotherapy."

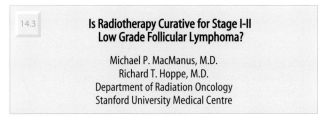

14.3 **Is Radiotherapy Curative for Stage I-II Low Grade Follicular Lymphoma?**

Michael P. MacManus, M.D.
Richard T. Hoppe, M.D.
Department of Radiation Oncology
Stanford University Medical Centre

The characteristics of 177 patients with Stage I and II follicular small cleaved cell or mixed low grade follicular lymphoma are summarized in [14.4]. There are 102 patients with Stage II disease. As expected, there is a male predominance, and the median age was 52 years. Follicular small cleaved cell histology was seen in 101 patients. The majority were treated with limited radiation, defined as radiation given to one side of the diaphragm – either a true involved field or regional radiotherapy. Extensive radiotherapy refers to subtotal or total lymphoid irradiation. Only 45 of the 177 patients underwent staging laparotomy.

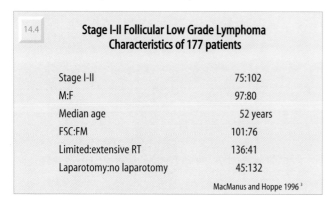

14.4	Stage I-II Follicular Low Grade Lymphoma Characteristics of 177 patients	
Stage I-II		75:102
M:F		97:80
Median age		52 years
FSC:FM		101:76
Limited:extensive RT		136:41
Laparotomy:no laparotomy		45:132
		MacManus and Hoppe 1996 [3]

The Kaplan-Meier plots for the overall freedom from relapse and survival [14.5] show a median overall survival of 13.8 years. At 10 years the actuarial frequency of patients who were free of recurrent lymphoma was about 45%.

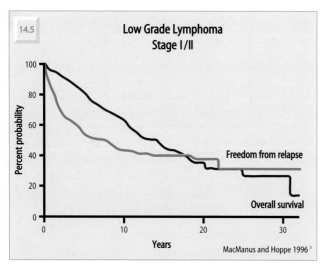

The incidence of recurrences declines after ten years but late events do occur. The data in [14.6] represent freedom from relapse actuarially plotted according to patient age. There is a significant difference in favor of younger patients. This confirms our earlier report, and many other reports in the literature, that younger patients are more likely to remain in remission.

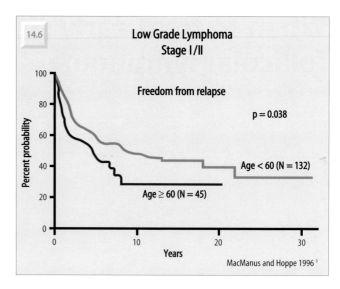

Shown in [14.7] are data on patients grouped according to whether or not a laparotomy was performed. Survival is better for patients who have had more extensive staging, that is to say laparotomy. Presumably this is because an occult disease was found in this group of patients, who were then assigned to a higher Stage. This may be relevant to reports, based on PCR analysis of peripheral blood, which indicate that circulating tumor cells are present in patients who were otherwise thought to have limited follicular low grade lymphoma.

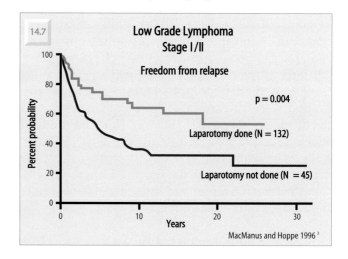

Freedom from relapse data is again shown in [14.8], in this case according to the extent of radiation – either both sides or one side of the diaphragm. The results do significantly favor more extensive radiation. However, if survival is reviewed, there is no difference according to the extent of radiation [14.9], which must mean that intercurrent deaths occur to explain these differences.

Overall survival according to age is shown in [14.10]. These curves contrast the observed versus the expected survival for patients aged over or under the age of 60, and these curves are matched with age and gender matched controls. It is quite apparent that survival is shorter than normal in each group when their limited stage low grade lymphoma was treated with radiation therapy with curative intent.

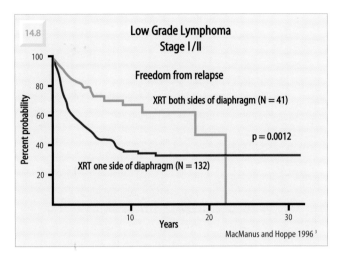

MacManus and Hoppe 1996 [3]

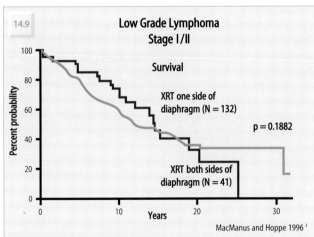

MacManus and Hoppe 1996 [3]

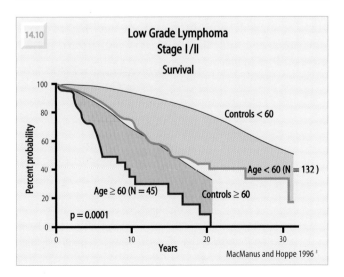

MacManus and Hoppe 1996 [3]

The causes of death in these patients need to be explored further, but it is clear that there has not been a single consistent cause. It is of interest to look at the

incidence of malignant solid tumors according to the radiation treatment volume. In [14.11] the cancers occurring in patients who received extensive total or subtotal nodal radiation are summarized. A total of seven tumors arose in 41 patients, an incidence of 17%.

14.11	Incidence of Malignant Solid Tumour According to Radiation Treatment Volume		
Total or subtotal nodal radiation patients			
Non small cell lung carcinoma	2	Both fatal
Squamous carcinoma esophagus	1	Fatal
Parotid carcinoma	1	Nonfatal
Oligodendroglioma	1	Fatal
Adenocarcinoma unknown primary	1	Fatal
Adenocarcinoma rectum	1	Nonfatal
Total of 7 tumors in 41 patients treated (17%); 5 fatalities (12%)			
		MacManus and Hoppe 1996 [3]	

The data for the larger group of 133 patients who received involved or extended field irradiation limited to one side of the diaphragm are shown in [14.12]. There were nine tumors, an incidence of 6.8%.

14.12	Incidence of Malignant Solid Tumor According to Radiation Treatment Volume		
Involved /extended field irradiation patients			
Nasal cavity carcinoma	1	Fatal
Prostate adenocarcinoma	1	Nonfatal
Prostate adenocarcinoma	1	Fatal
Stomach adenocarcinoma	1	Fatal
Carcinoma unknown primary	1	Fatal
Breast carcinoma	1	Nonfatal
Adenocarcinoma rectum	1	Nonfatal
Metastatic adenocarcinoma	1	Fatal
CNS tumor	1	Fatal
Total of 9 tumors in 133 patients treated (6.8%); 7 fatalities (5.2%)			
		MacManus and Hoppe 1996 [3]	

How do these results compare with those in the literature? [14.13] shows, in tabular form, data from the Princess Margaret Hospital, the MD Anderson Hospital, the Vancouver Group, the British National Lymphoma Investigation, and the Stanford series. All patients received some degree of radiotherapy. A significant proportion of the MD Anderson patients also received chemotherapy in the form of COP or CHOP. The patients had either Stage I or II disease but were relatively consistent between centers. The follicular lymphoma patients at the MD Anderson also included those with predominantly large cell neoplasms. Some series included small lymphocytic lymphoma, and the series from Britain included patients with diffuse small cell lymphoma.

14.13 Stage I-II Follicular Low Grade Lymphoma Comparison of Treatment Results			Overall survival		Freedom from relapse	
			10 y	15 y	10y	15y
PMH (285)	IFRT	FM, FSC, SL	65	57	52	48
MDA (144)	RT, CM	Foll	69	63	56	46
BCCC (78)	IFRT	FM, FSC, SL	80	-	59	-
BNLI (208)	RT	FM, FSC, SL	64	-	47	-
SUH (177)	RT	FM, FSC	64	44	44	40

If the actuarial percentages for overall survival and freedom from relapse at about ten and fifteen years are considered, the data are more similar than they are different. Overall survivals range from 64 to 80%, and the freedom from relapse at ten years was between 45 and 60%.

One additional point of interest is seen in [14.14] which summarizes survival for patients seen in our center with Stage I and II low grade lymphoma who, for a variety of reasons, were not treated. These were generally older patients or patients with less bulky disease. Few if any patients with limited stage disease have true constitutional symptoms. One can see that very few patients are at risk after more than five to ten years. Seventeen of the 31 patients have received some form of treatment for their lymphoma to date and the one very early death was associated with histologic transformation.

In conclusion [14.15], relapses are unlikely to recur after ten years in Stage I and II follicular low grade lymphoma patients who have received radiation therapy of any extent. The extent of radiotherapy does influence freedom from relapse, but not overall survival. Age is an important prognostic factor, both for freedom from relapse and overall survival, and

survival is shortened in patients receiving radiotherapy for early stage follicular lymphoma, without a single consistent cause.

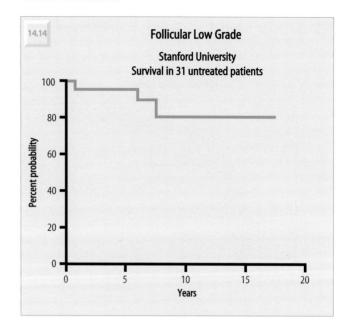

14.14 Follicular Low Grade
Stanford University
Survival in 31 untreated patients

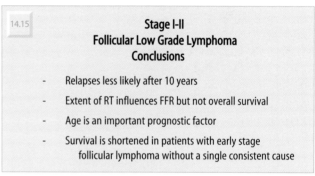

14.15 Stage I-II
Follicular Low Grade Lymphoma
Conclusions

- Relapses less likely after 10 years
- Extent of RT influences FFR but not overall survival
- Age is an important prognostic factor
- Survival is shortened in patients with early stage follicular lymphoma without a single consistent cause

My colleagues in the Radiotherapy Department would have included in this list the point that radiotherapy remains the choice of treatment for early stage low grade lymphoma. That may be true, but one can argue that "the jury is still out" regarding the cure and its price.

REFERENCES

1. The Non-Hodgkin's Lymphoma Pathologic Classification Project. National Cancer Institute sponsored study of classifications of non-Hodgkin's lymphomas: summary and description of a Working Formulation for clinical usage. *Cancer* 1982; **49**: 2112-35.

2. Paryani SB, Hoppe RT, Cox RS, Colby TV, Kaplan HS. The role of radiation therapy in the management of stage III follicular lymphomas. *J Clin Oncol* 1984; **2**: 841-8.

3. MacManus MP, Hoppe RT. Is radiotherapy curative for stage I and II low-grade follicular lymphoma? Results of a long-term follow-up study of patients treated at Stanford University. *J Clin Oncol* 1996; **14**: 1282-90.

Transformed follicular lymphoma

S J Horning

Any consideration of transformed follicular lymphoma has to address the problem of how to define "transformation" since this influences any assessment of its frequency as a complication of follicular lymphoma.

In the author's series transformation is diagnosed when a low grade lymphoma (as defined in the Working Formulation, i.e. follicular small cleaved and follicular mixed) evolves into a diffuse higher grade lymphoma [15.1]. We generally do not talk of transformation when the neoplastic cells become larger but the lymphoma retains its follicularity. Thus we require a change in not only cell morphology but also in architecture.

15.1	**Transformed Lymphoma** **Problems in Determination of Incidence**
	- Definition
	- Type of specimen
	- Biopsy policy
	- Discordant / composite histology
	- Clinical judgement

The diagnosis of transformation by these criteria is obviously dependent on the specimen available, since architecture is not apparent in fine needle aspirations, which are used ever more frequently. Assessment of the incidence of transformation also relates to the policy of biopsy, that is to say whether one always attempts to document transformation when it is suspected.

In practice policies on this are often quite inconsistent. For example, the author can recall a new patient conference at which a young woman was discussed who had presented with very extensive and bulky follicular small cleaved cell lymphoma, and who had achieved what appeared to be a complete remission. However, some eight months later lymphadenopathy recurred in other areas together with an elevated LDH. Her attending physician had no doubt that this was a transformed lymphoma, and she was treated accordingly. However, another physician might well have interpreted this quite differently and would not have recorded this case, at least without further investigation, as representing a transformation.

Another point relates to discordant and occasionally "composite" histology. There are many reports in the literature which indicate that, if multiple biopsies are done at the time of diagnosis, 20-30% of patients will show more than one histologic subtype. This is particularly important in the context of very early histologic transformations, since these may represent a previously unrecognized discordant lymphoma. It is obviously relevant that the most common discordance in follicular lymphoma involves the co-existence of small cleaved cell and diffuse large cell neoplasms.

Finally, we should consider variations in clinical judgement, since these will influence when one decides to do a biopsy and when one becomes suspicious of transformation. These decisions very much reflect the clinician's degree of familiarity with the disease.

The data in [15.2] are from a study published some years ago in which we analyzed the risk of histologic transformation in a group of patients who had participated in consecutive randomized trials at Stanford in the 1970s.[1] We compared the incidence of transformation in patients who were initially untreated with the risk in treated patients. These curves are remarkably similar, suggesting that histologic transformation is part of the natural history of the disease, rather than a consequence of the mutagenic effects of chemo- or radiotherapy. These data are also relevant to the argument, which is sometimes advanced, that histologic transformation is more frequent at our institution or seen later because patients have not been previously treated.

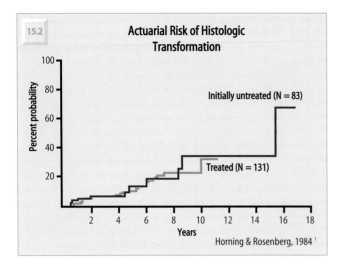

Actuarial Risk of Histologic Transformation

Initially untreated (N = 83)

Treated (N = 131)

Horning & Rosenberg, 1984 [1]

clinical remission for their low grade lymphoma following treatment, and who then relapse with histologic transformation. Fifty two of the 74 patients had received at least one prior chemotherapy regimen. A few were symptomatic with constitutional symptoms at the time of transformation, and the majority were ambulatory.

Transformed Lymphoma Characteristics of 74 patients	
LDH normal	31
LDH abnormal	33
Prior chemotherapy	
0	22
≥ 1 regimen	52
B symptoms present	11
B symptoms absent	62
ECOG PS-01	44
ECOG PS 2-4	12

Yuen *et al.* 1995 [2]

Dr. Yuen, a post-doctoral fellow at Stanford, has performed a retrospective analysis of a group of 74 patients with transformed lymphoma [15.3].[2] These patients had a median age of 58 years and the median time from diagnosis was 66 months, although there was a very wide range, from 7 to 300 months. The commonest diagnosis at the time of transformation was diffuse large cell lymphoma, but others were classified as diffuse mixed cell lymphoma and there was one lymphoblastic lymphoma and one high grade lymphoma.

The survival data are shown in [15.5]. The overall median survival of 22 months is about what one expects for advanced diffuse large cell lymphoma. A Cox regression analysis was performed to assess variables that might be prognostically significant. These included the re-stage category, and, difficult as it can be to assess, limited disease was a better prognostic feature than extensive disease. Prior chemotherapy was also relevant in that patients with no prior exposure to treatment did better than those who had received some treatment. A complete response to therapy at the time of transformation was preferable to a partial or no response.

Transformed Lymphoma Characteristics of 74 patients	
Median age	58 years (31-81)
Median time from diagnosis	66 months (7-300)
DLC	65
DM	7
LB / HG	2
Limited Stage	33
Advanced Stage	41

Yuen *et al.* 1995 [2]

Restaging at the time of transformation is another very difficult area unless multiple biopsies are performed. However, in essence we assess patients at the time of transformation and compare their disease to what has been noted during continuous previous follow-up. We then try to categorize patients as having either limited stage disease, when the diffuse aggressive component appears to be limited in the usual Ann Arbor sense, or as having more advanced disease.

Further characteristics in this retrospective study are shown in [15.4], including the distribution of normal versus abnormal LDH values. Twenty two of the 74 patients had not received prior chemotherapy, and it should be emphasized that sometimes histologic transformation is the first event. We have also seen numerous patients who are in apparent complete

Transformed Lymphoma Survival Analyses

Median survival = 22 months

Kaplan-Meier survival %	5 year	10 year	15 year	20 year
From diagnosis	70	48	32	17
From transformation	34	18	-	-

Cox regression analysis

Stage (limited vs extensive)	p = 0.01
Prior chemotherapy (none vs any)	p = 0.01
CR v PR/NR	p = 0.005

The Kaplan-Meier plots in [15.6] demonstrate that a subset of these patients achieve complete remission post-transformation, and a minority of patients should therefore survive ten or more years. Some recurrences represent reappearance of the transformed lymphoma, whereas others indicate recurrence of the original low grade lymphoma.

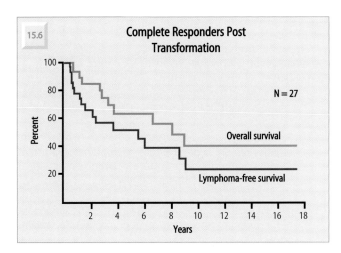

15.6 Complete Responders Post Transformation

N = 27

Overall survival

Lymphoma-free survival

How do these results compare with those in the literature? Other reported series have been relatively small compared to our experience in Stanford [15.7]. The median time to transformation is variable and the median survival tends to be short. However, it should again be emphasized that this is a heterogeneous group of patients, and that a small subset have a complete response clinically at the time of recurrence and enjoy a relatively prolonged survival.

15.7	Transformed Lymphoma Comparative Results		
Author (N)	Median time to HT (months)	Median survival	Median survival if CR (months)
Hubbard (19)[3]	25	11	41
Cullen (8)[4]	31	5	-
Oviatt (13)[5]	54	2.5	-
Ersbøll (23)[6]	53	4	-
Armitage (14)[7]	47	12	-
Yuen (74)[2]	66	22	88

The many genetic abnormalities that may occur secondarily to the (14;18) translocation are summarized in [15.8], and the clinical variation that we see no doubt reflects this underlying genetic heterogeneity of ongoing mutational events. Abnormalities of p53 and of chromosomes 6 and 7 have all been associated with progression from low grade to intermediate or high grade lymphoma.

In conclusion, histologic transformation is a clinically heterogeneous disease, probably reflecting different underlying genetic mechanisms [15.9]. Very early transformation may represent an occult discordant lymphoma or perhaps an early mutational event. Transformation may occur in patients who are in continuing full remission after treatment for low grade lymphoma, and for this reason we should continue to be vigilant in following our patients. Finally, good prognostic features include limited disease, no prior chemotherapy and disease which is responsive to therapy.

15.8	Transformed Lymphoma Abnormalities Secondary to t(14;18)	
Abnormality		Clinical association
Additional copies of chromosome 7		Diffuse histologic growth pattern; progression to intermediate- and high-grade NHL
Additional copies of 7q		Progression to intermediate- and high-grade NHL
Loss of chromosome 6 or deletion of 6q		Progression to intermediate- and high-grade NHL
Deletion of 6q with trisomy 7 and/or 12		Progression to follicular mixed small and large cell or follicular large cell NHL
Deletion of 13q32		Features of leukemia and acceleration of disease
Trisomy 2 or duplication of 2p		Acceleration of clinical course and poor prognosis
Mutation of p53 gene, or deletion of 17 or 17p		Progression to intermediate- and high-grade NHL

15.9 Transformed Lymphoma Conclusions

- Transformed lymphomas are clinically heterogeneous, probably representing genetic heterogeneity
- Very early transformation may represent discordant lymphoma
- Transformation may occur in patients who are in continuous remission after treatment for low grade lymphoma
- Limited extent of disease, no prior chemotherapy and responsive disease select a relatively favorable group

REFERENCES

1. Horning SJ, Rosenberg SA. The natural history of initially untreated low-grade non-Hodgkin's lymphomas. *N Engl J Med* 1984; **311**: 1471-5.

2. Yuen AR, Kamel OW, Halpern J, Horning SJ. Long-term survival after histologic transformation of low-grade follicular lymphoma. *J Clin Oncol* 1995; **13**: 1726-33.

3. Hubbard SM, Chabner BA, DeVita VT Jr *et al.* Histologic progression in non-Hodgkin's lymphoma. *Blood* 1982; **59**: 258-64.

4. Cullen MH, Lister TA, Brearley RI, Shand WS, Stansfeld AG. Histological transformation of non-Hodgkin's lymphoma: a prospective study. *Cancer* 1979; **44**: 645-51.

5. Oviatt DL, Cousar JB, Collins RD, Flexner JM, Stein RS. Malignant lymphomas of follicular center cell origin in humans. V. Incidence, clinical features, and prognostic implications of transformation of small cleaved cell nodular lymphoma. *Cancer* 1984; **53**: 1109-14.

6. Ersbøll J, Schultz HB, Pedersen-Bjergaard J, Nissen NI. Follicular low-grade non-Hodgkin's lymphoma: long-term outcome with or without tumor progression. *Eur J Haematol* 1989; **42**: 155-63.

7. Armitage JO, Dick FR, Corder MP. Diffuse histiocytic lymphoma after histologic conversion: a poor prognostic variant. *Cancer Treat Rep* 1981; **65**: 413-8.

Therapies for advanced and high-risk follicular lymphoma

A S Freedman

This chapter is concerned with therapy for advanced stage and high-risk follicular lymphoma and, more specifically, with the goals of treatment, the results of conventional therapy, and myelo-ablative treatment. A major question of interest from both the clinical and the research perspective is why we should attempt to treat patients with advanced stage follicular lymphoma. One obvious reason is to alleviate symptoms, but we also want to improve on conventional therapy and to develop new approaches - and for the true optimist, there is always the hope that one can cure patients with this disease.

When should we start therapy in advanced stage patients? The indications in [16.1] come from Stanford and NCI studies of a "watch and wait" approach. One should treat when there is evidence of progressive systemic and/or symptomatic disease. Other indications are the presence of B symptoms, effusions, extranodal disease, cytopenias, and symptomatic disease that is not treatable with radiation therapy. Finally, we should take into account the patient's insistence on further therapy.

16.1	When to Initiate Conventional Therapy in Advanced Stage Disease

Progressive systemic/symptomatic/bulk disease

B symptoms

Effusions, extranodal disease

Cytopenias

Symptomatic disease not treatable with XRT

Patient insistence

One consideration of importance when assessing different approaches for this disease is whether the treatment will have an impact on disease-free or progression-free survival and on overall survival, and this chapter focuses on that context.

If we consider conventional therapy, the response rate to single alkylating agents is in the range of 60 - 80%, with a complete remission rate of about 40%. Using combination chemotherapy, one sees similar response rates, of around 80%, and the median duration of response is around two and a half years. The data in [16.2] from Dr. Lister's group in London are representative of data from many other studies.

16.2	Conventional Treatment - Responses

Initial treatment

Single alkylating agent - 76% (38% CR)

Combination chemotherapy - 80%

Median duration of response - 31 months

Johnson *et al.* 1995 [1]

Does an increase in therapy alter the outcome? A study from Stanford [16.3], published some years ago, suggests that increasing the amount of therapy reduces the time to complete remission. Patients were randomized to either low dose TBI, single alkylating agent, or CVP. There was no significant difference in the complete remission rate, but the time to remission, particularly when the single alkylating agent was compared to CVP, was clearly shorter.

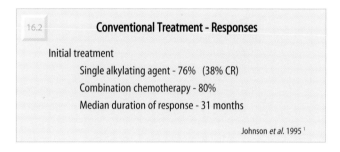

16.3	More CR - Shorter Time to CR	
	CR	Median time to CR
TBI (150 rad)	71%	3 months
Single agent (CPA, CHL)	64%	12 months
CVP	88%	5 months

Hoppe *et al.* 1981 [2]

The next question is whether more therapy gives better results when assessed in randomized trials of initial therapy for advanced stage patients. Data from three randomized trials are summarized in [16.4].[3-5] In an ECOG study comparing CVPP to cytoxan and prednisolone, and to another combination, a greater progression-free survival was found in follicular small cleaved cell lymphoma patients treated with CVPP, but there was no impact on overall survival. Another study, from SWOG, investigated the role of adriamycin, and showed no difference in the rate of complete remission, or in progression-free or overall survival. Finally, a CALGB study, which has unfortunately never been published except in abstract form, compared CHOP-bleomycin with cytoxan in low grade lymphoma as initial therapy, and reported an improved survival only in follicular lymphoma cases of mixed cell histology. This is reminiscent of the early NCI studies, which suggested that patients with follicular lymphomas of mixed histology may have a better outcome with combination chemotherapy. However, although combination chemotherapy has an impact on these diseases, its effect is limited.

What is the effect of treating patients at the time of first recurrence [16.6]? With conventional therapy, one sees a response rate of about 67% to the reinstitution of single agents. A similar response rate is achieved with combination chemotherapy. For example, in a series from Andrew Lister's group in London, the figure was 75%. However, the median duration of response was significantly less at 13 months. The Kaplan-Meier curves from that study [16.7] show that, with each subsequent relapse, the median duration of remission becomes shorter and shorter.

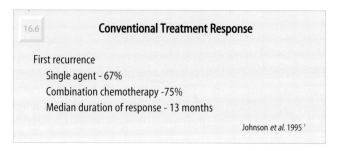

16.6   **Conventional Treatment Response**

First recurrence
    Single agent - 67%
    Combination chemotherapy -75%
    Median duration of response - 13 months

Johnson *et al.* 1995[1]

16.4   **Randomized Trials of Initial Therapy Is More Really Better?**

CVPP, CP, or BCVP
    Greater progression-free survival to FSC with PVPP
COP-BLEO, CHOP-BLEO or CHOP-BCG
    No difference in CR, progression-free or overall
    survival
CHOP-BLEO or CTX
    Improved survival in follicular mixed
Combination chemotherapy limited in impact

Ezdinli *et al.* 1985;[3] Jones *et al.* 1979;[4] Peterson *et al.* 1985[5]

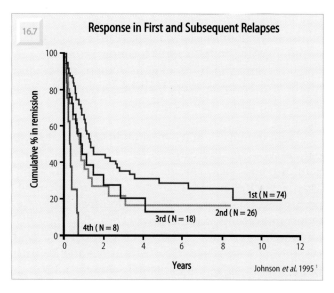

16.7   **Response in First and Subsequent Relapses**

1st (N = 74)
2nd (N = 26)
3rd (N = 18)
4th (N = 8)

Johnson *et al.* 1995[1]

Four randomized trials have shown improved progression-free survival through the addition of interferon-α, but no improvement in survival. One study that did show an influence on survival was a French-Belgian study published several years ago [16.5].[6] This demonstrated a higher response rate, event-free survival and overall survival for combination chemotherapy. However, despite this, the use of interferon remains limited and controversial.

The role of purine analogues has been investigated in both initial treatment and for recurrent disease in these patients [16.8]. With 2-CDA and with fludarabine one sees high response rates in previously untreated patients, the complete remission rate being around 30%.

16.5   **Randomized Trials of Initial Therapy Does Interferon Add to Conventional Therapy?**

4 randomized trials show improved progression free
    survival adding interferon-α, no impact on survival.

French-Belgian study demonstrated higher response rate,
    event-free survival, overall survival for COPA+ 1 vs COPA

Interferon - use remains limited and controversial

Solal-Celigny *et al.* 1993[6]

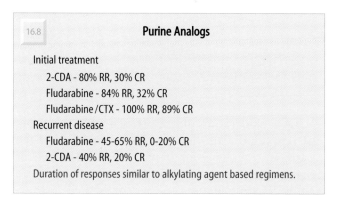

16.8   **Purine Analogs**

Initial treatment
    2-CDA - 80% RR, 30% CR
    Fludarabine - 84% RR, 32% CR
    Fludarabine /CTX - 100% RR, 89% CR
Recurrent disease
    Fludarabine - 45-65% RR, 0-20% CR
    2-CDA - 40% RR, 20% CR
Duration of responses similar to alkylating agent based regimens.

In recurrent disease, one again sees relatively good response rates, of 40 - 65%, with a lower percentage of complete remission, with both fludarabine and 2-CDA. However, the duration of responses to these purine analogs is similar to that seen with alkylating agent based regimens.

The next question that arises is whether there is a role for high dose therapy in low grade follicular lymphoma [16.9], an idea that appears to be largely based on the hypothesis that "more is better". In support of this is the dose response curve for these diseases with radiation therapy. As already shown, the time to complete remission decreases when more therapy is given. There is also a suggestion of a higher complete remission rate with more therapy. However, the major reason for adopting a strategy based on increased therapy is probably that it can be effective in other malignant diseases.

16.9   **Rationale for High Dose Therapy in Low Grade NHL**

      Hypothesis: more is better
        Dose response to XRT
        Shorter time to CR with more therapy
        Higher CR rate with more therapy (?)
        It works in other diseases

The data in [16.10] is from 142 consecutive patients with low grade lymphoma treated at our institution between 1985 and the early part of 1994.[7] They received high dose cyclophosphamide/total body radiation and transplantation with autologous bone marrow purged of B cells. The median age of these patients was 42, and 90% had follicular lymphoma, mostly of a small cleaved cell histology. Virtually all patients had bone marrow involvement and varying numbers had B symptoms, bulky disease and a history of extranodal disease outside the marrow.

16.10   **Patient Characteristics**
Relapsed Low Grade (N = 142)

Median age	42
Histology	
FSC	97 (68%)
FM	31 (22%)
Other	14 (10%)
(MCL-10, SL-3, Monocytoid-1)	
History of BM involvement	9 (70%)
B symptoms	28 (20%)
Mass > 10 cm	13 (9%)
Extranodal disease	47 (33%)

Freedman *et al.* 1997 [7]

All patients had received prior chemotherapy and about 30% had been treated previously with involved field radiation therapy [16.11]. About half of these patients had achieved complete clinical remission in response to therapy, but, at the time of bone marrow harvest and transplant, only a third were in complete clinical remission. The bone marrow was involved histologically in nearly half of the patients.

16.11   **Prior Therapy - Relapsed Low Grade**

Chemotherapy	142
Radiotherapy	39 (1 TBI)
Prior response	
PR	75 (53%)
CR	67 (47%)
Status at ABMT	
PR	99 (68%)
CR	43 (32%)
BM-positive histologically	65 (46%)

Freedman *et al.* 1997 [7]

When these 142 patients were analyzed, 79 were in complete clinical remission. There have been 59 relapses, the vast majority at sites of prior bulk disease. The Kaplan-Meier plot for disease-free survival is promising. Shown in [16.12], a figure of 45% at five years, and overall survival [16.13] is around 80% at five years.

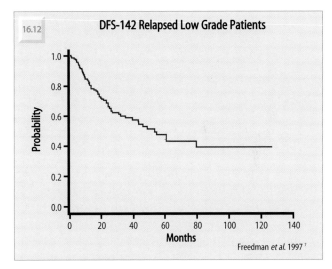

16.12   **DFS-142 Relapsed Low Grade Patients**

Freedman *et al.* 1997 [7]

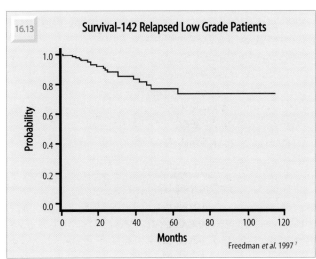

16.13   **Survival-142 Relapsed Low Grade Patients**

Freedman *et al.* 1997 [7]

We have also evaluated the role of high dose therapy as a component in the initial treatment of low grade follicular lymphoma. [16.14] is based on a study of 77 patients who received an autologous marrow transplant following CHOP induction.[8] The great majority had small cleaved cell histology, and most patients had advanced stage disease. A few patients had extranodal bulky disease and B symptoms.

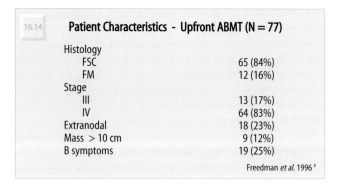

16.14	Patient Characteristics - Upfront ABMT (N = 77)	
Histology		
FSC	65 (84%)	
FM	12 (16%)	
Stage		
III	13 (17%)	
IV	64 (83%)	
Extranodal	18 (23%)	
Mass > 10 cm	9 (12%)	
B symptoms	19 (25%)	
	Freedman et al. 1996[8]	

At the time of transplant, after 6-8 cycles of CHOP, only about a third were in complete remission, and about half the patients had bone marrow involvement at the time of harvest [16.15].

16.15	Patient Characteristics - Upfront ABMT (N = 77)	
Status at ABMT		
PR	49 (64%)	
CR	28 (36%)	
BM histologically neg.	36 (46%)	
BM histologically pos.	41 (54%)	
	Freedman et al. 1996[8]	

There were two acute in-hospital deaths, and four late deaths in remission. A total of 47 patients are alive and disease-free with a median follow-up of 45 months. There have been 24 relapses. The disease-free survival for these patients, treated in first remission, is 63% at three years, with an overall survival of 89% [16.16]. The Kaplan-Meier plots for these patients, showing their disease-free survival [16.17] and their overall survival [16.18], are seen below.

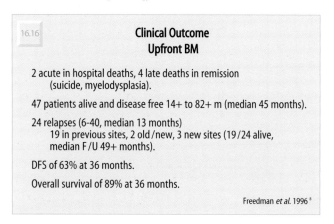

16.16	Clinical Outcome Upfront BM
2 acute in hospital deaths, 4 late deaths in remission (suicide, myelodysplasia).	
47 patients alive and disease free 14+ to 82+ m (median 45 months).	
24 relapses (6-40, median 13 months) 19 in previous sites, 2 old/new, 3 new sites (19/24 alive, median F/U 49+ months).	
DFS of 63% at 36 months.	
Overall survival of 89% at 36 months.	
	Freedman et al. 1996[8]

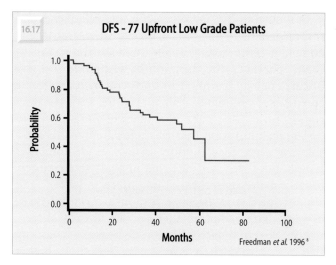

DFS - 77 Upfront Low Grade Patients

Freedman et al. 1996[8]

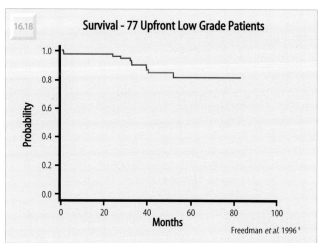

Survival - 77 Upfront Low Grade Patients

Freedman et al. 1996[8]

The important question, which many would like to answer but which unfortunately at the present time remains unresolved, is whether autologous bone marrow transplantation has any role to play in relapsed low grade non-Hodgkin's lymphoma. A collaborative study, between our institution and Dr. Lister's group at St. Bartholomew's Hospital in London, of follicular lymphomas with small cleaved and mixed cell histology has been performed [16.19]. Ninety two patients transplanted in second remission were reviewed, who had been treated with the same ablative regimen and B cell purged autologous marrow transplant. The results were compared to patients in second complete remission in the London database, who were treated with conventional therapy.

16.19	Does ABMT Have an Impact in Relapsed NHL
Relapsed low grade (retrospective DFCI/Barts data)	
Follicular small cleaved, follicular mixed.	
92 patients in CR2.	
CTX/TBI, anti-B cell Mab treated ABMT compared to conventionally treated patients in CR2.	

The disease-free survival for patients undergoing transplants in second remission was statistically better in this retrospective analysis than that of conventionally treated cases [16.20]. There was no benefit from transplantation if overall survival is considered [16.21]. However, the follow-up is significantly shorter for transplanted patients versus those receiving conventional therapy.

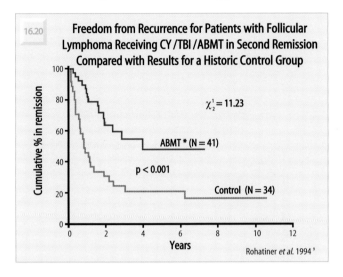

16.20 Freedom from Recurrence for Patients with Follicular Lymphoma Receiving CY/TBI/ABMT in Second Remission Compared with Results for a Historic Control Group

$\chi_2^1 = 11.23$

ABMT * (N = 41)

p < 0.001

Control (N = 34)

Rohatiner *et al.* 1994 [9]

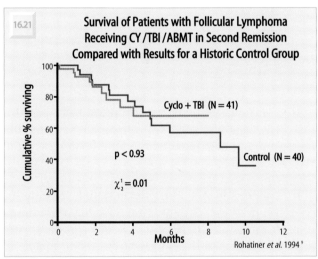

16.21 Survival of Patients with Follicular Lymphoma Receiving CY/TBI/ABMT in Second Remission Compared with Results for a Historic Control Group

Cyclo + TBI (N = 41)

p < 0.93

$\chi_2^1 = 0.01$

Control (N = 40)

Rohatiner *et al.* 1994 [9]

Listed in [16.22] is the criteria which define high risk patients. Relapsed patients with follicular lymphoma – and there are very good retrospective ECOG data on this – under the age of 60 whose first remission lasts less than a year, have a median survival of just over two years. These poor-prognosis patients constitute an appropriate group in which to study the impact of a strategy such as autologous marrow transplantation. When we consider untreated patients with low grade follicular lymphoma, one can identify those with a high tumor burden, with high LDH and/or β2-microglobulin (following the model from the MD Anderson Hospital), or with a high score on the International Prognostic Index, as being poorish subjects. It may be that in the future one will

be able to use factors such as the proliferation index or chromosomal and genetic abnormalities to identify subsets of patients.

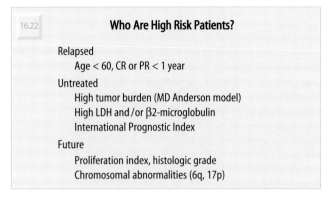

16.22 **Who Are High Risk Patients?**

Relapsed
    Age < 60, CR or PR < 1 year
Untreated
    High tumor burden (MD Anderson model)
    High LDH and /or β2-microglobulin
    International Prognostic Index
Future
    Proliferation index, histologic grade
    Chromosomal abnormalities (6q, 17p)

A paper published in the *Journal of Clinical Oncology* in 1994 applied the International Index to 100 patients with follicular lymphoma.[10] It was clear that patients could be stratified using this model in terms of complete remission rate and ten year survival [16.23]. However, the problem with such a study, and with applying such a method to identify high risk patients, lies in the low numbers involved, since only 11% of these patients fitted into the poor risk group.

16.23 **Outcome by Risk Groups in Low Grade NHL Defined by International Index**

Risk group (%)	Risk factors	CR	10-year survival
Low (36)	0.1	60%	74%
Low-int (32)	2	35%	45%
High-int (21)	3	23%	54%
High (11)	4,5	21%	0%

*Age, Stage, LDH, Performance status EN sites

Lopez-Guillermo *et al.* 1994 [10]

Taken from an article by Drs. Bastion and Coiffier which also applied these different models to a large number of patients,[11] and confirmed that β2-microglobulin, or LDH, or the International Index, identify subsets of follicular lymphoma patients who have different risks [16.24]. However, again there is a problem (if one wants to make an impact on outcome) inherent in the low numbers of patients in the very high risk group.

The next question relates to the parameters which we can use in a disease such as follicular lymphoma, which has such a long natural history and in which one has to carry out very long term studies in order to see any impact on survival. One approach is to study minimal residual disease [16.25]. We know that cells carrying the (14;18) translocation (as detected by PCR) persist in bone marrow and peripheral blood in patients who are in complete remission following conventional therapy.[12] Both early stage and advanced stage patients who are in remission can remain PCR-positive. However, in our own studies of transplanted patients, investigated by Dr. Gribben, PCR-detectable cells in follow-up bone marrow samples are highly predictive of clinical relapse.[13,14] So, at least within the context of bone marrow transplant, this provides a very good surrogate measure of future outcome. It therefore appears that achieving and maintaining a PCR-negative status is critical when we talk in terms of curing follicular lymphoma. The curves in [16.26] show an analysis of the disease-free survival in low grade lymphoma patients who have undergone transplant in first remission, separated according to the PCR status of the reinfused purged marrow [16.27 opposite]. At three years the disease-free survival is about 90% for those patients whose marrow was PCR-negative, compared to about 47% for those who received a PCR-positive marrow. If one then follows up these patients by monitoring serial bone marrow samples, those who were reinfused with PCR-positive marrow remain PCR-positive and virtually all eventually relapse.

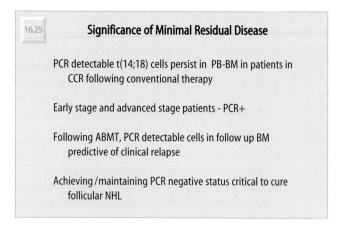

16.25   **Significance of Minimal Residual Disease**

PCR detectable t(14;18) cells persist in PB-BM in patients in CCR following conventional therapy

Early stage and advanced stage patients - PCR+

Following ABMT, PCR detectable cells in follow up BM predictive of clinical relapse

Achieving/maintaining PCR negative status critical to cure follicular NHL

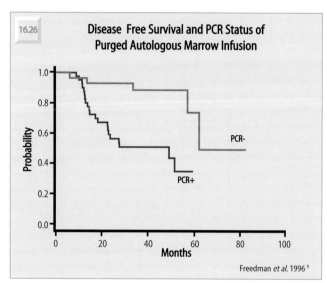

16.26   **Disease Free Survival and PCR Status of Purged Autologous Marrow Infusion**

Freedman *et al.* 1996 [8]

In contrast, patients whose reinfused marrow was PCR-negative, generally remained negative on follow-up, and also remained in long-term remission [16.28 opposite].

In conclusion [16.29], conventional therapy is effective in these patients, but not for very long. Interferon-a and high dose therapy probably do improve the disease-free survival, but their impact on overall survival is still unclear. The definition of cure is uncertain, although certainly molecular remissions are achievable through the use of autologous marrow transplants. Finally, current treatment is clearly inadequate, and new approaches are needed for these diseases.

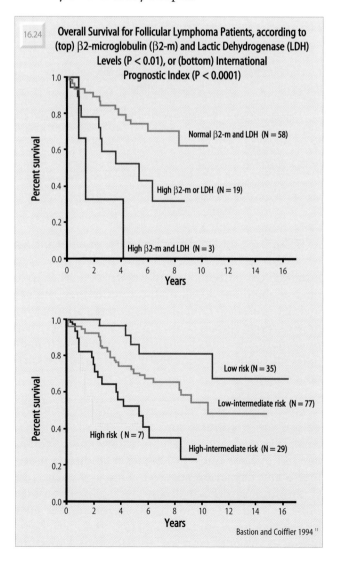

16.24   **Overall Survival for Follicular Lymphoma Patients, according to (top) β2-microglobulin (β2-m) and Lactic Dehydrogenase (LDH) Levels (P < 0.01), or (bottom) International Prognostic Index (P < 0.0001)**

Normal β2-m and LDH (N = 58)

High β2-m or LDH (N = 19)

High β2-m and LDH (N = 3)

Low risk (N = 35)

Low-intermediate risk (N = 77)

High risk (N = 7)

High-intermediate risk (N = 29)

Bastion and Coiffier 1994 [11]

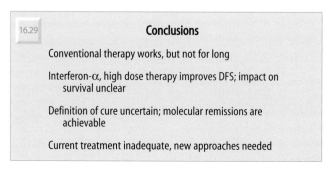

16.29   **Conclusions**

Conventional therapy works, but not for long

Interferon-α, high dose therapy improves DFS; impact on survival unclear

Definition of cure uncertain; molecular remissions are achievable

Current treatment inadequate, new approaches needed

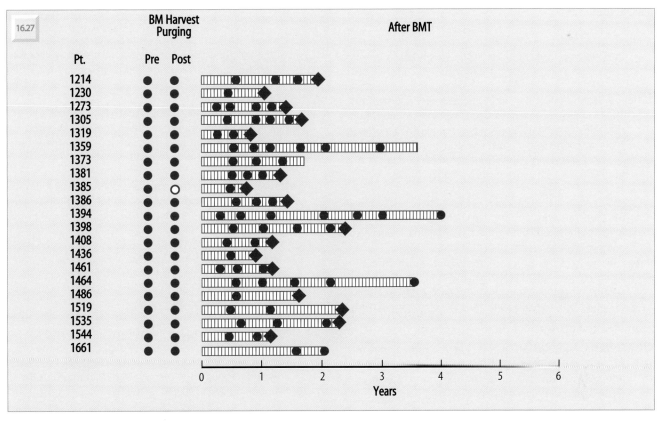

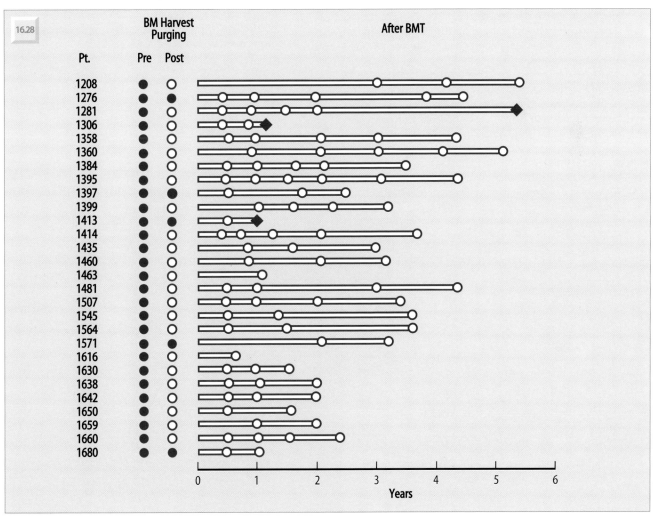

REFERENCES

1. Johnson PW, Rohatiner AZ, Whelan JS *et al.* Patterns of survival in patients with recurrent follicular lymphoma: a 20-year study from a single center. *J Clin Oncol* 1995; **13**: 140-7.

2. Hoppe RT, Kushlan P, Kaplan HS, Rosenberg SA, Brown BW. The treatment of advanced stage favorable histology non-Hodgkin's lymphoma: a preliminary report of a randomized trial comparing single agent chemotherapy, combination chemotherapy, and whole body irradiation. *Blood* 1981; **58**: 592-8.

3. Ezdinli EZ, Anderson JR, Melvin F, Glick JH, Davis TE, O'Connell MJ. Moderate versus aggressive chemotherapy of nodular lymphocytic poorly differentiated lymphoma. *J Clin Oncol* 1985; **3**: 769-75.

4. Jones SE, Grozea PN, Metz EN *et al.* Superiority of adriamycin-containing combination chemotherapy in the treatment of diffuse lymphoma: a Southwest Oncology Group study. *Cancer* 1979; **43**: 417-25.

5. Peterson BA, Anderson JR, Frizzera G *et al.* A comparative trial of cyclophosphamide (CTX) and cyclophosphamide, adriamycin, vincristine, prednisone and bleomycin (CAVPB). *Blood* 1985; **66** (Suppl): 216a.

6. Solal-Celigny P, Lepage E, Brousse N *et al.* Recombinant interferon alfa-2b combined with a regimen containing doxorubicin in patients with advanced follicular lymphoma. Groupe d'Etude des Lymphomes de l'Adulte. *N Engl J Med* 1993; **329**: 1608-14.

7. Freedman A, Gribben J, Neuberg D *et al.* Long term prologation of disease-free and overall survival following autologous bone marrow transplantation in patients with advanced relapsed follicular lymphoma. *Proc ASCO* 1997; **16**: 89a.

8. Freedman AS, Gribben JG, Neuberg D *et al.* High-dose therapy and autologous bone marrow transplantation in patients with follicular lymphoma during first remission. *Blood* 1996; **88**: 2780-6.

9. Rohatiner AZ, Johnson PW, Price CG *et al.* Myeloablative therapy with autologous bone marrow transplantation as consolidation therapy for recurrent follicular lymphoma. *J Clin Oncol* 1994; **12**: 1177-84.

10. Lopez-Guillermo A, Montserrat E, Bosch F, Terol MJ, Campo E, Rozman C. Applicability of the International Index for aggressive lymphomas to patients with low-grade lymphoma. *J Clin Oncol* 1994; **12**: 1343-8.

11. Bastion Y, Coiffier B. Is the International Prognostic Index for Aggressive Lymphoma patients useful for follicular lymphoma patients? *J Clin Oncol* 1994; **12**: 1340-2.

12. Gribben JG, Freedman AS, Wood SD *et al.* All advanced stage non-Hodgkin's lymphomas with a polymerase chain reaction amplifiable breakpoint of bcl-2 have residual cells containing the bcl-2 rearrangement at evaluation and after treatment. *Blood* 1991; **78**: 3275-80.

13. Gribben JG, Neuberg D, Freedman AS *et al.* Detection by polymerase chain reaction of residual cells with the bcl-2 translocation is associated with increased risk of relapse after autologous bone marrow transplantation for B-cell lymphoma. *Blood* 1993; **81**: 3449-57.

14. Gribben JG, Neuberg D, Barber M *et al.* Detection of residual lymphoma cells by polymerase chain reaction in peripheral blood is significantly less predictive for relapse than detection in bone marrow. *Blood* 1994; **83**: 3800-7.

FURTHER READING

Gallagher CJ, Gregory WM, Jones AE *et al.* Follicular lymphoma: prognostic factors for response and survival. *J Clin Oncol* 1986; **4**: 1470-80.

Morphologic, immunologic and genetic features of MALT lymphoma and the role of *Helicobacter*

17

P G Isaacson

Marginal zone B cell lymphomas of extranodal MALT type [17.1] recapitulate features of mucosa-associated lymphoid tissue (MALT), as exemplified by Peyer's patches. The neoplastic infiltrate starts in the marginal zone, around reactive B cell follicles, and the histologic hallmark is the formation of lymphoepithelial lesions in which the lymphoma infiltrates and destroys the associated glandular epithelium. The neoplastic cells are cytologically diverse - in most cases they look like small cleaved or centrocyte cells, but they can also be monocytoid or resemble small lymphocytes. An important feature is that there is always a scattering of transformed blasts within the infiltrate. A variable percentage of neoplastic cells show plasma cell differentiation, a phenomenon which is often masked by reactive plasma cells. The cells colonize reactive B cell follicles, and this may give a superficial resemblance to follicular lymphoma. These lymphomas are frequently multifocal, and they spread to marginal zones of adjacent lymph nodes. They only rarely involve the spleen, but, when they do so, the spread is again to marginal zones. And, finally, an important feature is their capacity to transform into high grade lymphomas.

Shown in [17.2] is a normal Peyer's patch, with a central follicle and a broad marginal zone. The B lymphocytes in the marginal zone infiltrate the overlying epithelium - the so-called dome epithelium - to form a lymphoepithelial structure, which is the defining feature of MALT.

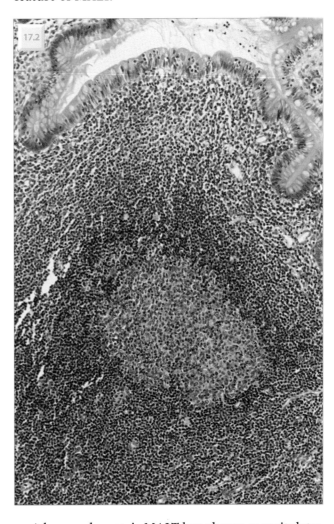

A low grade gastric MALT lymphoma recapitulates these features [17.3]. They are also seen in other organs, but the stomach is the commonest site for MALT lymphomas. A reactive B cell follicle is present,

---

17.1

Marginal Zone B Cell Lymphoma
Extranodal (MALT type)

- Recapitulate features of MALT (Peyer's patches)
- Infiltrate centered in marginal zone around reactive B cell follicles
- Lymphoepithelial lesions
- Cytology: CCL, monocytoid, lymphocytic with transformed blasts and plasma cell differentiation
- Follicular colonization
- Often multifocal
- Spread to nodal and splenic marginal zone
- May transform to high grade lymphoma

together with neoplastic B cells infiltrating around the follicle in the marginal zone [17.3]. Invasion of gastric glands is also seen, forming the neoplastic counterpart of lymphoepithelial structures.

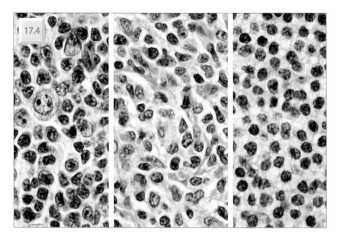

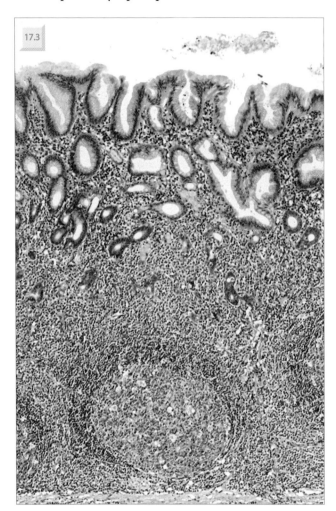

The cytologic features vary from case to case and within the same case. In the central panel in [17.4] the commonest appearance is seen, in which the neoplastic cells resemble centrocytes or small cleaved cells. On the right in [17.4], the cells have more abundant pale cytoplasm, and less irregular nuclei, and these resemble monocytoid B cells. In contrast, on the left in [17.4], the cells resemble small lymphocytes. In this field, one of the scattered transformed blast cells that appear in these lymphomas is also seen.

Plasma cell differentiation is best seen in an immunostained preparation, because of the difficulty in separating monoclonal plasma cell differentiation arising from the neoplasm from the reactive plasma cells that are frequently found beneath the surface epithelium. Plasma cell differentiation in a MALT lymphoma is often seen near the luminal surface, as if it were a response to antigenic stimulus in the epithelium or the lumen [17.5].

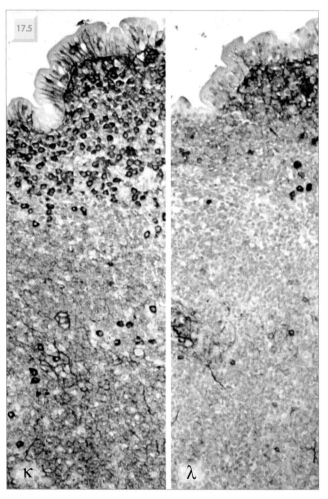

κ   λ

The gastric lymphoma in [17.6] shows infiltration of the entire lamina propria of the stomach, but the cells have also entered the reactive follicles that were present previously in this tissue. This phenomenon of follicular colonization can closely mimic follicular lymphoma.

The gastric lymph node in [17.7] shows that, when MALT lymphomas spread to adjacent nodes, they tend to infiltrate the marginal zones and then to spread outward to form a more diffuse interfollicular infiltrate.

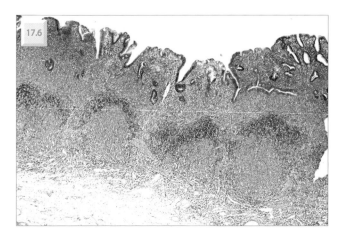

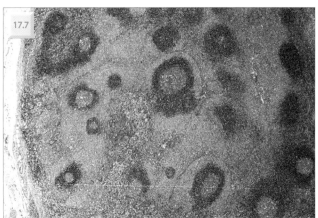

The immunophenotype of low grade MALT lymphomas [17.8] is very similar to that of marginal zone B cells. The main exceptions are that there is some difference in terms of the Ig heavy chain expressed, and about 50 - 70% of marginal zone MALT lymphomas express CD43.

17.8	MALT Lymphoma and Marginal Zone B Cell Immunophenotype	
	Marginal zone	MALT
Ig	M$^+$, D$^-$	M (G, A)$^+$, D$^-$
CD20	+	+
CD10	−	−
CD5	−	−
CD23	−	−
CD21	+	+
CD35	+	+
CD43	−	+/−
Cyclin D1	−	−

Immunoglobulin genes, as expected, show a monoclonal pattern of rearrangement [17.9]. Furthermore, they are mutated and show evidence for a bias towards those families that tend to include autoantibodies. The author's laboratory has shown that

the somatic mutations are "ongoing", and this may reflect the interaction of the neoplastic cells with reactive follicle centers.

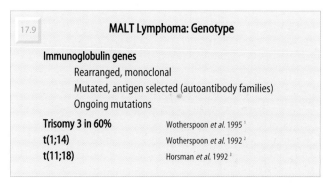

17.9	MALT Lymphoma: Genotype	
Immunoglobulin genes		
	Rearranged, monoclonal	
	Mutated, antigen selected (autoantibody families)	
	Ongoing mutations	
Trisomy 3 in 60%		Wotherspoon *et al.* 1995 [1]
t(1;14)		Wotherspoon *et al.* 1992 [2]
t(11;18)		Horsman *et al.* 1992 [3]

The author's group has also shown a high frequency of chromosome 3 trisomy in low grade MALT lymphomas at various sites. There have been reports of a number of translocations, but none of them is entirely characteristic.

Low grade MALT lymphomas can transform to high grade lymphomas [17.10]. We have published evidence for this in gastric lymphomas, in which low grade MALT and high grade neoplasms often occur simultaneously. In essence, the harder one looks, whether in low or high grade lymphomas, the more often one finds a neoplasm of the other grade. Our laboratory has shown by gene sequencing that the high and low grade components in these tumors share CDR3 sequences, and thus derive from the same clone.

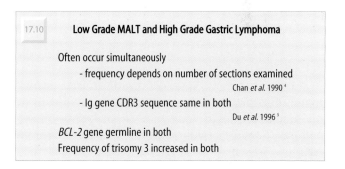

17.10	Low Grade MALT and High Grade Gastric Lymphoma
Often occur simultaneously	
- frequency depends on number of sections examined	
Chan *et al.* 1990 [4]	
- Ig gene CDR3 sequence same in both	
Du *et al.* 1996 [5]	
BCL-2 gene germline in both	
Frequency of trisomy 3 increased in both	

In contrast to high grade nodal lymphomas, extranodal high grade lymphomas in sites where MALT lymphomas are commonest virtually never show *BCL-2* gene rearrangement. Furthermore, there is some evidence that the frequency of trisomy 3 is also increased in high grade B cell lymphomas arising in sites where low grade MALT lymphomas are known to occur.

Shown in [17.11] is a low grade gastric MALT lymphoma with a lymphoepithelial lesion on the left, and a clearly transformed high grade lymphoma on the right.

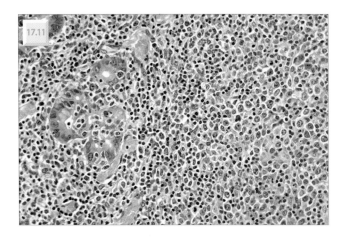

What is the normal cellular counterpart of MALT lymphoma [17.12]? These lymphomas infiltrate within marginal zones. When they spread to lymph nodes and spleen they also involve the marginal zone, and have an immunophenotype which resembles that of marginal zone cells. Immunoglobulin genes are mutated in both MALT lymphomas and splenic marginal zones. There are therefore good reasons for considering the marginal zone B cell as the counterpart of MALT lymphoma.

17.12	**MALT Lymphoma: Normal Cell Counterpart**

Lymphomas infiltrate in marginal zone

Spread to nodal and splenic marginal zones

Share marginal zone cell immunophenotype

Ig genes of MALT lymphoma and splenic marginal

    zone are mutated

Qin et al. 1995; [6] Dunn-Walters et al.1995; [7] Du et al. 1996 [5]

Shown in [17.13] is a low grade gastric MALT lymphoma that has disseminated to the spleen, as revealed by the restricted lambda light chain staining pattern. The selective involvement of the marginal zone is evident.

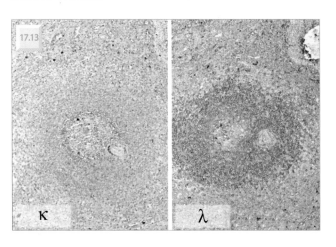

Turning to the clinical features of these tumors [17.14], there is often a history of chronic inflammatory diseases in the organ from which the lymphoma arises, usually of an autoimmune nature. These include *H. pylori* gastritis, which has an autoimmune component, and Sjögren's and Hashimoto's disease in salivary glands and thyroid respectively. In the course of these chronic inflammatory diseases the organ acquires lymphoid tissue which has the features of MALT.

17.14	**MALT Lymphoma: Clinical Features**

- History of chronic inflammatory (autoimmune) disease including *H. Pylori* gastritis, Sjögren's and Hashimoto's disease (acquired MALT)
- Usually present at Stage I_e or III_e
- Remain localized for prolonged periods
- Tendency to involve other "mucosal" sites
- Stage I_e may be curable with local treatment
- Growth may be antigen driven in early stages; removal of antigen (*H. pylori* in gastric lymphoma) may induce regression

These lymphomas usually present at early clinical stages, namely stages I_e or II_e. They tend to remain localized for prolonged periods and, when they do disseminate, there is a tendency to involve other sites where MALT lymphomas are known to occur. Stage I_e lymphomas may be curable with local treatment. There is evidence that tumor growth may be antigen driven in its early stages, and if the antigen is removed, for example *H. pylori* in gastric lymphoma patients, it may be possible to induce regression of the tumor.

Survival curves for high and low grade gastric MALT lymphoma [17.15], from a retrospective study from Kiel, show that survival is good in high grade disease. It is not affected by whether or not a low grade component is present, suggesting again that these are one and the same tumor. In low grade gastric MALT lymphoma, the survival curve is even more favorable. If this were a nodally based low grade lymphoma, the curve would decline steadily rather than reach a plateau.

What is the relationship of *H. pylori* to gastric lymphoma [17.16]? This question is important because it may provide lessons of relevance for other types of low grade lymphoma. There is no MALT in the normal stomach, and MALT is acquired as a specific response to H. pylori. Furthermore, one can find H. pylori in over 90% of gastric MALT lymphomas.

There is a higher incidence of gastric MALT lymphoma in places such as North Eastern Italy, where there is a high prevalence of H. pylori. It has been shown that a previous H. pylori infection is much more frequent in gastric lymphoma than in non-gastric lymphoma. In our own studies, gastric MALT lymphomas show a T cell mediated strain-specific response to *H. pylori*. Finally, if the organism is eradicated the lymphomas may regress.

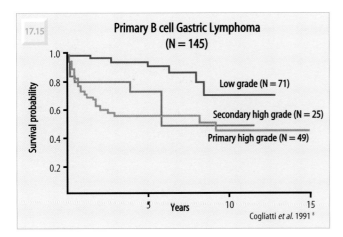

Primary B cell Gastric Lymphoma
(N = 145)

Low grade (N = 71)

Secondary high grade (N = 25)

Primary high grade (N = 49)

Cogliatti *et al.* 1991 [8]

H. pylori and Gastric MALT Lymphoma

No MALT in normal stomach
Acquisition of MALT a specific response to *H. pylori* infection
Wyatt *et al.* 1988 [9]
> 90% prevalence of *H. pylori* infection in gastric MALT lymphomas
Wotherspoon *et al.* 1991 [10]
Greater incidence of gastric lymphoma in NE Italy + high prevalence of
H. pylori   Doglioni *et al.* 1992 [11]
Previous *H. pylori* infection more likely in gastric lymphoma that
matched non-gastric lymphoma controls   Parsonnet *et al.* 1994 [12]
Gastric MALT lymphoma cells show T cell mediated strain specific responses
to *H. pylori*   Hussell *et al.* 1993 [13]
Eradication of *H. pylori* leads to regression of gastric MALT lymphoma
Wotherspoon *et al.* 1993 [14]

Shown in [17.17] is a gastric MALT lymphoma, diagnosed in September 1992. *H. pylori* was present, but eight months later [17.18], after eradication of the organism, the lymphoma had disappeared. Small aggregates of lymphoid tissue are seen, but no histologic evidence of lymphoma. This type of result has now been reported by many groups.

In conclusion, the other entity within the marginal zone B cell lymphomas may be considered. This is the nodal based lymphoma which is a provisional category in the REAL scheme [17.19] and it is also reviewed in Chapter 18. An important point is that many cases with this diagnosis, although certainly not all, represent secondary lymph node involvement by a cryptic MALT lymphoma, especially lymphomas arising in salivary glands.

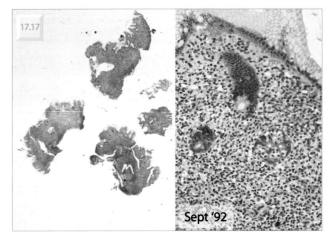

Sept '92

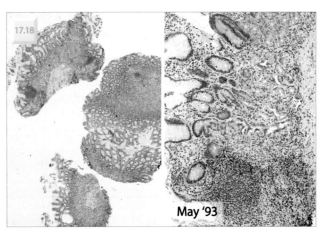

May '93

Provisional Entity: Nodal Marginal Zone B Cell Lymphoma

Most cases represent secondary lymph node involvement by (cryptic) MALT lymphoma especially salivary gland

Histology: as lymph nodes in MALT lymphoma

Cytology: CLL, monocytoid* or lymphocytic * hence "monocytoid B cell lymphoma"

Phenotype: as MALT lymphoma; genotype?

Normal cell counterpart is marginal zone B cell

Clinical behavior: as other low grade B cell lymphomas or Stage III MALT lymphoma

The histology is very similar to that seen in lymph nodes involved by MALT lymphoma, and the cytology is equally variable - centrocyte-like, monocytoid or lymphocytic. When it is monocytoid, the term "monocytoid B cell lymphoma" has been used, but this term is unsatisfactory because it doesn't take account of the other cytologic types.

The phenotype is the same as in MALT lymphoma. We know nothing about the genotype, and the probable normal cell counterpart is the marginal zone B cell. The clinical behavior appears to be that of low grade B cell lymphoma, and similar to Stage III or IV MALT lymphoma.

Represented in [17.20] is a cautionary tale. It shows one of the author's first cases of monocytoid B cell lymphoma, in which both a reactive follicle and lymphomatous infiltration with monocytoid B cells are seen. A cervical node [17.21] was diagnosed in 1993, but, when the patient's records were reviewed, it emerged that a parotid gland had been biopsied nineteen years previously. The diagnosis at the time was of a benign lymphoepithelial lesion, but we would now call it a salivary gland MALT lymphoma.

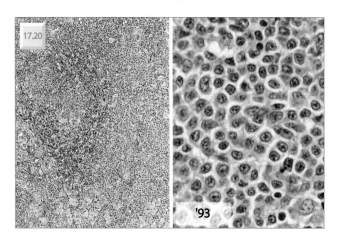

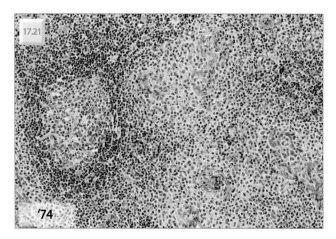

The cytologic features of the cells [17.22] are identical in the two biopsies nineteen years apart. Furthermore, molecular analysis [17.23] of the original parotid biopsy (track 1), of the neck node taken nineteen years later (track 2), and of a lymph node biopsy (track 3), revealed the same clone. This was thus an extremely indolent MALT lymphoma, which had reappeared after many years as a so-called "monocytoid B cell lymphoma".

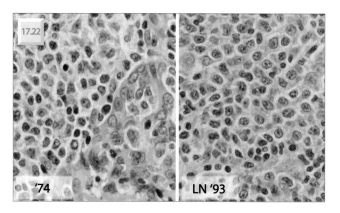

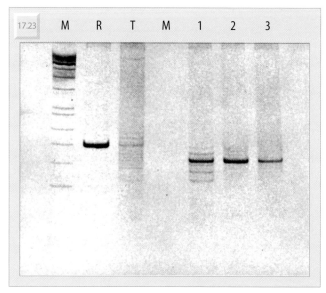

The lesson is that, when confronted with a lymph node which evokes a diagnosis of nodal marginal zone B cell lymphoma, the pathologist should remember to exclude primary MALT lymphoma. This entity should also not be confused with marginal zone differentiation in follicle center lymphoma, and mantle cell lymphoma should also be excluded since this can on occasion infiltrate in what appears to be a marginal zone pattern.

REFERENCES

1. Wotherspoon AC, Finn TM, Isaacson PG. Trisomy 3 in low-grade B cell lymphomas of mucosa-associated lymphoid tissue. *Blood* 1995, **85**: 2000-4.

2. Wotherspoon AC, Pan LX, Diss TC, Isaacson PG. Cytogenetic study of B-cell lymphoma of mucosa-associated lymphoid tissue. *Cancer Genet Cytogenet* 1992; **58**: 35-8

3. Horsman D, Gascoyne R, Klasa R, Coupland R. t(11;18)(q21;q21.1): a recurring translocation in lymphomas of mucosa-associated lymphoid tissue (MALT)? *Genes Chromosomes Cancer* 1992, **4**: 183-7.

4. Chan JK, Ng CS, Isaacson PG. Relationship between high-grade lymphoma and low-grade B-cell mucosa-associated lymphoid tissue lymphoma (MALToma) of the stomach. *Am J Pathol* 1990; **136**: 1153-64.

5. Du M, Diss TC, Xu C, Peng H, Isaacson PG, Pan L. Ongoing mutation in MALT lymphoma immunoglobulin gene suggests that antigen stimulation plays a role in the clonal expansion. *Leukemia* 1996; **10**: 1190-7.

6. Qin Y, Greiner A, Trunk MJF, Schmausser B, Ott MM, Müller-Hermelink HK. Somatic hypermutation in low-grade mucosa-associated lymphoid tissue-type B-cell lymphoma. *Blood* 1995; **86**: 3528-34.

7. Dunn-Walters DK, Isaacson PG, Spencer J. Analysis of mutations in immunoglobulin heavy chain variable region genes of microdissected marginal zone (MGZ) B cells suggests that the MGZ of human spleen is a reservoir of memory B cells. *J Exp Med* 1995; **182**: 559-66.

8. Cogliatti SB, Schmid U, Schumacher U *et al*. Primary B-cell gastric lymphoma: a clinicopathological study of 145 patients. *Gastroenterology* 1991; **101**: 1159-70.

9. Wyatt JI and Rathbone BJ. Immune response of the gastric mucosa to Campylobacter pylori. *Scand J Gastroenterol Suppl* 1988; **142**: 44-9.

10. Wotherspoon AC, Ortiz-Hidalgo C, Falzon MR, Isaacson PG. Helicobacter pylori-associated gastritis and primary B-cell gastric lymphoma. *Lancet* 1991; **338**: 1175-6.

11. Doglioni C, Wotherspoon AC, Moschini A, de Boni M, Isaacson PG. High incidence of primary gastric lymphoma in northeastern Italy. *Lancet* 1992; **339**: 834-5.

12. Parsonnet J, Hansen S, Rodriguez L *et al*. Helicobacter pylori infection and gastric lymphoma. *N Engl J Med* 1994; **330**: 1267-71.

13. Hussell T, Isaacson PG, Crabtree JE, Spencer J. The response of cells from low-grade B-cell gastric lymphomas of mucosa-associated lymphoid tissue to Helicobacter pylori. *Lancet* 1993; **342**: 571-4.

14. Wotherspoon AC, Doglioni C, Diss TC *et al*. Regression of primary low-grade B-cell gastric lymphoma of mucosa-associated lymphoid tissue type after eradication of Helicobacter pylori. *Lancet* 1993; **342**: 575-7.

FURTHER READING

Isaacson PG, Norton AJ. *Extranodal Lymphomas*. Edinburgh, London, Madrid, Melbourne, New York, Tokyo: Churchill Livingstone, 1994.

Isaacson PG, Spencer J. Malignant lymphoma of mucosa-associated lymphoid tissue. *Histopathology* 1987; **11**: 445-62.

Isaacson PG, Wotherspoon AC, Diss T, Pan L. Follicular colonization in B-cell lymphoma of mucosa-associated lymphoid tissue. *Am J Surg Pathol* 1991; **15**: 819-28.

Does nodal marginal zone lymphoma exist?

T M Grogan

When we consider the question of whether nodal marginal B cell lymphoma exists, the author is reminded of the Lewis Carroll poem, *The Hunting of the Snark*. In our retrospective study in the South West Oncology Group of indolent lymphomas diagnosed in the 1970s, we have gone into a jungle of boojum trees and yucca trees, but we have finally emerged triumphantly with some true primary nodal monocytoid B cell lymphomas.

This chapter can be begun by showing its major conclusion [18.1]. Although there is overlap with MALT lymphoma and also with follicular lymphomas, monocytoid B cell lymphomas, without mucosal involvement and without a follicular lymphoma component, do occur. We found eight such cases out of 376 as a result of spending about four days in Seattle going through every case in the South West Oncology Group. Accordingly, primary node based mono-cytoid B cell lymphoma should be given a separate status, after exclusion of extranodal involvement by MALT tumors and of follicular lymphoma. The author agrees with Prof. Isaacson's suggestion that it may take many years to make some of these exclusions, but luckily twenty year follow-up data were available for many of our cases.

> **18.1** **Does True Primary Nodal Monocytoid B Lymphoma (MCBL) Exist?**
>
> Although there is overlap with MALToma and follicular lymphomas, MCBL without mucosal involvement and without a follicular lymphoma component do occur (2%; 8/376 SWOG 7204, 7426, 7713). Accordingly, primary node based MCBL should be given *bona fide* separate status, after exclusion of extranodal involvement and of follicular lymphoma.

As part of the major study described elsewhere (Chapter 4), indolent lymphoma cases treated in the 1970s were reviewed [18.2]. This was an era of enthusiasm for using adriamycin-based drug regimes to treat indolent lymphoma. Cases were evaluated that were at Stage III or IV prior to therapy, with the aim of picking out MALT lymphomas or monocytoid B cell lymphomas. The pathologists involved were Dr. Banks and the author, who are both signatories to the REAL classification, and Dr. Nathwani, who has devoted much time and energy to describing monocytoid B cell lymphomas.[1]

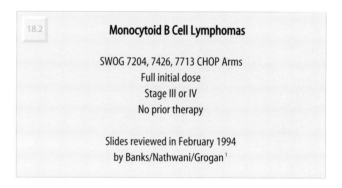

> **18.2** **Monocytoid B Cell Lymphomas**
>
> SWOG 7204, 7426, 7713 CHOP Arms
> Full initial dose
> Stage III or IV
> No prior therapy
>
> Slides reviewed in February 1994
> by Banks/Nathwani/Grogan[1]

Shown in [18.3] is a summary of what was found morphologically. In the right upper quadrant a lymph node is seen in which the pale area represents confluent sinuses (CS). Follicle centers (F) are present, one of which (FC) has undergone follicular colonization. One comes to recognize this pattern quite readily at low power. The lower part of the figure shows the morphology of the neoplastic cells, which are of medium size. They are seen best in a touch preparation (lower right), where their abundant cytoplasm is obvious. We had the opportunity to look at the spleens in a number of these patients (top left quadrant) and typically there was involvement of marginal zone regions (MR) which surround the mantle zones (MT).

The phenotype in some of these cases was analyzed using antigen retrieval techniques, and, in spite of their age, it was fairly straightforward to demonstrate heavy and light chain restriction. In the case shown in [18.4], the cells express kappa chains and pan-B antigens (such as CD20) but they also show dot-like staining for the monocyte-associated marker, CD11c. However, this was not a distinguishing feature from MALT lymphoma.

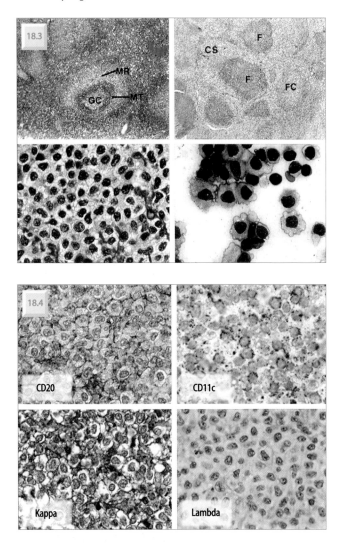

In this study, we also identified nodal involvement by MALT lymphomas, as described by Prof. Isaacson, and a crucial finding was the presence of lympho-epithelial lesions, as seen in [18.5]. These localized infiltrates are in some ways reminiscent of Pautrier's microabscess in the skin associated with mycosis fungoides. They arise in the context of a neoplastic proliferation, as seen in the upper left quadrant in the marginal zone region (MR). Typically, small slightly irregular lymphoid cells are seen, accompanied by a few larger transformed ones (lower right).

Occasionally, in MALT lymphomas monocytoid cells predominate. The pale areas seen in [18.6] are made up of these cells and naturally one wonders where the overlap occurs between a MALT lymphoma containing numerous monocytoid B cells, and primary nodal monocytoid B cell lymphoma. [18.7] shows a

MALT lymphoma containing many monocytoid B cells. The typical clustered invasion of epithelium by these monocytoid B cells is seen in [18.8], and this case gives a sense of how prominent monocytoid B cells may be in a MALT lymphoma. [18.9] shows a lymph node from the same case, in which there is typical marginal zone involvement. Prof. Isaacson has shown elsewhere (Chapter 17) an example of further progression, in which the neoplastic cells extend into the sinuses, but in the South West Oncology review, this was very much an exception to the rule, the common pattern being marginal zone involvement.

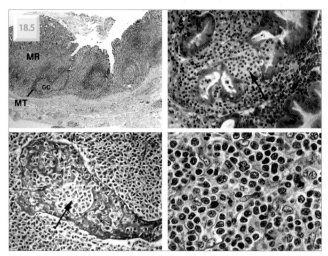

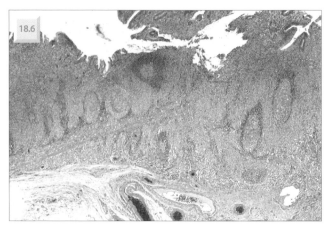

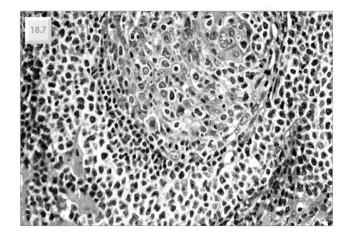

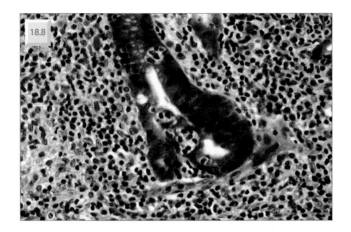

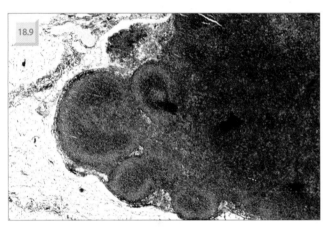

One interesting phenomenon was that follicles were commonly filled by small angular lymphoid cells, giving the superficial appearance of a follicular lymphoma [18.13] and [18.14]. In fact, we finally decided that some 13 of these 21 cases were composite with follicular lymphoma, and could not be pure monocytoid B cell lymphomas [18.15]. If we separate out a pure monocytoid B cell category, there were only eight cases. There is no obvious difference in survival between the composite and the non-composite cases, although the numbers are small. The main conclusion is that primary monocytoid B cell lymphoma is an indolent entity, whether or not it is a composite tumor.

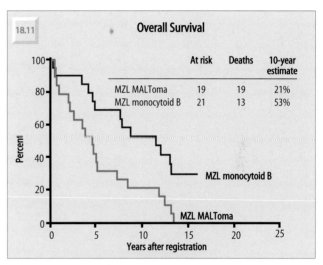

Shown in [18.10] is data on the 40 cases which were identified among the 376 samples, of which 21 were classified as monocytoid B cell neoplasms, and 19 as MALT lymphomas. It should be reiterated that the MALT lymphomas had to be Stage III and IV tumors and to have nodal involvement in order to qualify for the study. Of the 21 monocytoid B cell lymphomas, two showed involvement of epithelial surfaces. The median survival of the monocytoid B cell neoplasms approached twelve years [18.11]. The MALT lymphomas which had all already spread to lymph nodes, had a significantly shorter survival.

Characteristics of Marginal Zone Lymphoma		
	MALToma N = 19	Monocytoid N = 21
Median age (years)	56	44
Range	(23-67)	(24-76)
% Male	58%	47%
95% CI	(34%-80%)	(26%-70%)
% PS > 2	0%	10%
% Bone marrow	42%	48%
% GI disease	26%	10%
95% CI	(9%-51%)	(1%-30%)

18.10

Shown in [18.12] is a low power view of one of the lymph nodes involved by a monocytoid B cell lymphoma, with a clearly sinusoidal pattern of involvement.

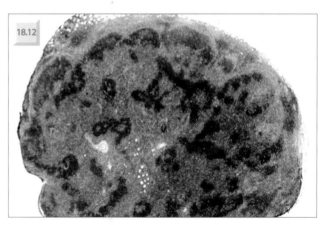

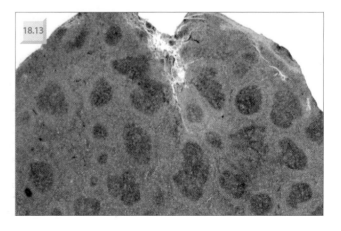

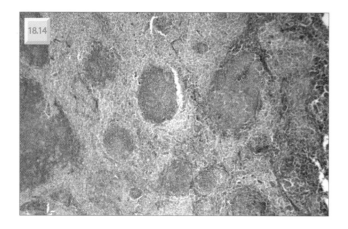

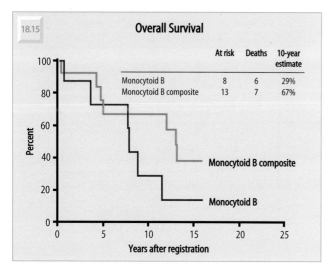

The important conclusions in terms of differential diagnosis [18.16] are that a MALT lymphoma can contain a predominance of monocytoid B cells and secondarily involve the lymph node, particularly in the marginal zone. By the same token, monocytoid B

Differential Diagnosis of MALTToma versus MCBL

- MALTToma may have a predominance of monocytoid B cells may involve lymph nodes in the marginal zone.

- MCBL may secondarily involve epithelial surfaces

- Follicular lymphoma may have a monocytoid B cell component.

- Therefore, *bona fide* 1° nodal MCBL excludes mucosal involvement and follicular lymphoma

cell lymphoma may involve epithelial surfaces, seen in two cases in our series. Examples of follicular lymphoma with a monocytoid B cell component can also be found. If these three exclusions are made, there were eight "pure" cases that had neither mucosal involvement nor an association with follicular lymphoma.

If we ignore the clinical features and rely on microscopy, how many cases were borderline cases between MALT lymphoma and monocytoid B cell lymphoma [18.17]? We could find only two out of the 40 cases, so that the two entities appear to be generally largely separable on a histologic basis without clinical information. The differences include microanatomic and distributional features, and the diseases also differ in their patterns of dissemination, and possibly in their survival. So for these reasons this provisional REAL category appears to be a true entity.

MALTToma versus MCBL

- Among 40 marginal zone lymphoma, overlap occurs in 5% of cases (2/40)

- MALTToma and MCBL were readily separable on a histologic basis (without prior knowledge of clinical data in 95% of cases - 38/40)

- Entities distinguished histologically:
  microanatomic, distributional differences

- Entities distinguished clinically:
  differ in dissemination
  differ in survival

Finally, although these entities are readily separable, there are many features, such as follicular colonization or the presence of a differentiated component, in which there is overlap. It is the author's belief that we have seen South West Oncology Group patients who have lived for 15, 20, or even 25 years with a monocytoid B cell lymphoma which arose in lymph node sinuses and spread to other lymph nodes and to the bone marrow, but which did not involve epithelial surfaces. These patients provide further evidence that monocytoid B cell lymphoma represents a true clinicopathologic entity.

REFERENCES

1. Fisher RI, Dahlberg S, Nathwani BN, Banks PM, Miller TP, Grogan TM. A clinical analysis of two indolent lymphoma entities: mantle cell lymphoma and marginal zone lymphoma (including the mucosa-associated lymphoid tissue and monocytoid B-cell subcategories): a Southwest Oncology Group study. *Blood* 1995; **85**: 1075-82.

FURTHER READING

Nathwani BN, Mohrmann RL, Brynes RK, Taylor CR, Hansmann ML, Sheibani K. Monocytoid B-cell lymphomas: an assessment of diagnostic criteria and a perspective on histogenesis. *Human Pathol* 1992; **23**: 1061-71.

Ngan BY, Warnke RA, Wilson M, Takagi K, Cleary ML, Dorfmann RF. Monocytoid B-cell lymphoma: a study of 36 cases. *Human Pathol* 1991; **22**: 409-21.

Nizze H, Cogliatti S, von Schilling C, Feller AC, Lennert K. Monocytoid B-cell lymphoma: morphologic variants and relationship to low-grade B-cell lymphoma of the mucosa-associated lymphoid tissue. *Histopathology* 1991; **18**: 403-14.

Piris M, Rivas C, Morente M, Cruz MA, Rubio C, Oliva H. Monocytoid B-cell lymphoma, a tumour related to the marginal zone. *Histopathology* 1988; **12**: 383-92.

Sheibani K, Burke JS, Swartz WG, Nademanee A, Winberg CD. Monocytoid B-cell lymphoma. Clinicopathologic study of 21 cases of a unique type of low-grade lymphoma. *Cancer* 1988; **62**: 1531-8.

Clinical features and treatment of MALT lymphoma

P M Mauch

This chapter covers three aspects of extranodal MALT lymphomas, notably pulmonary, small bowel and gastric tumors.

Papers published in *Histopathology* in 1995 [1] and a clinical report published in *Chest* two years earlier,[2] represent a review of 69 French patients with pulmonary non-Hodgkin's lymphoma [19.1]. Of the 69 cases, 61 (88%) were low grade neoplasms, and 54 (78%) of the overall group were MALT lymphomas.

19.1	**Primary Pulmonary NHL**
	French Combined Study of 69 Patients

88% low grade; 12% high grade
78% were MALT lymphomas
96% survival (5-year)

Fiche *et al.* 1995;[1] Cordier *et al.*1993[2]

As seen from the upper curve in [19.2], these patients have an excellent survival, with 90% of patients alive at five years and 60 - 70% at ten years. They were treated in a variety of ways. About 70% had surgical resection, followed in some cases by chemotherapy or radiation. Chemotherapy alone was given to 26% of the patients, and 5% received no treatment. Relief of symptoms was an important marker in this group of patients and was associated with an excellent prognosis. In the patients with pulmonary lymphoma, about 40% presented with no pulmonary symptoms, and 40% presented with a cough. About 25% had weight loss, 20% dyspnoea, and about 10% hemoptysis. There was some information in this report about the efficacy of chemotherapy, and good results were obtained with the single agent chlorambucil. It was noted that this approach appeared to be as effective as more aggressive combination regimens.

There are also data in the literature on intestinal and gastric MALT lymphoma. A study from the Danish Lymphoma Study Group reported on 306 patients with non-Hodgkin's lymphoma of the gastrointestinal tract [19.3].[3] In this series, 68% of the gastric and 52% of the intestinal lymphoma patients were Stage I or II, and about 30% of the gastric neoplasms and less than 10% of the intestinal tumors were of low grade. Univariate analysis was used in this study to identify factors which might predict for survival. For early stage gastric tumors, radiotherapy gave a favorable outcome, and surgical resection was of benefit for the gastrointestinal group. Chemotherapy did not improve the disease-free or overall survival in either subgroup.

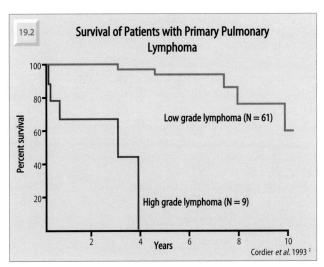

19.2 **Survival of Patients with Primary Pulmonary Lymphoma**

Low grade lymphoma (N = 61)

High grade lymphoma (N = 9)

Cordier *et al.* 1993 [2]

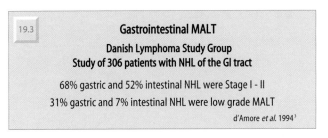

19.3	**Gastrointestinal MALT**

Danish Lymphoma Study Group
Study of 306 patients with NHL of the GI tract

68% gastric and 52% intestinal NHL were Stage I - II
31% gastric and 7% intestinal NHL were low grade MALT

d'Amore *et al.* 1994 [3]

A BNLI study of 175 patients with primary gastrointestinal lymphoma was published in 1993 [19.4].[4] The majority were Stage I or II. The frequency of MALT lymphomas was a little higher than in the

Danish study, with 50% and 27% of gastric and intestinal neoplasms respectively falling into this category. The commonest sites for intestinal MALT tumors were the jejunum and the ileocecal region. The authors compared the survival of MALT and non-MALT tumors, and the results were much better for MALT than for non-MALT lymphomas of the stomach [19.4].

For the intestinal tumors, the results were much poorer than for the gastric neoplasms, and there were no significant differences between the MALT and non-MALT lymphomas [19.4].

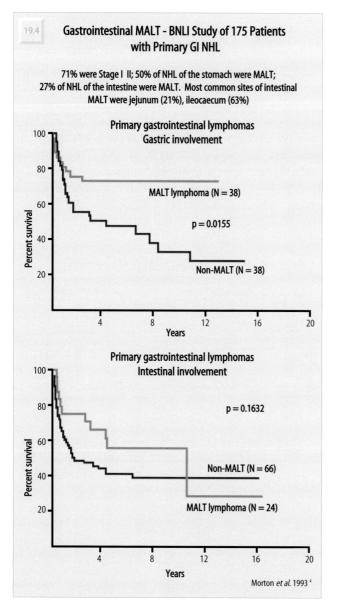

In a retrospective study from the Netherlands, 119 patients were seen over a twenty year period [19.5].[5] There was a mixture of histologic categories, but this study is important because it contains data on treatment outcomes, and makes it possible to ask the question of whether surgical resection adds anything

to radiation therapy in the treatment of gastric lymphoma [19.5]. About 50% of the Stage I gastric tumors were low grade MALT lymphomas, and about 25% were Stage II. The top two curves in [19.5] show partial gastrectomy plus radiation versus radiation alone, and there were essentially no differences in outcome.

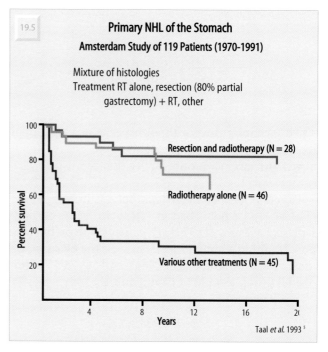

Two studies from the Harvard Medical School [19.6] are of interest. Dr. Fung (Massachusetts General Hospital) has investigated, in collaboration with Dr. Cook and Dr. Harris from the Department of Pathology, the outcome in 20 patients with gastric MALT lymphoma. Of this group, 15 had Stage I disease [19.6], of whom four received partial gastrectomy alone, six had either total or partial gastrectomy combined with radiation, two had radiation alone, two had chemotherapy, and one had no treatment. Of the patients who had gastrectomy or partial gastrectomy, none were up-staged to Stage II.

The graph in [19.6] shows the relapse-free survival curve, with a median follow-up of about six and a half years for Stage I patients; only one patient has relapsed. At nine years the relapse-free and overall survivals were 92% and 65% respectively [19.6].

We have reviewed our own experience in the treatment of twelve patients with localized gastric MALT lymphoma. Three were treated with partial gastrectomy and radiation, seven with radiation alone, and two with antibiotics alone [19.7]. Of the radiation alone group, three patients had been treated previously with antibiotics, but had persistent MALT lymphoma and therefore went on to receive radiation.

All of the ten patients treated with radiation alone are free from recurrence, at eight to forty-eight months after treatment.

19.6

Gastric MALT Lymphoma

Patients

Twenty patients with primary gastric MALT lymphoma 4/78 - 2/95

9 males, 11 females

Stage: 15 clinical Stage I
2 clinical Stage II, 1 PS II
1 clinical Stage III
1 clinical Stage IV

Treatment

Stage I patients:
4 surgery alone (partial gastrectomy) 12
6 surgery plus RT (1 total and 5 partial gastrectomy) local therapy
2 RT alone only
1 partial gastrectomy plus chemotherapy
1 chemotherapy and RT
1 untreated due to advanced age

Advanced Stage patients:
Combinations of gastrectomy, RT, and chemotherapy

Relapse-free survival (Stage I)

(N = 15)

Percent Survival / *Years*

Treatment results in Stage I

One of 14 csl patients relapsed.
Median follow-up 6.5 years

9-year actuarial Kaplan-Meier results:

Relapse-free survival	92%
Disease-free survival	100%
Overall survival	65%

19.7 **JCRT Experience**
Localized Gastric MALT

12 patients
Partial gastrectomy + RT (3)
RT alone (7), 3 treated previously with antibiotics
Antibiotics alone (2)
10/10 patients treated with RT are free from relapse at 8 - 48 months

A prospective trial has now been started at the Harvard Medical School in collaboration with the Massachusetts General Hospital, Brigham and Women's Hospital, the Beth Israel Hospital and the New England Deaconess Hospital. The trial was in part based on the observations of Dr. Isaacson and others that *H.pylori*-positive MALT lymphoma patients often demonstrate significant regression of their tumor with antibiotic treatment. In a study in the *Lancet* in 1995,[6] 33 patients with low grade MALT lymphoma in the German MALT Lymphoma Study Group were treated with two weeks of antibiotics [19.8]. 70% of the group had complete remission, 12% achieved partial remission, and 18% had no response to treatment. PCR showed complete disappearance of monoclonality in 13 of the 16 patients. There was a median follow-up of one year, and no recurrences were seen among the patients who achieved complete remission.

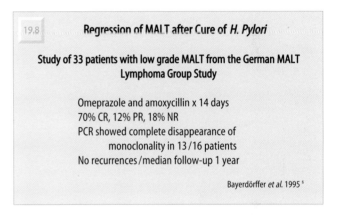

19.8 **Regression of MALT after Cure of *H. Pylori***

Study of 33 patients with low grade MALT from the German MALT Lymphoma Group Study

Omeprazole and amoxycillin x 14 days
70% CR, 12% PR, 18% NR
PCR showed complete disappearance of monoclonality in 13/16 patients
No recurrences/median follow-up 1 year

Bayerdörffer *et al.* 1995 [6]

It is interesting that of the six patients who achieved less than a partial response, five went on to surgery. Four of these patients who had total or partial gastrectomy were found to have high grade lymphoma [19.9].

In the current Harvard Medical School study, patients are enrolled who have a confirmed diagnosis of MALT lymphoma [19.10]. If they are *H.pylori*-negative, they go on to receive radiation therapy, with a three or four field technique to the entire stomach. If they are *H.pylori*-positive, they receive a course of antibiotics, and are then observed and re-endoscoped after three months. If they are negative for *H.pylori* at that point and have achieved complete remission of the lymphoma, they are observed. If they achieve partial remission, we continue to watch them for another three months to see if they undergo further regression. If they go into complete remission, they are observed further, but, if they do not demonstrate a complete response, they receive radiotherapy. Patients who achieve less than partial remission go on to radiation without further observation. If they are still *H.pylori*-positive, they undergo a second course of antibiotics before a decision is made about treatment as long as there is no tumor progression.

19.9 **Relation Between Baseline Characteristics and Outcome**	Complete regression	Partial regression	No change
Number (%)	23 (70%)	4 (12%)	6 (18%)
Tumor stage (by histology)			
EI_1	23	4	2 *
$\geq EII$	0	0	4 †
Endoscopic appearance			
Tumor	13	3	2
Ulcer	7	0	2
Erosions	1	0	0
Atypical mucosal relief	2	1	2
Tumor size (cm) ‡	2 (1-10)	4 (3-8)	5 (2-8)
Time after eradication of			
H.pylori (months)	4.0 (0.5-8.5)	8.5 (4.0-12.0)	4.0 (3.5-6.0)
Age (years)	58.0 (31-74)	58.5 (32-84)	47.5 (35-78)
Male /female	12/11	2/2	4/2

Data are number of patients or median (range).

* 1 patient also had a high grade T-cell lymphoma, and 1 was primarily treated by chemotherapy, so the exact tumor stage could not be determined.

† Pretreatment staging EI_1 found to be incorrect on histologic examination of resected stomach, when 5 of 6 patients in this group were diagnosed as high grade lymphoma.

‡ Largest dimension measured on endoscopy with biopsy forceps.

Bayerdörffer *et al.* 1995 [6]

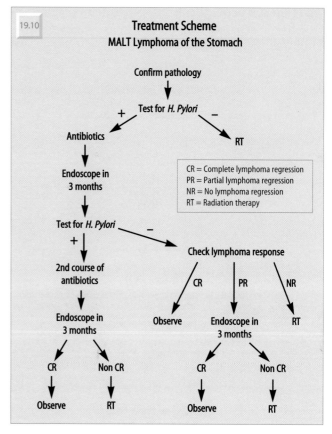

Some of the objectives of this study are to try to determine the percentage of patients whose tumor will completely regress, to establish the durability of their regressions, to understand the significance of PCR-positivity in patients who undergo a clinical complete response, and to define which follow-up studies are appropriate.

REFERENCES

1. Fiche M, Caprons F, Berger F *et al*. Primary pulmonary non-Hodgkin's lymphomas. *Histopathology* 1995; **26**: 529-37.

2. Cordier JF, Chailleux E, Lauque D *et al*. Primary pulmonary lymphomas. A clinical study of 70 cases in non-immuno-compromised patients. *Chest* 1993; **103**: 201-8.

3. d'Amore F, Brincker H, Gronbaek K *et al*. Non-Hodgkin's lymphoma of the gastrointestinal tract: a population-based analysis of incidence, geographic distribution, clinicopathologic presentation features, and prognosis. Danish Lymphoma Study Group. *J Clin Oncol* 1994; **12**: 1673-84.

4. Morton JE, Leyland MJ, Vaughan Hudson G *et al*. Primary gastrointestinal non-Hodgkin's lymphoma: a review of 175 British National Lymphoma Investigation cases. *Br J Cancer* 1993; **67**: 776-82.

5. Taal BG, Burgers JM, van Heerde P, Hart AA, Somers R. The clinical spectrum and treatment of primary non-Hodgkin's lymphoma of the stomach. *Ann Oncol* 1993; **4**: 839-46.

6. Bayerdörffer E, Neubauer A, Rudolph B *et al*. Regression of primary gastric lymphoma of mucosa-associated lymphoid tissue type after cure of Helicobacter pylori infection. MALT Lymphoma Study Group. *Lancet* 1995; **345**: 1591-4.

FURTHER READING

Gospodarowicz MK, Sutcliffe SB, Clark RM *et al*. Outcome analysis of localized gastrointestinal lymphoma treated with surgery and postoperative irradiation. *Int J Radiat Oncol Biol Phys* 1990; **19**: 1351-5.

Horstmann M, Erttmann R, Winkler K. Relapse of MALT lymphoma associated with Helicobacter pylori after antibiotic treatment. *Lancet* 1994; **343**: 1098-9.

Stolte M, Eidt S. Healing gastric MALT lymphoma by eradicating H pylori? *Lancet* 1993; **342**: 568.

Stolte M. Helicobacter pylori gastritis and gastric MALT lymphoma. *Lancet* 1992; **339**: 745-6.

Wotherspoon AC, Doglioni C, Isaacson PG. Low-grade gastric B-cell lymphoma of mucosa-associated lymphoid tissue (MALT): a multifocal disease. *Histopathology* 1992; **20**: 29-34.

Therapy of gastric lymphoma of MALT type, including antibiotics

P Koch and W Hiddemann

This chapter addresses the systemic therapy of marginal B cell lymphoma, a category which comprises MALT-type lymphomas and monocytoid B cell lymphomas [20.1]. These two different subtypes are approximately equal in frequency,[1] but this chapter restricts its scope to lymphomas of the stomach.

20.1	Marginal Zone B Cell Lymphomas	
-	Lymphoma of mucosa-associated lymphoid tissue (MALT)	
-	Monocytoid B cell lymphoma	
	MALT	19 (44%)
	MCBC	21 (49%)
	Unclassified	3 (7%)
		Fisher et al. 1995[1]

The first question to consider is whether this is really an indolent lymphoma [20.2]. This question is important for treatment strategies, and should also be of relevance from the viewpoint of the pathologist because many MALT-type lymphomas, at least in the stomach, are histologically of high grade. These comprise "secondary" neoplasms (i.e. that appear to arise from a low grade tumor), and those that are categorised as apparently "primary" (although it is likely that in some cases, a low grade component is present but not evident in the biopsy).

20.2	Extranodal Marginal Zone B cell Lymphoma
	A REAL INDOLENT LYMPHOMA?
Gastric lymphoma:	
- majority high grades	
- considerable proportion secondary high grades	

This is evident from published studies, which show that more than 50% of primary and secondary gastric MALT lymphomas are of high grade [20.3].

The significance of this is still unclear. Prof. Isaacson has argued that many high grade MALT-type lymphomas arise from a low grade neoplasm, but we are still uncertain about the relevance of these histologic features to the clinical picture and to the choice of treatment.

20.3	Gastric Marginal Zone B Cell Lymphoma - Patho-histologic Grading			
Authors	N	Low grade	Secondary high grade	High grade
Montalban et al. 1995[2]	143	84 (58%)	59 (42%)	
Kath et al. 1995[3]	41	19 (46%)	15 (37%)	7 (17%)
Cogliatti et al. 1991[4]	145	71 (49%)	25 (17%)	49 (34%)
Johnsson et al. 1992[5]	72	22 (31%)	43 (69%)	
Castrillo et al. 1992[6]	56	20 (36%)	11 (19%)	25 (45%)
Chan et al. 1990[7]	48	12 (25%)	10 (21%)	26 (54%)

For this reason a multicenter trial of primary gastric and intestinal NHL was performed in Germany to investigate some of these questions [20.4]. This trial was opened in October 1992, and we have enrolled more than 300 patients, of whom approximately 250 are evaluable in terms of their clinical features [20.5].

20.4	German Multicenter Study on Primary Gastrointestinal Lymphoma
Evaluation of:	Histology
	Clinical features
	Treatment modalities
	Therapeutic outcome

More than half of all patients had high grade lymphomas, which were either primary, or secondary to a low grade component [20.6].

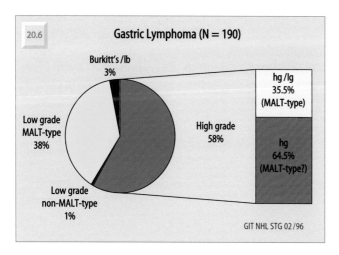

20.5   German Multicenter Study on Primary Gastrointestinal Lymphoma

Activated	October '92
Patients enrolled	**323**
- excluded (secondary GI-NHL, relapse)	15
- insufficient data	50
Evaluable for clinical features	**258**
- excluded according to protocol (age, 2nd malignancies, protocol violations)	62
- insufficient data	42
Evaluable for therapeutic outcome	**154**

GIT NHL STG 02/96

20.6   Gastric Lymphoma (N = 190)

Burkitt's /lb 3%
Low grade MALT-type 38%
Low grade non-MALT-type 1%
High grade 58%
hg /lg 35.5% (MALT-type)
hg 64.5% (MALT-type?)

GIT NHL STG 02/96

When the distribution by clinical stage is reviewed [20.7], we see that the low grade lymphomas tend to have localized disease, whereas more disseminated disease is associated with the high grade neoplasms, both primary and secondary. The same phenomenon was reported by Montalban *et al.* [20.8],[8] in a paper which also showed a lower incidence of higher Stages in the low grade lymphomas and *vice versa*. Consequently, when considering systemic therapies, we need to discriminate between low and high grade tumors.

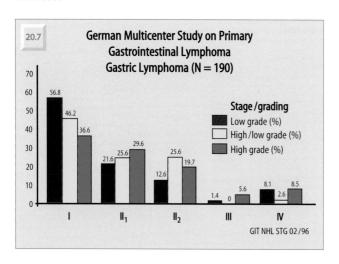

20.7   German Multicenter Study on Primary Gastrointestinal Lymphoma
Gastric Lymphoma (N = 190)

Stage /grading
- Low grade (%)
- High /low grade (%)
- High grade (%)

Stage	Low grade	High/low grade	High grade
I	56.8	46.2	36.6
II₁	21.6	25.6	29.6
II₂	12.6	25.6	19.7
III	1.4	0	5.6
IV	8.1	2.6	8.5

GIT NHL STG 02/96

20.8   Gastric Lymphoma Patho-Histologic Grade and Stage

	I	II₁	II₂	III	IV
Low grade	63	17	7	2	10
High grade	27	24	17	9	24

Montalban *et al.* 1995[8]

An obvious question when we consider the low grade lymphomas concerns the role of antibiotics in *H. pylori*-positive cases [20.9]. As you know, there have been several reports that eradication of *H. pylori* is associated with regression of MALT-type lymphoma [20.10]. However, one finds in reviewing these studies that, although *H. pylori* was eradicated in almost all patients, the number in whom the MALT lymphoma regressed was consistently less than the number in whom the infection was eradicated.

20.9   Extranodal Low Grade Marginal Zone B Cell Lymphoma

Stage	Treatment option
I (*H. pylori*-pos.)	Antibiotics
I (*H. pylori*-neg.)	Radiotherapy vs Resection
II₁	Radiotherapy vs Resection
II₂	Radiotherapy (resection?)
III	Chemotherapy
IV	Chemotherapy

20.10   Antibiotic Treatment in Stage I *H. pylori*-positive Low Grade Lymphoma

	H. pylori eradication	Lymphoma regression	Relapse
Roggero, 1995 *	36/37 (97%)	22/36 (61%)	2/22 (9%)
Bayerdörffer, 1996 **	59/59	CR 45/59 (100%) PR 12/59 (20%)	- (76%)
Fischbach, 1996 **	18/19 (94%)	15/18 (83%)	-

* First Workshop on Gastrointestinal Lymphoma, Münster 09/95
** Workshop on Gastric Malignancies, Münich 02/96

One of the reasons might be found in the updated study by Bayerdörffer *et al.* which was published in the *Lancet* [20.11].[9] This showed complete regression of the lymphoma in 72% of the 74 patients, but in 15% of cases there was not even partial response. Eight of these 11 non-responsive patients went on to surgery, and in six of them a high grade lymphoma was found.

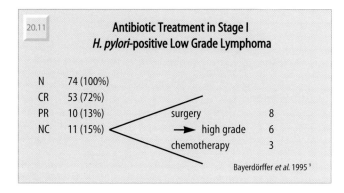

Antibiotic Treatment in Stage I
H. pylori-positive Low Grade Lymphoma

N	74 (100%)
CR	53 (72%)
PR	10 (13%)
NC	11 (15%)

surgery 8
high grade 6
chemotherapy 3

Bayerdörffer *et al.* 1995 [9]

This suggests that, when we use antibiotic therapy to treat patients with low grade MALT-type lymphomas, a high grade component may have been overlooked, even when multiple biopsies have been taken. Therefore a second lesson from this study is that eradication of *H. pylori* may no longer have any effect once a low grade MALT-type lymphoma has progressed towards a high grade lymphoma.

The most important question of course concerns the long term benefit of antibiotic therapy. Does eradication of *H. pylori* and tumor regression in low grade MALT-type lymphoma really offer the prospect of a true cure? This question remains unresolved and is relevant when we consider four cases reported by Montalban *et al.* in the *Lancet* [20.12].[10] In all of these cases, antibiotic therapy was effective in eradicating *H. pylori*, but lymphoma was still present in follow-up biopsies, as evidenced by the presence of a mono-clonal pattern of Ig gene rearrangement. In some cases this monoclonal population was present despite normal biopsy histology. This poses the question of the significance of monoclonality detected by this means. Do these cases really have persisting lymphoma, or does it represent some other phenomenon, for example an anomalous immune reaction?

How should patients with low grade lymphoma of MALT type be treated [20.9]? In low stages (i.e. I, II), surgery is generally considered the most appropriate approach. However, these patients are often in the older age group, and surgery is therefore not always possible.

We tried to address this question in our multicenter study. This is not a randomized trial, but one in which the different institutions can choose to use surgery or simply conservative management, including local radiation. The follow-up is still short, but we cannot at the present time see any difference in Stage I and II patients for conservative management versus surgery [20.13].

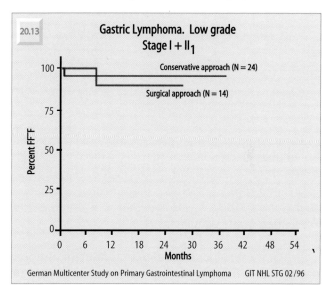

Gastric Lymphoma. Low grade
Stage I + II₁

German Multicenter Study on Primary Gastrointestinal Lymphoma   GIT NHL STG 02 / 96

Similar results are seen in a study, also published by Montalban *et al.*, which investigated the role of surgery compared to chemotherapy [20.14].[2] Chemotherapy is probably not the most appropriate treatment for low grade lymphoma, and it is therefore not surprising that patients treated with chemotherapy had a poorer outcome, at least in localized disease. However, surgery was clearly effective, although it was also evident that patients with more advanced disease had a worse prognosis. A question which we have to address in the future is therefore whether chemotherapy has some role in more advanced disease, and whether it can improve prognosis.

Antibiotic Therapy in MALT-type lymphoma

Patient	Time after H. pylori therapy	Endoscopy	Biopsy	IgH gene / FR2 / FR3	Treatment
1	1	Gastritis	Lymph	M	
	4	Gastritis	Lymph	M	
	5		Lymph	M	Surgery
	13	Normal	Normal	P	
2	2	Normal	Gastritis	P	Anti-*H. pylori*
	5	Normal	Normal	M	
	10	Normal	Normal	M	
3	2	Gastritis	Normal	M	Anti-*H. pylori*
4	2	Gastritis	Normal	M	Anti-*H. pylori*
	7	Normal	Normal	P	

Montalban *et al.* 1995 [10]

Gastric Lymphoma
Survival in Low Grade Lymphomas

	N	5 -year survival	
Stage			
I–II₂	68	0.95	p < 0.001
III /IV	11	0.34	
Treatment			
Surgery	34	1.0	
Chemotherapy	17	0.34	p < 0.001
Surgery + CT	26	1.0	

Montalban *et al.* 1995 [2]

The problem with Stage III and IV disease is that the number of patients is very limited. For example, in our own trial, there are very few such cases, and this makes it impossible to present any meaningful results [20.15].

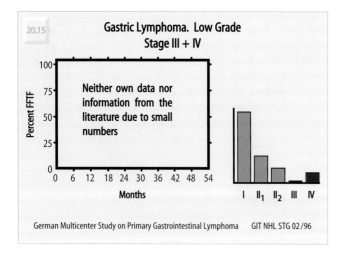

German Multicenter Study on Primary Gastrointestinal Lymphoma   GIT NHL STG 02/96

Returning to the high grade lymphomas, it should be emphasized again that there is a mixture of high grade lymphomas and high grade lymphomas associated with a low grade component [20.6]. There is therefore a bias towards higher clinical stages in these high grade neoplasms [20.7].

When we consider the different treatment options, the first question is whether there is a difference in clinical outcome for patients with only a low grade component, with only a high grade component, or with a mixture. The results of two published trials are shown in [20.16] and [20.17]. In both series there is a significant difference between low grade and high grade lymphomas, but in the study by Cogliatti *et al.*, the secondary high grade lymphoma had the same outcome as the primary high grade lymphomas. In contrast, in the study from Radaszkiewicz *et al.*, the primary low grade lymphomas and the secondary high grade lymphomas shared the same outcome, whereas the high grade lymphomas had a poorer prognosis.

In our own trial [20.18], we have yet to see any difference between these three groups, but the follow-up is shorter than in the two other studies.

These findings have to be taken into account when considering the treatment of these patients. An important question concerns the benefit of conservative management versus the surgical approach, and in our own trial we saw no difference in outcome between chemotherapy plus local radiotherapy compared to surgery combined with chemo/radiotherapy [20.19].

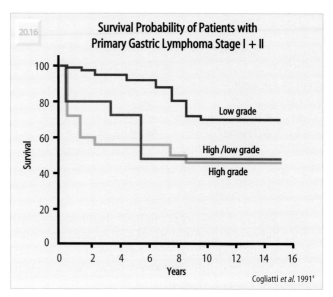

Cogliatti *et al.* 1991[4]

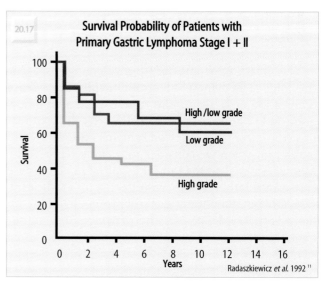

Radaszkiewicz *et al.* 1992[11]

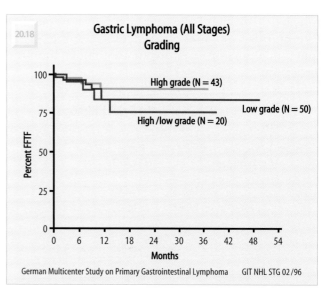

German Multicenter Study on Primary Gastrointestinal Lymphoma   GIT NHL STG 02/96

In another trial published by Dr. Montalban [20.20], there was essentially no difference for Stage I and II patients between surgery and chemotherapy, again suggesting that chemotherapy is as effective as the surgical approach. However, it should be noted that these results are inferior to our own results, in which systemic chemotherapy was always combined with local radiotherapy, the latter to cure the possible low grade component. Dr. Montalban also showed that patients with Stage III and IV disease had a clearly poorer prognosis. Similar results are also seen in a study by Gobbi et al.[12] in Stages III, IV [20.21] (the green line compares results in nodal lymphomas [13]). The reason for that might be that no local radiotherapy was given.

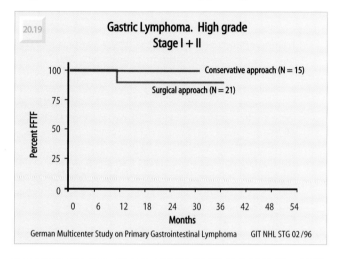

20.19

Gastric Lymphoma. High grade
Stage I + II

German Multicenter Study on Primary Gastrointestinal Lymphoma   GIT NHL STG 02/96

20.20

Gastric Lymphoma
Survival in High Grade Lymphomas

	N	5-year survival	
Stage			
I-II$_2$	37	0.80	p < 0.0027
III/IV	16	0.46	
Treatment			
Surgery	15	0.73	
Chemotherapy	11	0.62	n.s
Surgery + CT	27	0.70	

Montalban et al. 1995 [2]

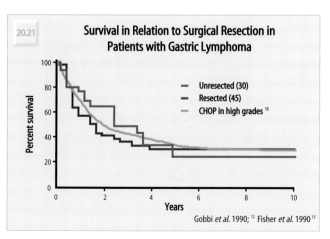

20.21

Survival in Relation to Surgical Resection in
Patients with Gastric Lymphoma

Gobbi et al. 1990;[12] Fisher et al. 1990[13]

To summarize, it now appears clear that in Stage I low grade lymphomas of MALT type antibiotics are able to eradicate *H. pylori*, and that this eradication is associated with a regression of the lymphoma. Whether this constitutes a true cure is not so clear. In Stage I and II disease, radiotherapy and maybe also surgery can cure a high proportion of patients. In more advanced stages, chemotherapy can only be of palliative value.

For high grade lymphomas of MALT type, the treatment of choice in all cases is chemotherapy, which should be combined with radiotherapy to provide a curative approach for the potential low grade component [20.22].

20.22

Extranodal Marginal Zone B Cell Lymphoma Low Grade
and (?) High Grade

Stage	Low grade	Goal	High grade	Goal
I (*H. pylori*-pos.)	Antibiotics	Cure (?)	Chemotherapy + Radiotherapy	Cure
I (*H. pylori*-neg.)	Radiotherapy	Cure	Chemotherapy + Radiotherapy	Cure
II	Radiotherapy	Cure	Chemotherapy + Radiotherapy	Cure
III + IV	Chemotherapy	Palliation	Chemotherapy + Radiotherapy	Cure

A question which remains open concerns the significance of histologic grade. Consideration should be given to the incorporation of cytologic grading into the REAL classification, and to the development of corresponding treatment strategies [20.23].

20.23

Extranodal Marginal Zone B Cell Lymphoma
Conclusion

Refinement of histologic categorisation:
low grade
high/low grade
high grade
=> cytologic grading
Definition of treatment strategy

Finally, the authors would like to thank the other members of the steering committee of the German Gastrointestinal Study Group who were responsible for the central reviews of pathology (Dr. Tiemann, Lymph Node Registry, Kiel), radiotherapy (Dr. Willich, University Münster), surgery (Dr. Reers, University Münster), and statistical analysis (Dr. Grothaus-Pinke).

REFERENCES

1. Fisher RI, Dahlberg S, Nathwani BN, Banks PM, Miller TP, Grogan TM. A clinical analysis of two indolent lymphoma entities: mantle cell lymphoma and marginal zone lymphoma (including the mucosa-associated lymphoid tissue and monocytoid B-cell subcategories): a Southwest Oncology Group study. *Blood* 1995; **85**: 1075-82.

2. Montalban C, Castrillo JM, Abraira V *et al.* Gastric B-cell mucosa-associated lymphoid tissue (MALT) lymphoma. Clinicopathological study and evaluation of the prognostic factors in 143 patients. *Ann Oncol* 1995; **6**: 355-62.

3. Kath R, Donhuijsen K, Hayungs J, Albrecht K, Seeber S, Hoffken K. Primary gastric non-Hodgkin's lymphoma: a clinico-pathological study of 41 patients. *J Cancer Res Clin Oncol* 1995; **121**: 51-6.

4. Cogliatti SB, Schmid U, Schumacher U *et al.* Primary B-cell gastric lymphoma: a clinicopathological study of 145 patients. *Gastroenterology* 1991; **101**: 1159-70.

5. Johnsson A, Brun E, Akerman M, Cavallin-Stahl E. Primary gastric non-Hodgkin's lymphoma. A retrospective clinico-pathological study. *Acta Oncol* 1992; **31**: 525-31.

6. Castrillo JM, Montalban C, Obeso G, Piris MA, Rivas MC. Gastric B-cell mucosa associated lymphoid tissue lymphoma: a clinicopathological study in 56 patients. *Gut* 1992; **33**: 1307-11.

7. Chan JK, Ng CS, Isaacson PG. Relationship between high-grade lymphoma and low-grade B-cell mucosa-associated lymphoid tissue lymphoma (MALToma) of the stomach. *Am J Pathol* 1990; **136**: 1153-64.

8. Montalban C, Manzanal A, Castrillo JM, Escribano L, Bellas C. Low grade gastric B-cell MALT lymphoma progressing into high grade lymphoma. Clonal identity of the two stages of the tumour, unusual bone involvement and leukemic dissemination. *Histopathology* 1995; **27**: 89-91.

9. Bayerdörffer E, Neubauer A, Rudolph B *et al.* Regression of primary gastric lymphoma of mucosa-associated lymphoid tissue type after cure of Helicobacter pylori infection. MALT Lymphoma Study Group. *Lancet* 1995; **345**: 1591-4.

10. Montalban C, Manzanal A, Boixeda D, Redondo C, Bellas C. Treatment of low-grade gastric MALT lymphoma with Helicobacter pylori eradication. *Lancet* 1995; **345**: 798-9.

11. Radaszkiewicz T, Dragosics B, Bauer P. Gastrointestinal malignant lymphomas of the mucosa-associated lymphoid tissue: factors relevant to prognosis. *Gastroenterology* 1992; **102**: 1628-38.

12. Gobbi PG, Dionigi P, Barbieri F *et al.* The role of surgery in the multimodal treatment of primary gastric non-Hodgkin's lymphomas. A report of 76 cases and review of the literature. *Cancer* 1990; **65**: 2528-36.

13. Fisher RI. CHOP chemotherapy as standard therapy for treatment of patients with diffuse histiocytic lymphoma. *Important Adv Oncol* 1990; 217-25.

POST-SCRIPT

Considering the latest data from our study, we would like to stress that from the clinician's point of view a cytologic grading for marginal zone lymphoma should be incorporated in the REAL classification. With nearly one third of high grade gastric lymphomas showing simultaneous low grade components with typical features of MALT-type NHL, one has to ask if all high grade NHL in the stomach originate from the marginal zone. In that case grading is of great importance.

After closing our study in December 1996, the final analysis of the data is in progress, and publications are also in progress concerning clinical features and treatment outcome. In Stages I and II, a high grade histology with a low grade component is now a significant prognostic factor if event-free survival is assessed (p = 0.0168) [PS.1]. Considering all Stages, there is only a trend (p = 0.0720) [PS.2]. No difference in overall survival has yet emerged [PS.3].

Looking at the failures, four of five relapses in secondary high grade NHL were of typical low grade MALT type. In addition, one high grade NHL also relapsed as a marginal zone lymphoma. All relapses occurred only in the stomach.

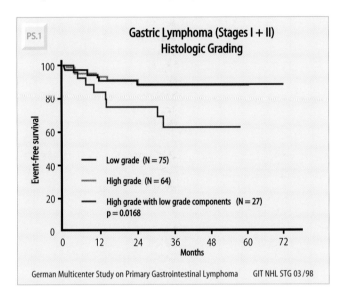

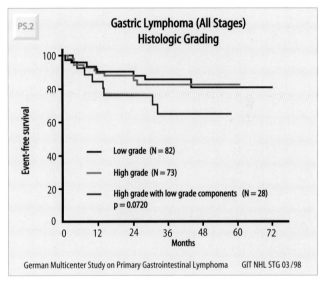

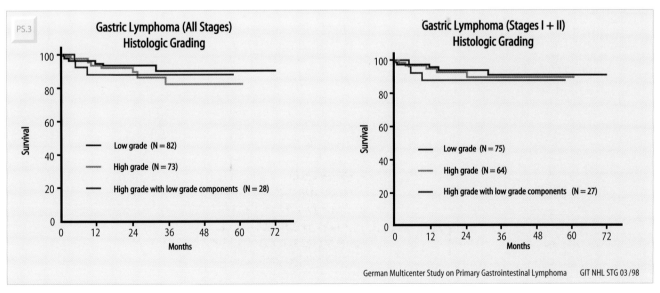

POST-SCRIPT

FURTHER READING

del Valle F, Hiddemann W, Willich N *et al.* (for the German Multicenter Study Group on GI-NHL). Clinical presentation of 371 primary gastrointestinal lymphoma: Results of a prospective multicenter study. *Blood* 1997; **90** (Suppl 1), 338a (abstract 1507).

Koch P, del Valle F, Hiddemann W *et al.* (for the German Multicenter Study Group on GI-NHL). Primary gastrointestinal (GI) lymphoma in 371 patients: Data from a prospective multicentre study. *Blood* 1997; **90** (Suppl 1): 586a (abstract 2608).

Koch P, Grothaus-Pinke B, Hiddemann W *et al.* (for the German Multicenter Study Group on GI-NHL). Primary lymphoma of the stomach: Three-year results of a prospective multicenter study. The German Multicenter Study Group on GI-NHL. *Ann Oncol* 1997; **8** (Suppl 1): S85-8.

Morphologic, immunologic and genetic features of lymphoproliferative disorders associated with immunodeficiency

D M Knowles

It has been known for a long time that the incidence of malignant lymphoma is greatly increased in individuals who are immunosuppressed, whether this is because of congenital, iatrogenic or acquired immunodeficiency. This chapter is concerned with two categories - those lymphomas which occur following transplantation, and those that are associated with HIV infection [21.1].

21.1	Post-transplantation Lymphoproliferative Disorders
Initially believed to represent EBV-associated malignant lymphomas	
Almost universally contain EBV	
Frequent extranodal location	
Diffuse pleomorphic histology	
Associated with high and rapid mortality	

Lymphoproliferative disorders occurring after transplantation were initially considered to be Epstein-Barr (EB) virus-associated malignant lymphomas. This was because they almost always contain EB virus, and are also morphologically rather pleomorphic. They occur in a variety of extranodal and unusual sites, and are usually associated with a rapid and high mortality. This concept was challenged by a paper published in 1984 in the *Lancet* (Starzl *et al.*[1]), which reported that a number of lymphoproliferative disorders that were thought to be monoclonal, and which had morphologic features of malignant lymphoma, appeared to be reversible when immunosuppressive therapy was reduced.

As a result, pathologists faced the challenge of finding criteria that would subdivide these cases morphologically into those lesions that would regress when immunosuppressive therapy was stopped and those that would not. The two most widely cited sets of criteria are those of Frizzera,[2] based on his experience in Minnesota, and those of Nalesnik,[3] from Pittsburg [21.2]. An important point to make is that the terminology was not based on any of the existing classifications, for the very good reason that these lesions are very difficult to classify using existing morphologic criteria. Consequently, the terms "polymorphic" and "monomorphic" have appeared in the literature in defining these lesions.

21.2	Histopathologic Classification of Post-transplant Lymphoproliferative Disorders	
	Frizzera *et al.* 1981 [2]	Nalesnik *et al.* 1988 [3]
	Polymorphic B cell hyperplasia	Polymorphic
	Polymorphic B cell lymphoma	Monomorphic
	Immunoblastic lymphoma	(Minimal polymorphism)
		(Plasmacytic hyperplasia)

Frizzera's concept was that the lesions are predominantly polymorphic, but that, using a variety of criteria, he could distinguish between hyperplasia and lymphoma. Nalesnik did not use the terms hyperplasia and lymphoma - he simply called them "polymorphic" or "monomorphic". Frizzera also recognized the concept of immunoblastic lymphoma, and Nalesnik had a few other miscellaneous categories that in practice are difficult to define.

If one goes back to the literature, one finds that Frizzera's criteria have not been widely used, and no large clinical series is available to review. Nalesnik's criteria have been used by his group, but they have not in practice made it possible to forecast clonality and clinical behavior. Shown in [21.3] is the largest series he has published, and one sees that about half of the lesions which were called "polymorphic" turned out to be polyclonal, and half to be monoclonal. Sometimes these lesions regressed, sometimes they resolved, sometimes there was no response. It is therefore clearly difficult, using these classification schemes, to forecast either clonality or clinical behavior.

		Clinical behavior		
Histology	**Clonality**	**Regression**	**Resolution**	**N response**
Polymorphic	17 polyclonal	5	8	2
	14 monoclonal	2	6	2
Monomorphic	5 monoclonal	0	3	1
Minimal	4 polyclonal	0	1	0
polymorphism	18 monoclonal	2	1	1

21.3   Correlation of Histopathology, Clonality and Clinical Behavior Among Post-transplantation Lymphoproliferative Disorders

Nalesnik *et al.* 1988 [3]

The author's own study[4] represented an attempt to correlate morphologic and molecular features. Nalesnik was probably correct when he surmised that some of his tumors which exhibited *c-MYC* rearrangement did very badly, but in 1988 knowledge of the genetic alterations that may occur in these lesions was limited. We tried to build on their experience and to analyze a series of cases both morphologically and in terms of molecular changes. For the morphologic evaluation we collaborated with Dr. Frizzera, who analyzed all cases without knowledge of the molecular studies. These were performed by Dr. Cesarman who analyzed a very wide range of features including immunoglobulin gene rearrangement, EB virus, *BCL-2*, *BCL-6*, *c-MYC*, *RAS*, *p53*.

To begin with, we used Frizzera's terminology, except for "plasmacytic hyperplasia", a term borrowed from Nalesnik. We also added multiple myeloma, since we found some cases of this disease [21.4]. Shown in [21.5] is an example of what Nalesnik called plasmacytic hyperplasia. In reality it is not strikingly plasmacytic in appearance, but it is clearly a benign lesion and could not be confused with a malignant lymphoma. There is a proliferation of small lymphocytes, some plasmacytoid cells, some plasma cells, occasional immunoblastic cells, but no tissue destruction or invasion. In all respects it is a benign looking lesion.

21.4   Histologic Categories of Post-transplant Lymphoproliferative Disorders

Plasmacytic hyperplasia
Polymorphic B cell hyperplasia
Polymorphic B cell lymphoma
Immunoblastic lymphoma
Multiple myeloma

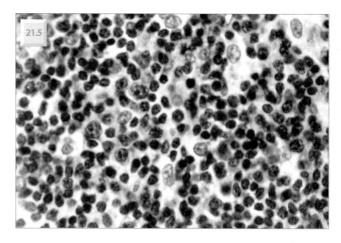

The lesion from the lung in [21.6] would fall into Frizzera's category of polymorphic B cell hyperplasia. It contains small lymphocytes and shows considerable plasmacytic differentiation. The three criteria Frizzera would use to distinguish it from lymphoma are plasmacytic differentiation, as seen here, and the lack of necrosis or significant cytologic atypia.

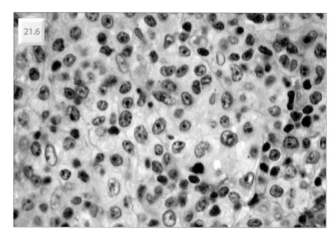

The lesion in [21.7] would be called polymorphic lymphoma. It lacks plasmacytic differentiation. There is considerable cytologic atypia, with large atypical immunoblasts [21.8], and there are large areas of necrosis [21.9].

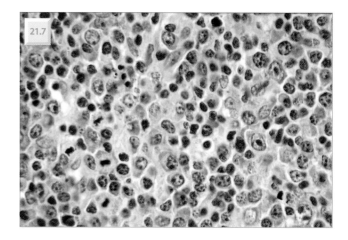

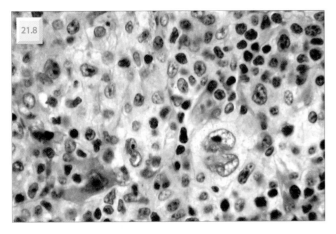

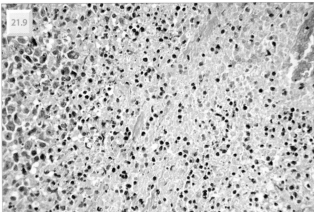

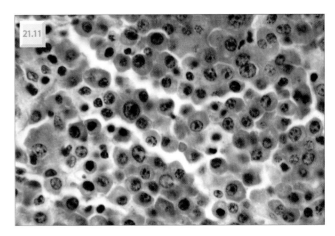

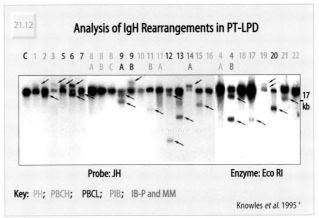

Analysis of IgH Rearrangements in PT-LPD

Probe: JH   Enzyme: Eco RI

Key: PH; PBCH; PBCL; PIB; IB-P and MM

Knowles et al. 1995 ⁴

Shown in [21.10] is obviously a high grade aggressive malignant lymphoma and such cases were easily identified in the study. It would probably correspond to a monomorphic lesion, using the Nalesnik criteria.

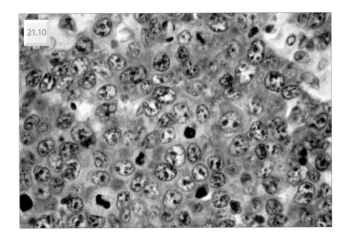

Shown in [21.11] is an example of multiple myeloma, which was associated with classical features of multiple myeloma, including IgA κ paraprotein and bone lesions.

[21.12] shows some of the immunoglobulin gene rearrangement studies performed by Dr Cesarman. The lanes corresponding to plasmacytic hyperplasia are devoid of rearrangements. The only exception is the first lane, in which there is a very faint band.

Every other pathologic type of lesion however showed evidence of monoclonality, having both heavy chain and, in other studies not shown here, light chain gene rearrangement. Samples 11A and 11B represent two different samples from the same patient. The first showed a plasmacytic hyperplasia and no evidence of clonality, whereas in sample 11B there was a clear rearrangement, so that this lesion was presumably clonal. Patient 9 also had two lesions, one in the brain and one in the breast. Although they were excised only six days apart they showed different immunoglobulin gene rearrangement patterns, suggesting that they are different tumors.

The cases were also analyzed for EB virus [21.13]. When one performs Southern blot using terminal repeat probes, one sees a smeared hybridization pattern when there are numerous infectious events with different EB viruses. In contrast, one sees a solitary band when a single virus has infected a cell and then propagated in the clonal progeny of the cell. The results in [21.13] show a range of patterns, from hybridization smears to single infection events, but in most cases EB virus is present.

There are two types of EB virus, types A and B, of which the latter is highly associated with immune deficiency states. We therefore used a PCR-based assay to distinguish between the two types. Two cell lines which contain type A EB virus, and two which contain type B were used as controls. It is evident from [21.14] that, whenever EB virus was present in post-transplant lymphoproliferative disorders it was of type A. This has been a consistent finding, and type B EB virus is only rarely involved in these post-transplant lymphoproliferative disorders.

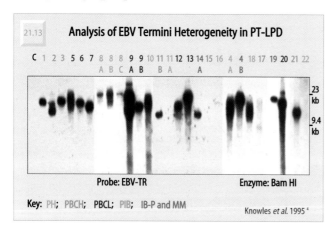

21.13 Analysis of EBV Termini Heterogeneity in PT-LPD

Probe: EBV-TR   Enzyme: Bam HI

Key: PH; PBCH; PBCL; PIB; IB-P and MM

Knowles *et al.* 1995 [4]

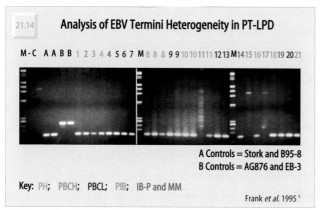

21.14 Analysis of EBV Termini Heterogeneity in PT-LPD

A Controls = Stork and B95-8
B Controls = AG876 and EB-3

Key: PH; PBCH; PBCL; PIB; IB-P and MM

Frank *et al.* 1995 [5]

These investigations and the other studies are summarized in [21.15].[4] Among examples of the plasmacytic hyperplasia, only one had evidence of clonal immunoglobulin gene rearrangement, and this was a very faint band. Two lacked EB virus, three showed a smear pattern, and five had evidence of a clonal population. None showed any other genetic alterations.

21.15 Results of Molecular Genetic Analysis of 28 PT-LPDs Occurring in 22 Patients

| Histopathology | N | Southern blot analysis | | | SSCP | |
		Clonal Ig.	EBV	C-MYC	N-RAS	p53
PH	10	1 (faint)	Negative, 2 Smear, 3 Clonal, 5	0	0	0
PBCH	5	5	Negative, 2 Clonal, 3	0	0	0
PBCL	8	8	Clonal, 8	0	0	0
PIB	2	1*	Clonal, 1*	0*	0	2
IB-P, MM	3	3	Clonal, 3	1	3	0

*Only one specimen evaluated because of insufficient tissue

Knowles *et al.* 1995 [4]

The polymorphic lesions, regardless of whether they were called hyperplasia or lymphoma, were all monoclonal on the basis of EB virus analysis, except for two cases that lacked EB virus. All of these cases lacked rearrangements of genes such as *c-MYC* or other genetic alterations. One might argue that many of these polymorphic lesions are simply diffuse large cell lymphomas, but it is of interest that they are consistently negative for *BCL-6* gene rearrangement.

The last two cases, the ones that were obvious high grade malignancies - myeloma or pleomorphic immunoblastic lymphoma - were also clonal. They contained EB virus, but interestingly they had additional genetic alterations, either *p53* mutations, *c-MYC* rearrangement, or *RAS* mutations.

Based on this data, it appears that there are three categories of disease [21.16]. Firstly, there are the plasmacytic hyperplasias, which appear to be benign lesions and are only rarely clonal. Secondly, there are polymorphic lesions, which, although one can refer to them on morphologic grounds as hyperplasia or lymphoma, appear to be a single entity, all being monoclonal and lacking other genetic alterations. And finally, there are true high grade aggressive lymphomas, which exhibit a variety of genetic alterations.

21.16 Conclusion

1. PT-LPDs are divisible into three separate clinicopathologic categories based on clinical, morphologic and genetic characteristics

    Plasmacytic hyperplasia

    Polymorphic PT-LPD (PBCH/PBCL)

    Malignant lymphoma/myeloma

These findings can be fitted into a simple scheme, as shown in [21.17]. B cells are infected with EB virus, either before or after transplantation. This patient is then immunosuppressed and a polyclonal or oligoclonal proliferation of EB virus-infected B cell clones occurs. This stage would correspond to the plasmacytic hyperplasia as just described. In this environment, one or more of these clones have a slight growth advantage and eventually one or possibly two clones of EB virus-infected cells become dominant, and we see the polymorphic lesions, in which cells are both clonal and EB virus-infected. At some stage other genetic events then occur which may give rise to aggressive, high-grade true malignant lymphomas.

The other topic covered in this chapter is HIV-associated lymphoma. A number of years ago, we reported a series of AIDS-associated lymphomas and demonstrated, using Working Formulation criteria, that the largest single category, accounting for about 40% of cases comprised small non-cleaved Burkitt's and Burkitt-like lymphomas [21.18]. Most of the other cases were evenly divided between large cell immunoblastic and diffuse large cell lymphomas. Other groups, both in Europe and the United States, have made essentially the same observations.

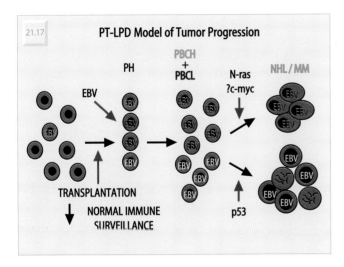

21.17 **PT-LPD Model of Tumor Progression**

The Burkitt-type lymphomas in these patients may resemble classical Burkitt's lymphoma, as seen in the non-immunosupressed general population. Shown in [21.19] is the typical morphology, with a starry sky appearance due to the presence of tingible body macrophages. The neoplastic cells have round regular nuclei, usually clumped chromatin, two to four nucleoli, and a small rim of cytoplasm.

21.18	**Histopathology of 89 AIDS-related NHLs**	
Small non-cleaved cell	36 (40%)
Large cell, immunoblastic, plasmacytoid	25 (28%)
Diffuse large cell	28 (32%)
Total	**89**

Knowles *et al.* 1988 [6]

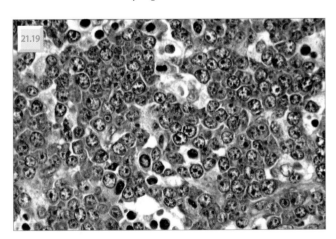

Many cases, however, have a morphology which is "Burkitt-like" rather than identical to classical Burkitt's lymphoma. There is much more variation in nuclear size and shape, and more cells have single nucleoli, which are large and sometimes centrally localized, as shown in [21.20].

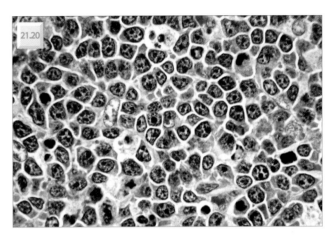

The large cell lymphomas have the features of large cell lymphomas as seen in the general population [21.21]. The immunoblastic lymphomas have a large vesicular nucleus, a paranuclear *hof*, and a prominent centrally placed nucleolus [21.22]. Some cases have an exceedingly pleomorphic morphology [21.23], but this is uncommon.

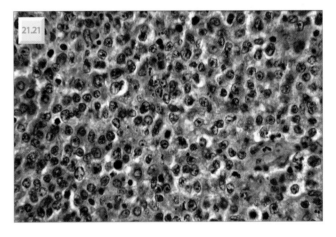

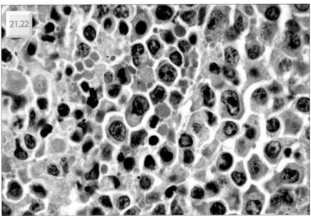

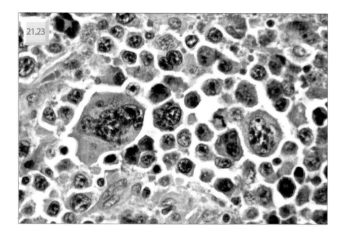

In our hands virtually all of these cases are B cell neoplasms, and they exhibit clonal rearrangement of immunoglobulin heavy and light chain genes [21.24].[7] There has been some controversy over this because of studies from UCSF by McGrath *et al.* which suggested that up to 40% of AIDS-associated lymphomas are polyclonal[8] since they showed a germline Ig gene configuration; they were also EB virus-negative.

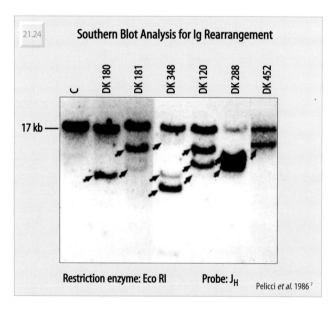

Southern Blot Analysis for Ig Rearrangement

17 kb —

Restriction enzyme: Eco RI   Probe: J_H

Pelicci *et al.* 1986 [7]

We have looked at this carefully and have not been able to confirm these findings. The cases we studied came from the West coast of the United States, so that they should resemble the UCSF cases [21.25]. We investigated specifically those cases which had a germline immunoglobulin heavy chain gene configuration, but they appeared to be clonal, based on EB virus detection. There were a few cases that were apparently germline, but it is still debatable whether or not these cases are truly polyclonal.

More recently, we have identified evidence of the Kaposi's sarcoma-associated herpes virus (KSHV) in a subset of AIDS-related lymphomas which had

previously been referred to as "body-cavity-based lymphomas" [21.26]. This is a type of lymphoma which we identified a number of years ago,[9] as did a number of other individuals, including Dr. Said and co-workers. These cases are unusual in that the lymphoma presents as a massive effusion without a tumor mass. In contrast, cases in which there is a pleura-based tumor mass, such as the pyothorax-associated lymphomas reported from Japan for example, are KSHV-negative. Furthermore lymphomas with a Burkitt-type morphology and *c-MYC* rearrangements which present as large effusions, are also KSHV-negative [21.27].

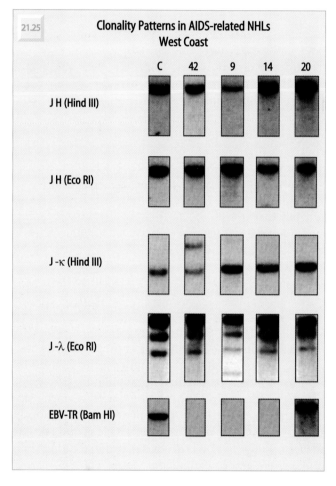

Clonality Patterns in AIDS-related NHLs West Coast

C   42   9   14   20

J H (Hind III)

J H (Eco RI)

J-κ (Hind III)

J-λ (Eco RI)

EBV-TR (Bam HI)

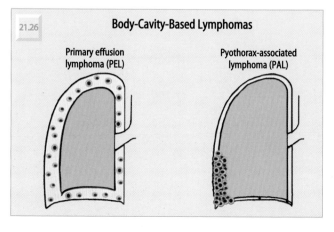

Body-Cavity-Based Lymphomas

Primary effusion lymphoma (PEL)   Pyothorax-associated lymphoma (PAL)

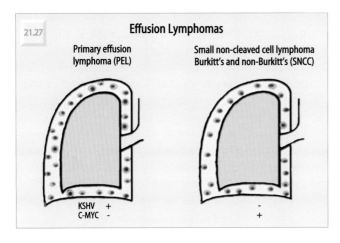

Effusion Lymphomas

Primary effusion lymphoma (PEL)

Small non-cleaved cell lymphoma Burkitt's and non-Burkitt's (SNCC)

KSHV	+	-
C-MYC	-	+

Hence the tumors we have identified represent a subset of lymphomas, usually, but not always, associated with AIDS, in which KSHV is present and *c-MYC* is not rearranged. These tumors appear to arise as primary neoplasms in body cavities, where they form large effusions, usually without serosal involvement.

The cytologic appearance of these lymphomas in a cytospin preparation is seen in [21.28].[10] The neoplastic cells are very large and they have some features of immunoblastic lymphomas, such as a paranuclear *hof* and deep blue cytoplasm. However, one can also see features reminiscent of Reed-Sternberg cells or anaplastic large cell lymphoma, with large prominent nucleoli and large cell size [21.29].[10]

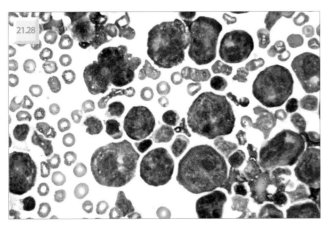

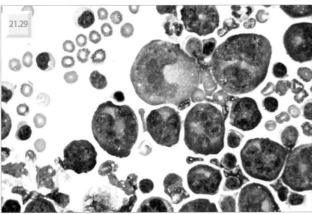

These cases are rare, probably constituting only 2-3% of all AIDS-associated lymphomas [21.30]. However all of the 17 cases we have been able to study in detail occurred in men, and only one of the 35 to 40 cases in the literature occurred in a woman. In our hands 15 of the 17 patients were HIV-positive, and this was associated with homosexuality. The two HIV-negative patients were in their early 80s. In nearly every case the patient presented with massive effusion. The disease was usually restricted to the body cavity and had the immunoblastic/anaplastic morphology already illustrated.

Primary Effusion Lymphoma

Epidemiology similar to Kaposi's sarcoma	
Male predominance	17/17
HIV-seropositive	15/17
Homosexuality as a risk factor	15/15
HIV-positive 43 years vs HIV-negative 82 years	
Initial presentation as an effusion	16/17
Disease remains restricted to body cavity	13/15
Immunoblastic/anaplastic large cell cytology	17/17
Median survival 5 months	

The phenotypic features of these cells are distinctive [21.31]. They usually express leucocyte common antigen (CD45), but in most cases they lack B cell antigens and immunoglobulin. However, they are usually of B cell origin as shown by gene rearrangement studies. In addition to KSHV, they virtually always also contain EB virus. In our experience they never show *c-MYC* rearrangement.

Primary Effusion Lymphoma

CD45 (leukocyte common antigen)	17/17
Absence of B cell associated antigens	15/17
Clonal immunoglobulin gene rearrangements	16/17
Epstein-Barr virus	16/17
Absence of *c-MYC* gene rearrangements	14/14
Presence of KSHV (KHV-8)	17/17

There have been suggestions in the literature, based on reports from Europe and from the United States, that AIDS-associated lymphomas have different clinical features depending on their anatomic site and their histopathology [21.32]. The systemic lymphomas appear to be most common in patients with higher numbers of CD4 T cells. There is a lower incidence of prior diagnosis of AIDS. Within the spectrum of histologic types already mentioned, Burkitt's or Burkitt-type lymphomas are fairly common.

Primary CNS lymphomas, in contrast, arise in patients who are usually much more immunosuppressed, as evidenced by very low CD4 T cell counts.

Most of these patients have already been diagnosed as having AIDS and usually the morphology is that of a large cell or immunoblastic lymphoma. It is also interesting that the primary CNS AIDS lymphomas are virtually always EB virus-positive, whereas this is true for only about half of the systemic ones. C-MYC rearrangement is very frequent in the systemic cases but virtually always absent in primary CNS lymphomas.

21.32	Principal Differences Among AIDS-related NHLs According to Anatomic Site of Origin		
Parameter	Systemic	CNS	Primary effusion
Prior AIDS	37%	70%	60%
CD4 Cells/mm^3	189	30	84
Histology	40% BL	LC/IB	IB/ALCL
EBV	50%	100%	100%
c-MYC gene	60%	0	0

The primary effusion lymphomas are often seen in patients with a prior diagnosis of AIDS, and who are very immunosuppressed. Usually, EB virus is present and c-MYC rearrangement is absent.

One can also note clinical differences when patients are separated according to histologic category [21.33]. In general, the patients with Burkitt-type lymphomas tend to be younger and commonly have a prior diagnosis of AIDS and high CD4 counts. Dr. Raphael and her colleagues in the French Lymphoma Study Group have shown that there is a statistically significant difference in the sites of involvement by Burkitt-type lymphomas versus immunoblastic and large cell type lymphomas.[11] The latter types preferentially involve the CNS and gastrointestinal tract.

21.33	Principal Clinical Differences Among AIDS-related NHLs According to Histopathology		
Parameter	BL	IB	LC
Patient age	Younger	Older	?
Prior AIDS	Uncommonly	Frequently	?
CD4 cells	Higher	Lower	?
Disease sites	Lymph nodes, Muscles Marrow	CNS Oral GI tract	CNS Oral GI tract
Survival	Intermediate	Worse	Best

Data from Dr. Dalla-Favera's laboratory suggest that different molecular genetic events account for the different morphologic disease categories [21.34].[12] If one investigates systemic AIDS-associated lymphomas, one finds a spectrum of genetic alterations. However, if one looks at these cases according to

morphology, the genetic alterations are different. For example, the Burkitt-type lymphomas virtually always have c-MYC rearrangements and lack BCL-6 rearrangement. p53 mutations are found in a high percentage of cases, whereas EB virus is found in only a few. In contrast, in immunoblastic lymphomas EB virus is commonly found, c-MYC rearrangement is present in only a quarter of cases, BCL-6 rearrangement, which is associated with large cell lymphomas, occurs in only a small percentage, and p53 mutations are usually absent. Thus it appears that not only clinical characteristics but also molecular genetic events differ between the morphologic categories.

21.34	Genetic Lesions in AIDS-related NHLs			
		Histopathologic subtypes		
Genetic lesion	All cases	BL	LC	IB
EBV	42%	31%	25%	100%
c-MYC	79%	100%	50%	25%
BCL-1	0	0	0	0
BCL-2	0	0	0	0
BCL-6	14%	0	25%	19%
RAS	15%	19%	0	20%
p53	37%	63%	0	0
RB-1	0	0	0	0

Ballerini et al. 1993;[12] Gaidano et al. 1994[13]

In conclusion, AIDS-associated lymphomas vary in their anatomic sites and histologic features [21.35]. If one compares AIDS-associated lymphomas with the post-transplant lymphoproliferative disorders described earlier, there appear to be more differences than similarities. Polymorphic lesions are only occasionally seen in AIDS-associated lymphomas. Furthermore, EBV is found frequently in post-transplant lymphoproliferative disorders but it is present in only a subset of AIDS-associated lymphomas. Burkitt-type lymphomas and the associated c-MYC rearrangement are common in AIDS-associated lymphomas, and uncommon in tumors arising following transplantation.

21.35	Categories of AIDS-related NHL	
Anatomic site	Histopathology	
Systemic	Burkitt, Burkitt-like	
Central nervous system	Immunoblastic	
Body cavity	Large cell	

The features of the immunosuppressed state that allow these different forms of lymphoma, associated with very different molecular alterations, to arise in the two clinical settings remain unclear and represent a challenge for the future.

ACKNOWLEDGEMENTS

The following figures are reproduced by copyright permission of W. B. Saunders:
[21.5], [21.6], [21.9], [21.12], [21.13] and [21.15] - reproduced from *Blood* 1995; **85**: 552-65;
[21.28] and [21.29] - reproduced from *Blood* 1996; **88**: 645-56.

Figure [21.24] is reproduced from *The Journal of Experimental Medicine* 1986; **164**: 2049-60 by copyright permission of The Rockefeller University Press.

REFERENCES

1. Starzl TE, Nalesnik MA, Porter KA *et al*. Reversibility of lymphomas and lymphoproliferative lesions developing under cyclosporin-steroid therapy. *Lancet* 1984; **1**: 583-7.

2. Frizzera G, Hanto DW, Gajl-Peczalska KJ *et al*. Polymorphic diffuse B-cell hyperplasias and lymphomas in renal transplant recipients. *Cancer Res* 1981; **41**: 4262-79.

3. Nalesnik MA, Jaffe R, Starzl TE *et al*. The pathology of post-transplant lymphoproliferative disorders occurring in the setting of cyclosporine A-prednisone immunosuppression. *Am J Pathol* 1988; **133**: 173-92.

4. Knowles DM, Cesarman E, Chadburn A *et al*. Correlative morphologic and molecular genetic analysis demonstrates three distinct categories of posttransplantation lymphoproliferative disorders. *Blood* 1995; **85**: 552-65.

5. Frank D, Cesarman E, Liu YF, Michler RE, Knowles DM. Posttransplantation lymphoproliferative disorders frequently contain type A and not type B Epstein-Barr virus. *Blood* 1995; **85**: 1396-403.

6. Knowles DM, Chamulak GA, Subar M *et al*. Lymphoid neoplasia associated with the acquired immunodeficiency syndrome (AIDS). The New York University Medical Center experience with 105 patients (1981-1986). *Ann Intern Med* 1988; **108**: 744-53.

7. Pelicci PG, Knowles DM 2nd, Arlin ZA *et al*. Multiple monoclonal B cell expansions and c-myc oncogene rearrangements in acquired immune deficiency syndrome-related lymphoproliferative disorders. Implications for lymphomagenesis. *J Exp Med* 1986; **164**: 2049-60.

8. McGrath MS, Shiramizu B, Meeker TC, Kaplan LD, Herndier B. AIDS-associated polyclonal lymphoma: identification of a new HIV-associated disease process. *J Acquir Immune Defic Syndr* 1991; **4**: 408-15.

9. Cesarman E, Chang Y, Moore PS, Said JW, Knowles DM. Kaposi's sarcoma-associated herpesvirus-like DNA sequences in AIDS-related body-cavity-based lymphomas. *N Engl J Med* 1995; **332**: 1186-91.

10. Nador RG, Cesarman E, Chadburn A *et al*. Primary effusion lymphoma: a distinct clinicopathologic entity associated with the Kaposi's sarcoma-associated herpes virus. *Blood* 1996; **88**: 645-56.

11. Raphael M, Gentilhomme O, Tulliez M, Byron PA, Diebold J. Histopathologic features of high-grade non-Hodgkin's lymphomas in acquired immunodeficiency syndrome. The French Study Group of Pathology for Human Immunodeficiency Virus-Associated Tumors. *Arch Pathol Lab Med* 1991; **115**: 15-20.

12. Ballerini P, Gaidano G, Gong JZ *et al*. Multiple genetic lesions in acquired immunodeficiency syndrome-related non-Hodgkin's lymphoma. *Blood* 1993; **81**: 166-76.

13. Gaidano G, Lo Coco F, Ye BH *et al*. Rearrangements of the BCL-6 gene in acquired immunodeficiency syndrome-associated non-Hodgkin's lymphoma: association with diffuse large-cell subtype. *Blood* 1994; **84**: 397-402.

POST-SCRIPT

Since this chapter was prepared, an exciting new development concerning the pathogenesis of post-transplantation lymphoproliferative disorders has occurred. We have discovered that mutations involving the BCL-6 gene in the absence of rearrangement of this gene occur in almost 50% of these disorders. Moreover, the frequency of BCL-6 gene mutation segregates according to the clinicopathologic category of disease and correlates with clinical behavior. BCL-6 gene mutations are absent from the plasmacytic hyperplasias and occur in approximately 40% of the polymorphic lesions, including those classifiable as hyperplasia and those classifiable as lymphoma according to Frizzera, and in about 90% of those lesions classifiable as malignant lymphoma or multiple myeloma. Furthermore, the presence of BCL-6 gene mutations predicts shorter survival and refractoriness to reduced immunosuppression and/or surgical excision. These findings suggest that the BCL-6 gene structure is a reliable indictor for the categorization of PT-LPDs into hyperplasia and malignant lymphoma. BCL-6 gene mutation may prove to be a useful clinical marker to determine whether a reduction in immunosuppressive therapy should be attempted or more aggressive chemotherapy should be instituted in the management of patients with these lesions.

REFERENCE

Cesarman E, Chadburn A, Liu YF, Migliazza A, Dalla-Favera R, Knowles DM. BCL-6 gene mutations in posttransplantation lymphoproliferative disorders predict response to therapy and clinical outcome. *Blood* 1998; **92**: 2294-302.

Clinical aspects of AIDS-associated lymphomas

D T Scadden

It is clear from a number of studies [22.1] that there is an increased incidence of neoplastic complications in HIV disease. In the Concorde and the ACTG019 studies of patients with early HIV disease, from Europe and the U.S. respectively, about a quarter of all patients developed a malignancy as their AIDS-defining illness. In the ACTG196 study of patients with more advanced immunosuppression who were receiving a prophylactic anti-mycobacterial agent, there was approximately the same frequency of death from a neoplastic disease. Furthermore, as infectious disease physicians become more successful in controlling opportunistic infection, the frequency of neoplasms is rising. It is estimated that as many as 40% of HIV-positive patients will develop a malignancy at some stage. These lesions represent a link between infectious disease and oncology, since each of the major tumor types seen in HIV-positive patients is associated with at least one infectious agent. Non-Hodgkin's lymphomas are associated not only with Epstein-Barr (EB) virus, but also with the herpes virus, HHV-8, which has also been associated with Kaposi's sarcoma. The list in [22.2] is probably incomplete and it is likely that other infectious agents will in the future be implicated in subsets of AIDS-associated tumors.

About a quarter of these malignancies were lymphomas, and it is estimated that in 6 - 10% of patients with AIDS death is due to lymphoma. A very dramatic increase in the incidence of lymphoma was noted in the early 1980s in particular geographic areas and demographic subsets, and as a result non-Hodgkin's lymphoma was designated in 1987 as an AIDS-defining illness [22.3].

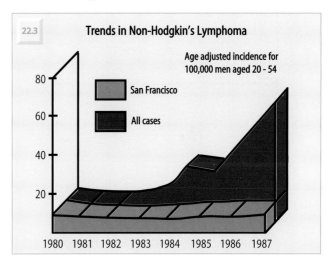

22.3 Trends in Non-Hodgkin's Lymphoma

Age adjusted incidence for 100,000 men aged 20 - 54

San Francisco
All cases

There have been varying estimates of the frequency with which AIDS patients will develop non-Hodgkin's lymphoma. The most comprehensive of these studies is from Moore *et al.* [22.4] who estimated the incidence of non-Hodgkin's lymphoma in patients with symptomatic HIV disease to be 1.6% per year.[1] This is fairly consistent over time. However, other estimates have been as high as 8% per year. Lymphomas are more common in patients who have late HIV disease, but risk is not exclusively restricted to patients with advanced immunosuppression, and lymphoma may indeed be the presenting manifestation of HIV infection.

HIV disease differs in its epidemiology from Kaposi's sarcoma, whose occurrence may be related to particular sexual practices, since it is generally

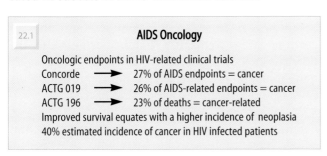

22.1 AIDS Oncology

Oncologic endpoints in HIV-related clinical trials
Concorde → 27% of AIDS endpoints = cancer
ACTG 019 → 26% of AIDS-related endpoints = cancer
ACTG 196 → 23% of deaths = cancer-related
Improved survival equates with a higher incidence of neoplasia
40% estimated incidence of cancer in HIV infected patients

22.2 Infectious Agents Associated with AIDS-Related Tumors

Tumor	Pathogen
Non-Hodgkin's lymphoma	Epstein-Barr virus
Squamous cell	Papillomavirus
Kaposi's sarcoma	Human herpes virus-8 (HHV-8)

restricted to homosexual or bisexual partners of homosexual men. In contrast, there is a fairly even distribution of risk of lymphomas regardless of the mode of HIV transmission [22.5]. However, there are some minor differences between patient groups that may reflect aspects of care, such as the reduced incidence in IV drug abusers, perhaps due to higher likelihood of death from infection in this group. In addition, there are some patients, such as hemophiliacs, in whom there may be an increased incidence, possibly reflecting true biologic differences. One hopes that more detailed analysis of differences between these groups may shed light on the pathophysiologic mechanisms underlying these neoplasms.

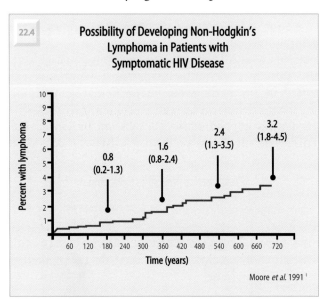

22.4 Possibility of Developing Non-Hodgkin's Lymphoma in Patients with Symptomatic HIV Disease

0.8
(0.2-1.3)

1.6
(0.8-2.4)

2.4
(1.3-3.5)

3.2
(1.8-4.5)

Moore *et al.* 1991 [1]

22.5	Relative Risk of Lymphoma by Transmission	
HIV transmission group	**Relative risk (95% CR)**	
Haemophiliac or clotting disorder	1.66	
Homosexual or bisexual men	1.13	
Transfusion recipient	1.0	
Children infected perinatally	0.90	
Heterosexual contact, except those born in the Caribbean or Africa	0.77	
Intravenous drug user	0.6	
Heterosexual contact born in the Caribbean or Africa	0.41	

Beral *et al.* 1991 [2]

Unlike Kaposi's sarcoma, which has little impact on the overall survival of HIV infected individuals, lymphoma is the most lethal complication of HIV infection [22.6]. This observation suggests that if we could control these lymphomas we would significantly affect the outcome for a subset of AIDS patients.

22.6	Relative Risk of Death Following AIDS	
Initial AIDS illness	**RR**	**p**
KS	1.0	
PCP or PCP and KS	1.19	0.006
NHL	1.79	< 0.0005
Other	1.37	< 0.0005

Luo *et al.* 1995 [3]

There are two distinct clinical subsets of patients with AIDS lymphoma: those who present with a parenchymal mass lesion exclusively restricted to the CNS, and patients who have systemic involvement that may or may not also include the CNS [22.7]. The patients who present with primary CNS lymphoma typically have more advanced stage HIV disease, lower CD4 counts, and a higher frequency of opportunistic infections or other AIDS-defining illness. The lymphomas in these patients are virtually all of immunoblastic type and they are associated with the presence of the EB virus genome. The EB virus latency genes expressed in these tumors EBNA2 through 5 and LMP1 and 2 are similar to those seen in post-transplant lymphomas.

22.7	AIDS Lymphoma	
	Primary CNS	**Systemic**
Median CD4/mm^3	30	189*
Prior OI or KS	73%	37%*
Immunoblastic histology	100%	~30%
EB virus genome	100%	38-68%
Median survival	2.5 months	6.0 months*

*Levine *et al.* 1991 [4]

In contrast, the systemic lymphoma patients tend to have higher CD4 counts and a lower incidence of prior AIDS-defining illnesses [22.7]. Immunoblastic lymphoma is not the only subtype and the EB genome is less frequently found. Furthermore, the EB virus latency genes expressed within this subset of lymphoma vary, about half of the cases expressing EBNA2 and virtually all expressing EBNA1.

Summarized in [22.8] are 12 different studies which have reviewed the histologic subtypes of lymphomas in AIDS patients. The great majority are of large cell, immunoblastic or anaplastic large cell type, but fully a third of patients have neoplasms with a small non-cleaved cell or Burkitt-like histology. This spectrum of histologic types differs not only from age-matched controls in the world population, but also from immunosuppressed transplant patients who develop lymphomas [22.9]. In iatrogenic (as in post-transplantation) or congenitally immuno-suppressed patients the incidence of EB virus genome is much higher, and small non-cleaved cell histology is much rarer. At the moment we have no clear understanding of the unique aspects of immune dysfunction in these two clinical settings which account for differences in the types of lymphoma seen.

22.8 Histologic Grade of Non-Hodgkin's Lymphoma in AIDS Patients				
Study	Patients	SNCC	Histology IBS/ALC	LC
Levine et al. 1985 [5]	27	10	13	-
Kalter et al. 1985 [6]	14	7	1	5
Gill et al. 1987 [7]	22	16	6	-
Knowles et al. 1988 [8]	89	36	25	25
Ziegler et al. 1984 [9]	90	32	24	17
Bermudez et al. 1989 [10]	31	8	6	10
Lowenthal et al. 1988 [11]	43	16	8	16
Kaplan et al. 1989 [12]	84	29	36	17
Kaplan et al. 1991 [13]	30	7	16	3
Levine et al. 1991 [14]	42	17	14	4
Remick et al. 1993 [15]	18	0	7	10
Raphael et al. 1991 [16]	113	41	33	35
TOTAL	603	219 (36%)	189 (31%)	142 (24%)

SNCC - Small non-cleaved cell; IBL - Immunoblastic; ALC - Anaplastic large cell; LC - Large cell

22.9 NHL in Immunosuppression		
	Organ transplantation	AIDS
EB virus genome	~100%	38-64%
SNCC histology	~ 1%	50%
MYC-translocation	NO	30-50%
Polyclonal phase	YES	?

If we consider the pattern of organ involvement in patients with HIV disease, we see that extranodal involvement is the rule rather than the exception [22.10]. Fully 90% of patients in some studies have been diagnosed by tissue biopsy of extranodal lesions, and up to 50% of these patients have disease exclusively restricted to extranodal sites. The most common sites are gastrointestinal tract, CNS and bone marrow, and particular histologic subtypes are associated with each of these sites. Large cell immunoblastic lymphomas are associated with gastro-intestinal involvement, whereas meningeal and marrow involvement are typically associated with small non-cleaved cell histology. The frequency of CNS involvement over time has been estimated to be as high as two thirds of patients, indicating the

importance of evaluating the CNS in the initial staging of these patients, using both imaging techniques and CSF sampling. This feature has also resulted in the common practice of intrathecal chemotherapy prophylaxis of the CNS. This practice has become standard within the AIDS Clinical Trials Group lymphoma trials, although, in view of the high association of meningeal CNS lymphoma with small non-cleaved cell histology, it might be more reasonable to confine it to patients with this histologic subtype.

22.10 Location and Stage of NHL in AIDS Patients Summary of 12 Clinical Trials							
		Extranodal sites				Stage	
	Patients	GI	Liver	CNS	Marrow	I or II	III or IV
Totals	603	124	78	133	138	128	339
		21%	13%	22%	23%	27%	73%

There are particular features which may be useful in defining prognostic subsets of patients, and comprehensive data has been published by the AIDS Clinical Trials Group [22.11]. In the ACTG 142 study, which compared full-dose m-BACOD with a half-dose m-BACOD regimen, 192 patients were treated prospectively and 18 different variables were evaluated in terms of their effect on prognosis. The disease-free survival was adversely affected by the small non-cleaved histology, and by a CD4 count of less than one hundred.

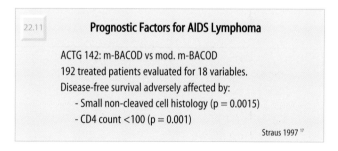

22.11 Prognostic Factors for AIDS Lymphoma
ACTG 142: m-BACOD vs mod. m-BACOD 192 treated patients evaluated for 18 variables. Disease-free survival adversely affected by: - Small non-cleaved cell histology (p = 0.0015) - CD4 count <100 (p = 0.001)

Straus 1997 [17]

This and other studies documented that overall survival is affected by a low CD4 count (<100 cells/mm^3), and also identified Stage and age as prognostically significant [22.12]. Interestingly, LDH has little impact as a prognostic variable in most studies. The effect of the CD4 count on prognosis indicates the importance of evaluating the overall immune status of patients before embarking on intensive chemotherapy. Such therapy with curative intent is rational in these patients, but it clearly must be done in the context of their underlying immuno-suppression. For a subset of patients, in whom the advanced nature of their HIV generally compromises both their ability to tolerate therapy and their longevity, palliative care alone is appropriate.

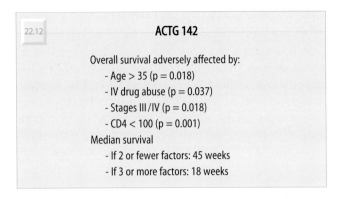

22.12	**ACTG 142**

Overall survival adversely affected by:
- Age > 35 (p = 0.018)
- IV drug abuse (p = 0.037)
- Stages III/IV (p = 0.018)
- CD4 < 100 (p = 0.001)

Median survival
- If 2 or fewer factors: 45 weeks
- If 3 or more factors: 18 weeks

22.14	**ACTG 142: Treatment Regimens** **m-BACOD**	
Agent	**Standard-dose**	**Low-dose**
Methotrexate	200 mg/m², day 15	200 mg/m², day 15
Bleomycin	4 U/m², day 1	4 U/m², day 1
Doxorubicin	45 mg/m², day 1	25 mg/m², day 1
Cyclophosphamide	600mg/m², day 1	300 mg/m², day 1
Vincristine	1.4 mg/m², day 1	1.4 mg/m², day 1
Dexamethasone	6 mg/m², day 1-5	3 mg/m², day 1-5
GM-CSF	5 mcg/kg, day 4-13	5 mcg/kg, day 4-13

Kaplan *et al.* 1997 [18]

These patients respond to standard lymphoma regimens at a rate comparable to other populations with a similar histologic diagnosis. Early on in the epidemic in the U.S., dose intensification was attempted because of the aggressive course of these lymphomas. However, the results were generally very poor, partly because of the high incidence of opportunistic infections. That led to an effort to try to define minimally intensive chemotherapy regimens, and the efficacy of a half-dose regimen was shown in a pilot study by Dr. Levine of the University of Southern California [22.13]. In contrast, in Europe efforts have been directed at intensive therapy regimens and the results have been approximately equivalent.

22.15	**ACTG 142: Results**		
Parameter	**Standard-dose**	**Low-dose**	**p-value**
Complete response	42/81 (52%)	39/94 (41%)	NS
Time to progression	30 wks	39 wks	NS
Median survival	31 wks	35 wks	NS
Time to gr 3/4 toxicity	12 wks	not reached	0.001
Gr 4 neutropenia	39% cycles	24% cycles	0.007
NHL at death	57%	70%	NS
AIDS 1° cause death	30%	26%	NS

Kaplan *et al.* 1997 [18]

22.13	**Response to Therapy** **AIDS Lymphoma**	
		CR (%)
Kaplan *et al.* 1997 [18]	CHOP	67
Gill *et al.* 1987 [7]	m-BACOD	54
Levine *et al.* 1991 [14]	mod m-BACOD	46
Gisselbrecht *et al.* 1993 [19]	LNH-84	63
Remick *et al.* 1993 [15]	ORAL	39
Sparano *et al.* 1996 [20]	CDE	56

In the U.S., a study has recently been completed by the AIDS Lymphoma Trials Group, evaluating standard m-BACOD versus a half-dose m-BACOD regimen [22.14]. The standard dose chemotherapy group included GM-CSF, while this growth factor was used on an "as needed" basis in the low-dose arm. It was important to note that all patients received *Pneumocystis carinii* pneumonia prophylaxis, and this should be a part of every treatment regimen for these patients.

This study has revealed no significant difference in terms of response rate, time to progression or median survival, all being poor using either full-dose or half-dose chemotherapy [22.15]. The main difference was in the incidence of hematologic complications.

Thus it was considered that a low-dose chemotherapy regimen was appropriate for patients with AIDS lymphoma, and this regimen was adopted as a standard for the treatment of these patients. However, the advent of highly active anti-retroviral therapy (HAART) has radically changed the overall outlook for patients with HIV disease and their tolerance for chemotherapy. It is now considered appropriate to use modified or low-dose therapy for those patients who have failed HAART or who have advanced AIDS. For those patients tolerating HAART with good HIV-1 suppression, standard dose chemotherapy regimens such as CHOP are being used and high-dose regimens are again being tested.

Alternative strategies for enhancing anti-tumor activity while seeking to avoid the immunosuppressive effects of intensive chemotherapy include the use of monoclonal antibody-based reagents. We evaluated a modified m-BACOD chemotherapy regimen in conjunction with an immunotoxin. The agent was an anti-CD19 monoclonal antibody, developed by Dr. Nadler, covalently linked to a modified ricin molecule, generated by Immunogen. We treated all patients with standard chemotherapy and, after they had responded to their first cycles of chemotherapy, gave seven day continuous infusions of the monoclonal antibody during cycles 3 and 4 [22.16]

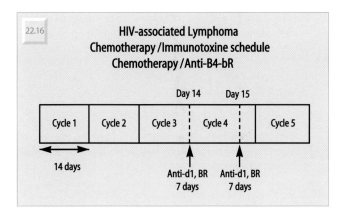

HIV-associated Lymphoma
Chemotherapy /Immunotoxine schedule
Chemotherapy /Anti-B4-bR

We enrolled 46 patients in this multi-center trial. Our findings so far are that we can safely administer the CD19 immunotoxin in conjunction with standard chemotherapy with tolerable toxicity; that the combination does not impair the delivery of the full-dose chemotherapy; and that the outcome in these patients is favorable compared to other results using chemotherapy alone [22.17]. Further trials comparing chemotherapy alone versus chemotherapy plus an immunoglobulin are under development.

Finally, it may be mentioned that the National Cancer Institute of the U.S. has established an AIDS Malignancy Consortium [22.18]. This is a co-operative oncology group that interacts with the AIDS Clinical Trials Group, and other co-operative groups of the NCI. It is composed of 13 centers in 12 geographic locations. The focus of the trials conducted by this group will be the rapid testing of pathophysiologic based therapies.

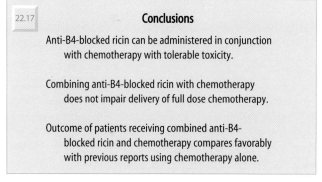

Conclusions

Anti-B4-blocked ricin can be administered in conjunction with chemotherapy with tolerable toxicity.

Combining anti-B4-blocked ricin with chemotherapy does not impair delivery of full dose chemotherapy.

Outcome of patients receiving combined anti-B4-blocked ricin and chemotherapy compares favorably with previous reports using chemotherapy alone.

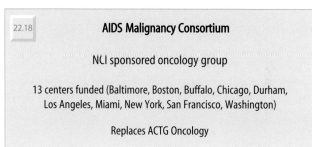

AIDS Malignancy Consortium

NCI sponsored oncology group

13 centers funded (Baltimore, Boston, Buffalo, Chicago, Durham, Los Angeles, Miami, New York, San Francisco, Washington)

Replaces ACTG Oncology

REFERENCES

1. Moore RD, Kessler H, Richman DD, Flexner C, Chaisson RE. Non-Hodgkin's lymphoma in patients with advanced HIV infection treated with zidovudine. *JAMA* 1991; **265**: 2208-11.

2. Beral V, Peterman T, Berkelman R, Jaffe H. AIDS-associated non-Hodgkin lymphoma. *Lancet* 1991; **337**: 805-9.

3. Luo K, Law M, Kaldor JM, McDonald AM, Cooper DA. The role of initial AIDS-defining illness in survival following AIDS. *AIDS* 1995; **9**: 57-63.

4. Levine AM, Sullivan-Halley J, Pike MC *et al.* Human immunodeficiency virus-related lymphoma. Prognostic factors predictive of survival. *Cancer* 1991; **68**: 2466-72.

5. Levine AM, Gill PS, Meyer PR *et al.* Retrovirus and malignant lymphoma in homosexual men. *JAMA* 1985; **254**: 1921-5.

6. Kalter SP, Riggs SA, Cabanillas F *et al.* Aggressive non-Hodgkin's lymphomas in immunocompromised homosexual males. *Blood* 1985; **66**: 655-9.

7. Gill PS, Levine AM, Krailo M *et al.* AIDS-related malignant lymphoma: results of prospective treatment trials. *J Clin Oncol* 1987; **5**: 1322-8.

8. Knowles DM, Chamulak GA, Subar M *et al.* Lymphoid neoplasia associated with the acquired immunodeficiency syndrome (AIDS). The New York University Medical Center experience with 105 patients (1981-1986). *Ann Intern Med* 1988; **108**: 744-53.

9. Ziegler JL, Beckstead JA, Volberding PA *et al.* Non-Hodgkin's lymphoma in 90 homosexual men. Relation to generalized lymphadenopathy and the acquired immunodeficiency syndrome. *N Engl J Med* 1984; **311**: 565-70.

10. Bermudez MA, Grant KM, Rodvien R, Mendes F. Non-Hodgkin's lymphoma in a population with or at risk for acquired immunodeficiency syndrome: indications for intensive chemotherapy. *Am J Med* 1989; **86**: 71-6.

11. Lowenthal DA, Straus DJ, Campbell SW, Gold JW, Clarkson BD, Koziner B. AIDS-related lymphoid neoplasia. The Memorial Hospital experience. *Cancer* 1988; **61**: 2325-37.

12. Kaplan LD, Abrams DI, Feigal E *et al.* AIDS-associated non-Hodgkin's lymphoma in San Francisco. *JAMA* 1989; **261**: 719-24.

13. Kaplan LD, Kahn JO, Crowe S *et al.* Clinical and virologic effects of recombinant human granulocyte-macrophage colony-stimulating factor in patients receiving chemotherapy for human immunodeficiency virus-associated non-Hodgkin's lymphoma: results of a randomized trial. *J Clin Oncol* 1991; **9**: 929-40.

14. Levine AM, Wernz JC, Kaplan L *et al.* Low-dose chemotherapy with central nervous system prophylaxis and zidovudine maintenance in AIDS-related lymphoma. A prospective multi-institutional trial. *JAMA* 1991; **266**: 84-8.

15. Remick SC, McSharry JJ, Wolf BC *et al.* Novel oral combination chemotherapy in the treatment of intermediate-grade and high-grade AIDS-related non-Hodgkin's lymphoma. *J Clin Oncol* 1993; **11**: 1691-702.

16. Raphael M, Gentilhomme O, Tulliez M, Byron PA, Diebold J. Histopathologic features of high-grade non-Hodgkin's lymphomas in acquired immunodeficiency syndrome. The French Study Group of Pathology for Human Immunodeficiency Virus-Associated Tumors. *Arch Pathol Lab Med* 1991; **115**: 15-20.

17. Straus DJ. Human immunodeficiency virus-associated lymphomas. *Med Clin North Am* 1997; **81**: 495-510.

18. Kaplan LD, Straus DJ, Testa MA *et al.* Low-dose compared with standard-dose m-BACOD chemotherapy for non-Hodgkin's lymphoma associated with human immunodeficiency virus infection: National Institute of Allergy and Infectious Diseases AIDS Clinical Trials Group. *N Engl J Med* 1997; **336**: 1641-8.

19. Gisselbrecht C, Oksenhendler E, Tirelli U *et al.* Human immunodeficiency virus-related lymphoma treatment with intensive combination chemotherapy. French-Italian Co-operative Group. *Am J Med* 1993; **95**: 188-96.

20. Sparano JA, Wiernik PH, Hu X *et al.* Pilot trial of infusional cyclophosphamide, doxorubicin and etoposide plus didanosine and filgrastim in patients with human immunodeficiency virus-associated non-Hodgkin's lymphoma. *J Clin Oncol* 1996; **14**: 3026-3

FURTHER READING

Levine AM, Tulpule A, Tessman D *et al.* Mitoguazone therapy in patients with refractory or relapsed AIDS-related lymphoma: results from a multicenter phase II trial. *J Clin Oncol* 1997; **15**: 1094-1103.

Levine AM, Tulpule A, Espina B *et al.* Low dose methotrexate, bleomycin, doxorubicin, cyclophosphamide, vincristine, and dexamethasone with zalcitabine in patients with acquired immunodeficiency syndrome-related lymphoma. Effect on human immunodeficiency virus and serum interleukin-6 levels over time. *Cancer* 1996; **78**: 517-526.

Scadden DT, Schenkein DP, Bernstein Z *et al.* Combined immunotoxin and chemotherapy for AIDS-related non-Hodgkin's lymphoma. *Cancer* (in press).

R A Warnke

Diffuse large B cell lymphoma is a major entity in the REAL scheme by virtue of its frequency in clinical practice [23.1]. If we relate it to the Working Formulation, it includes both cleaved and non-cleaved large cell lymphoma, and immunoblastic lymphoma. In the updated Kiel classification it includes both the centroblastic and B cell immunoblastic categories.

23.1 **Diffuse Large B Cell Lymphoma Definition**

Diffuse large B cell lymphoma is characterized by a diffuse proliferation of large neoplastic lymphoid cells with nuclear size exceeding that of normal macrophages. In the Working Formulation, it includes diffuse large cell (cleaved or non cleaved) and immunoblastic. In the updated Kiel classification, it includes centroblastic lymphoma (diffuse) and immunoblastic lymphoma (B cell type).

The architectural pattern can be quite variable [23.2], although most examples diffusely replace the lymph node and may extend into the soft tissue. However, some cases show paracortical or partial involvement or even sinusoidal involvement, and a variety of other patterns may be encountered.

23.2 **Diffuse Large B Cell Lymphoma Morphology**

Architectural features variable
Nuclear and cytoplasmic features of large cells highly variable
Cellular composition variable
Mitotic figures easily identified

The nuclear and cytoplasmic features of the large cells are also highly variable, so this is a heterogeneous morphologic category, and the background cellular composition is also variable. One may see numerous reactive T cells, many macrophages, and other cells including plasma cells (some of which may be part of the tumor), and eosinophils. Mitotic figures are usually easy to find.

A typical low power view of a diffuse large B cell lymphoma is shown below [23.3]. It is often hard to tell where the lymph node ends and the soft tissue begins in these tumors, unless some patent subcapsular sinuses remain.

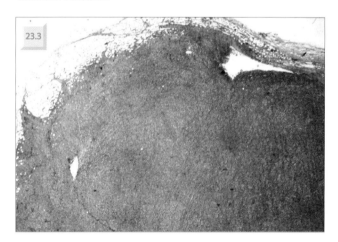

23.3

The lymphoma is composed of non-cleaved cells or "centroblasts" [23.4]. Many contain multiple nucleoli, some of which are adjacent to the nuclear membrane. However, one can also often find occasional cells with single more central nucleoli. Shown in [23.5] is a lymphoma with a much more "immunoblastic" appearance, in which many of the cells have prominent central nucleoli and abundant amphophilic cytoplasm. This would be called a "plasmacytoid immunoblastic lymphoma" in the Working Formulation.

Many pathologists have great difficulty in distinguishing between Working Formulation large cell and immunoblastic categories. Data relating to this was obtained in a reproducibility study in the early

1980s at Stanford [23.6].[1] The agreement between four hematopathologists was reasonable if one considers the raw figures. However, the kappa statistic eliminates agreement by chance alone, and when that is taken into account, results are less satisfactory. The results were also disappointing when the same case was looked at twice by the same pathologist [23.7].

It may be noted that these were the cases from Stanford that were included in the Working Formulation study, but that this was a separate reproducibility project. However, a considerable amount of very interesting reproducibility data was generated as part of the Working Formulation study, but never published.

The problem of reproducibility represents one reason to combine the two categories of "immunoblastic" and "large cell" lymphoma. The other reason emerges from studies, such as one performed at Stanford, which have shown that the two putative lymphoma types have exactly the same survival and freedom from relapse [23.8].[2]

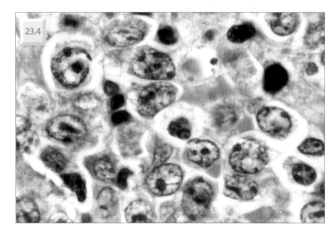

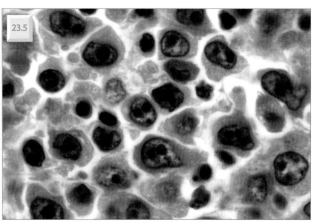

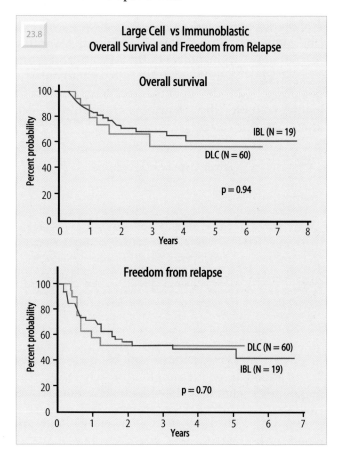

23.6	Large Cell vs Immunoblastic	
Observer	**% agreement**	**Kappa**
1 vs 2	65	40
1 vs 3	61	36
1 vs 4	61	35
2 vs 3	63	36
2 vs 4	68	44
3 vs 4	51	22

23.7	Large vs Immunoblastic Same Case - Second Look	
	% agreement	**Kappa**
Observer 1	60	38
Observer 2	78	64
Observer 3	78	60
Observer 4	72	54

As already indicated, the morphologic spectrum in these lymphomas is very wide. Occasionally, the tumor cells have multilobated nuclei [23.9]. In other instances the tumor cells are exceptionally large – the example shown in [23.10] is from a case seen in the mid-1970s, which was diagnosed as giant cell carcinoma of the thyroid. This case also shows how many reactive small lymphoid cells may be present in the background.

Some large cell lymphomas are extremely pleomorphic, and one may encounter cells resembling bizarre lacunar cells from Hodgkin's disease [23.11].

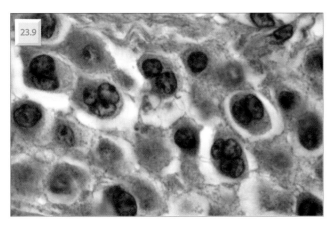

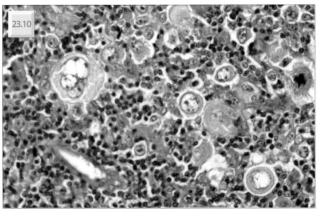

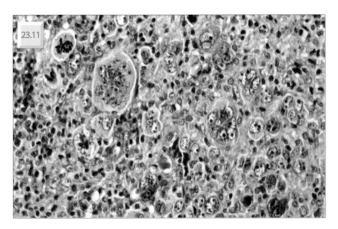

23.12	Diffuse Large B Cell Lymphoma Immunology	
Surface Ig		+/-
Cytoplasmic Ig		-/+
CD5		-/+
CD10		-/+
CD19, 20, 22. 79a		+

About two thirds to three quarters of large cell lymphomas have surface or cytoplasmic immunoglobulin and the most common heavy chain is μ, although γ is not uncommon and occasional cases express α chain [23.12]. A subset of cases, probably 10 - 20%, express CD5, and a similar number express CD10. Dr. Knowles and his associates[3] have investigated the molecular features of these cases to see if they might represent transformed small lymphocytic lymphomas, but they found no such relationship. Nevertheless, a number of these large B cell lymphomas represent progression or transformation of an underlying low grade lymphoma. Finally, large cell lymphomas express a variety of pan-B markers, although occasionally a case will lack one or more of these antigens.

[23.13] is compiled from a complete listing of the genetic abnormalities that are seen. About 20 - 30% of cases carry the t(14;18) translocation. Some of those patients will be known to have an underlying low grade lymphoma, or relapse with an underlying low grade lymphoma, but this is certainly not always the case. About 10-12% have rearrangement of *BCL-6* due to a reciprocal translocation involving 3q27 and a variety of chromosomal partners, frequently including immunoglobulin loci. Some cases have *c-MYC* translocation and others have RB inactivation.

23.13	Diffuse Large B Cell Lymphoma Genetic Features	
t(14;18)(q32;q21) (*BCL-2*)		20-30%
t(3q27;14q32, 2p12, 22q11...) (*BCL-6*)		10-12%
c-MYC translocation		10-20%
RB inactivation		10-20%

Much effort has been expended in looking for morphologic, immunologic or genetic features that may relate to prognosis in large cell lymphoma [23.14]. In general the cytology of the neoplastic cells shows little association with clinical behavior, although the data in the literature are mixed. Several large studies, especially from Dr. Grogan and the Southwest Oncology Group,[4] have shown that a high growth fraction is associated with a worse prognosis. Some molecular or genetic features are said to be associated with a worse outcome, others with a better outcome. The commoner ones, for example *BCL-6* rearrangement, appear to confer a somewhat better prognosis, whereas the t(14;18) translocation is said to be associated with a poorer outcome.

A second category of large B cell neoplasia to consider is primary mediastinal lymphoma [23.15]. This tumor usually presents in the anterior mediastinum, and in a number of cases one can show an origin from the thymus. These cases are often indistinguishable cytologically from other large B cell lymphomas. However, the International Lymphoma Study Group, when they compiled the REAL scheme, felt that these neoplasms merited separate consideration because of their distinctive clinicopathologic features, and also because of some immunohistochemical and molecular differences.

23.14	Diffuse Large B Cell Lymphoma Morphologic, Immunologic and Genetic Features that May Affect Prognosis	
Cytology of large cells		No effect
High proliferative fraction		Worse
Genetic features		
- > 4 marker chromosomes		Worse
- 1q21-23 and 17 abnormalities		Worse
- trisomy 5, 6, or 18		Worse
- 2p breaks or duplicated 3p		Better
- 3q27 (*BCL-6*)		Sl. better
- t(14;18) (*BCL-2*)		Sl. worse

23.15	Primary Mediastinal Large B Cell Lymphoma Definition
	Mediastinal large B cell lymphoma is a diffuse large cell lymphoma presenting primarily with anterior mediastinal involvement. An origin in the thymus gland can be demonstrated in at least a proportion of cases. Although some mediastinal large B cell lymphomas may be cytologically indistinguishable from large cell lymphomas of other sites, they merit separate consideration because of their distinctive clinicopathologic as well as immunohistochemical features.

Sclerosis is frequently seen in these tumors. The nuclear and cytoplasmic features, and also the cellular composition, are variable [23.16].

23.16	Primary Mediastinal Large B Cell Lymphoma Morphology
	Sclerosis frequent
	Nuclear and cytoplasmic features of large cells variable
	Cellular composition variable

Normal thymus is seen in [23.17] on the right, but on the left, a lobe has been replaced by a large cell lymphoma, containing a large area of necrosis. In [23.18], the thymus is also on the right (and contains epithelial lined cysts, as are often seen in the uninvolved thymus) and the large cell lymphoma is on the left. At higher power [23.19] it looks indistinguishable from other large cell lymphomas. It is infiltrating in this area around a residual Hassall's corpuscle. Many cases, especially if they spread into soft tissue, show fine sclerosis that can compartmentalize the tumor into clusters of lymphoma cells [23.20].

Some cases have very multilobated nuclei [23.21]. In other cases they are cleaved. Clear cytoplasm, although emphasized in some papers, is an inconstant feature.

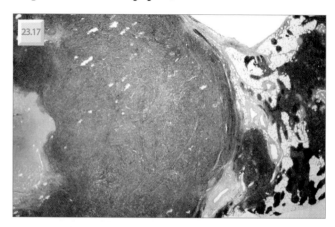

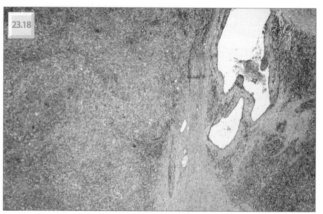

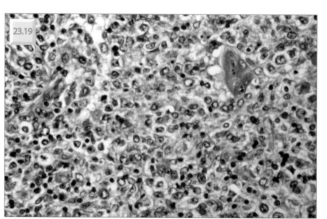

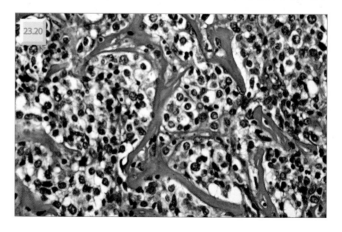

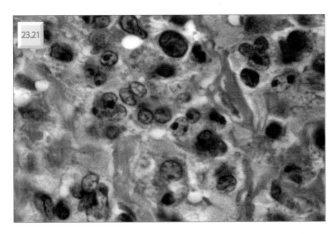

Most of these tumors are unusual among B cell neoplasms in that they lack surface and cytoplasmic immunoglobulin [23.22]. They also usually lack CD5 and CD10, but they express a variety of useful markers, including the immunoglobulin associated polypeptide, CD79a (mb-1). They also lack CD21, which is found on some other large cell lymphomas but which is absent from normal B cells in the thymic medulla. [23.23] shows the pan-B marker CD22 on the left, and staining for Ig μ chains on the right, and is a good example of a case that lacks immunoglobulin.

23.22	Primary Mediastinal Large B Cell Lymphoma Immunology	
Surface and cytoplasmic Ig		-/+
CD5		-
CD10		-
CD19, 20, 22, 79a		+
CD21		-

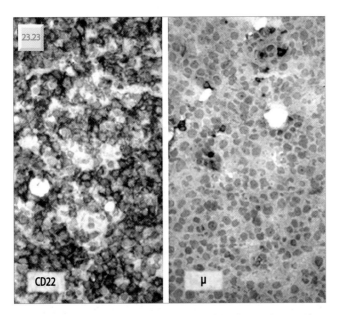

CD22   μ

These lymphomas never carry the t(14;18) translocation or 3q27 abnormalities [23.24]. Figures for the frequency of c-MYC rearrangements are variable.

23.24	Primary Mediastinal Large B Cell Lymphoma Genetic Features	
t(14;18) (BCL-2)		No
3q27 (BCL-6)		No
c-MYC		Variable

Turning finally to small non-cleaved cell lymphomas, the author's personal bias is that many diagnosed as "non-Burkitt's" neoplasms in children in reality represent true Burkitt's lymphoma. In contrast, many small non-cleaved cell lymphomas in adults are probably diffuse large cell lymphoma [23.25]. Survival curves [23.26] from Stanford adult patients show that the small number of Burkitt's cases had a relatively good survival, although none of the survival curves were statistically different. The important point is that curves for the non-Burkitt and large cell lymphomas are very similar.

23.25	Working Formulation	REAL Classification
		B cell neoplasms
Small noncleaved cell Non-Burkitt's		Burkitt's Diffuse large B cell

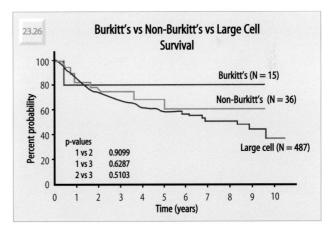

Finally, one other lymphoma category that falls into the REAL diffuse large cell lymphoma group is made up of many of the cases that were formerly called diffuse mixed lymphoma, and which represent T cell-rich large B cell lymphomas [23.27].

23.27	Working Formulation	REAL Classification
		B cell neoplams
Diffuse mixed small and large cell		Diffuse large B cell

REFERENCES

1. Warnke RA, Strauchen JA, Burke JS, Hoppe RT, Campbell BA, Dorfman RF. Morphologic types of diffuse large-cell lymphoma. *Cancer* 1982; **50**: 690-5.

2. Kwak L, Wilson M, Weiss L, Horning S, Warnke R, Dorfman R. Clinical significance of morphologic subdivision in diffuse large cell lymphoma. *Cancer* 1991; **68**: 1988-93.

3. Matolcsy A, Chadburn A, Knowles DM. De novo CD5-positive and Richter's syndrome-associated diffuse large B cell lymphomas are genotypically distinct. *Am J Pathol* 1995; **147**: 207-16.

4. Miller TP, Grogan TM, Dahlberg S *et al.* Prognostic significance of the Ki-67-associated proliferative antigen in aggressive non-Hodgkin's lymphomas: a prospective Southwest Oncology Group trial. *Blood* 1994; **83**: 1460-6.

FURTHER READING

Addis B, Isaacson P. Large cell lymphoma of the mediastinum: a B-cell tumor of probable thymic origin. *Histopathology* 1986; **10**: 379-90.

Bastard C, Deweindt C, Kerckaert JP *et al.* LAZ3 rearrangements in non-Hodgkin's lymphoma: correlation with histology, immunophenotype, karyotype, and clinical outcome in 217 patients. *Blood* 1994; **83**: 2423-7.

Delabie J, Vandenberghe E, Kennes C *et al.* Histiocyte-rich cell lymphoma. A distinct clinicopathologic entity possibly related to lymphocyte predominant Hodgkin's disease, paragranuloma subtype. *Am J Surg Pathol* 1992; **16**: 37-48.

Horning SJ, Doggett RS, Warnke RA, Dorfman RF, Cox RS, Levy R. Clinical relevance of immunologic phenotype in diffuse large cell lymphoma. *Blood* 1984; **63**: 1209-15.

Jacobson J, Aisenberg A, Lamarre L *et al.* Mediastinal large cell lymphoma: an uncommon subset of adult lymphoma curable with combined modality therapy. *Cancer* 1988; **62**: 1893-8.

Lamarre L, Jacobson J, Aisenberg A, Harris N. Primary large cell lymphoma of the mediastinum. *Am J Surg Pathol* 1989; **13**: 730-9.

Offit K, Lo Coco F, Louie DC *et al.* Rearrangement of the *BCL-6* gene as a prognostic marker in diffuse large cell lymphoma. *N Engl J Med* 1994; **331**: 74-80.

O'Hara C, Said J, Pinkus G. Non Hodgkin's lymphoma, multi-lobated B cell type. *Hum Pathol* 1986; **17**: 593-9.

Scarpa A, Bonetti F, Menestrina F. Mediastinal large cell lymphoma with sclerosis. Genotypic analysis establishes its B nature. *Virchows Arch* [A] 1987; **412**: 17-21.

Yousem SA, Weiss LM, Warnke RA. Primary mediastinal non-Hodgkin's lymphomas: a morphologic and immunologic study of 19 cases. *Am J Clin Pathol* 1985; **83**: 676-80.

POST-SCRIPT

One of the most difficult and controversial areas relates to the category of Burkitt-like (small non-cleaved non-Burkitt's) lymphomas. In children and in the setting of immunodeficiency (typically HIV infection), Burkitt-like lymphomas often have the clinical, phenotypic and molecular features of Burkitt's lymphoma. Although several studies suggest that Burkitt-like lymphomas in immuno-competent adults are more closely related to large cell lymphoma (e.g. BCL-2+ or having a t(14;18)) than to Burkitt's lymphoma, some of the Burkitt-like lymphomas do have the molecular features of Burkitt's and some have molecular features of both large cell lymphoma and Burkitt's lymphoma. These latter cases are often associated with progression of an underlying follicular lymphoma and unpublished data from the Vancouver group suggest an unusually aggressive behavior.

Clinical and biological prognostic factors in diffuse large B cell lymphoma

M A Shipp

Large B cell lymphomas are very different, from a clinician's point of view, from the indolent malignancies. A significant percentage can be cured with currently available combination chemotherapy regimens, but the problem remains that the majority of patients will die of their disease. It is therefore of crucial importance to find ways of distinguishing between patients who can be cured with standard therapy and those who require new treatment approaches. Only in this way can we hope to improve upon the present situation.

A number of investigators have identified clinical prognostic factors that predict overall survival [24.1].[1] Some of these features reflect the tumor's growth or invasive potential. Others reflect the patient's response to the tumor, or reflect the patient's ability to tolerate aggressive therapy. Although the same clinical prognostic factors were identified repeatedly over many years, the models that were established on the basis of these prognostic factors differed.

24.1	**Prognostic Features in Univariate Analyses**

The tumor's growth and invasive potential (LDH, stage, mass size, number of nodal and extranodal sites, bone marrow involvement).

The patient's response to the tumor (performance status, B symptoms).

The patient's ability to tolerate aggressive therapy (performance status, bone marrow involvement, age).

Shipp 1994 [1]

As a result, a large collaborative project was undertaken several years ago, the International Non-Hodgkin's Lymphoma Prognostic Factors Project, in which sixteen groups pooled data on more than three thousand patients suffering from aggressive non-Hodgkin's lymphoma.[2] This project identified factors that had independent prognostic significance for survival [24.2]: age; stage of disease; number of extranodal sites; performance status; and serum LDH at diagnosis. These factors are all associated with similar relative risks for shortened survival, and this has the practical advantage that it leads to a prognostic model based simply on the number of risk factors present at diagnosis.

24.2	**International NHL Prognostic Factors Project** **Significant Features in Regression Analysis -** **Training Sample Patients**	
Variable	**Relative risk**	**p-value**
Age ($\leq$ 60 vs > 60)	1.80	$< 10^{-3}$
Stage (I / II vs III / IV)	1.50	$< 10^{-3}$
No. of extranodal sites (0,1 vs > 1)	1.45	$< 10^{-3}$
Performance Status (0,1 vs 2, 3, 4)	1.83	$< 10^{-3}$
LDH ($\leq$ nl vs > nl)	1.88	$< 10^{-3}$

Shipp MA, Harrington DP, Anderson JR *et al.* (The International Non-Hodgkin's Lymphoma Prognostic Factors Project). A predictive model for aggressive non-Hodgkin's lymphoma. *New Engl J Med* 1993; **329**: 987-94. Copyright ©1993 Massachusetts Medical Society. All rights reserved. Adapted with permission 1998.

This prognostic model, termed the International Index, comprises four risk groups: low; low-intermediate; high-intermediate; and high [24.3]. These risk groups have very different five year survivals, ranging from 72% to 26%. The two major factors that contribute to these large differences in survival are differences in the initial complete response rate, and differences in the durability of attained complete responses.

24.3	**International Index** **Model - All Analyzable Cases**				
Risk category	**N risk factors**	**Cases (%)**	**CR rate**	**RFS of CRs 5-year**	**5 -year survival**
Low	0,1	35%	87%	70%	72%
Low-Int.	2	27%	67%	50%	50%
High-Int.	3	22%	55%	48%	43%
High	4,5	16%	44%	40%	26%

Shipp MA, Harrington DP, Anderson JR *et al.* (The International Non-Hodgkin's Lymphoma Prognostic Factors Project). A predictive model for aggressive non-Hodgkin's lymphoma. *New Engl J Med* 1993; **329**: 987-94. Copyright ©1993 Massachusetts Medical Society. All rights reserved. Adapted with permission 1998.

One of the goals of the Prognostic Factors Project was to identify patients who would be the most appropriate candidates for new intensive regimens. It was therefore important to look more closely at patients aged less than sixty, because it was felt that these patients should be best able to tolerate such regimens. Previous analyses also indicated that patients over sixty years of age had significantly different outcomes [24.2].

Three factors were identified that retained significance in patients who were less than sixty years of age - stage of disease, performance status, and serum LDH [24.4]. These features conferred comparable relative risks for shortened survival.

24.4	**International NHL Prognostic Factors Project** **Significant Features in Regression Analysis -** **Patients ≤ 60 years**		
Variables		**Relative risk**	**p-value**
Advanced Stage (III/IV)		2.05	< 10⁻³
> 1 Extranodal disease site		1.20	0.134
Non-ambulatory performance status (2-4)		1.76	< 10⁻³
Elevated serum LDH		1.94	< 10⁻³

It was then possible to use these factors to develop a simple model based on the number of risk factors present at diagnosis [24.5]. As before, patients fall into four risk categories - low, low-intermediate, high-intermediate, and high. The overall survivals for these groups are dramatically different, ranging from 83% in low risk patients, to 32% in high risk patients. These differences in overall survival also reflect differences in patients' ability to achieve an initial complete response, as well as the durability of this response. The predictive value of the International Index and the Age Adjusted Index have now been validated in several other large studies of patients with aggressive non-Hodgkin's lymphoma.

24.5	**International Index** **Model - Patients ≤ 60 years**				
Risk category	**N risk factors**	**Cases (%)**	**CR rate**	**RFS of CRs 5-year**	**5-year survival**
Low	0	22%	92%	85%	83%
Low-int.	1	32%	78%	66%	69%
High-int.	2	32%	57%	52%	46%
High	3	14%	46%	58%	32%

In consequence, it is now possible to identify, on the basis of clinical prognostic factors, aggressive non-Hodgkin's lymphoma patients who are more or less likely to do well with our standard therapeutic regimens. We can therefore begin to develop risk-related approaches to the treatment of patients [24.6]. In particular, low-risk patients, who might be more appropriate candidates for standard therapeutic approaches, can be identified, as can high-intermediate and high risk patients who have a less than 50% predicted overall survival with standard therapy. There is a general consensus that these patients should be candidates for dose-intensive experimental approaches. For the low and low-intermediate risk groups it is more difficult to provide definitive guidelines. The oncologist's approach to these patients depends on whether the results associated with currently available approaches are judged acceptable.

24.6	**Aggressive B Cell Lymphomas Can Be Grouped for** **Risk-related Therapy**
-	Low risk - standard therapy (combination chemotherapy +/- RT)
-	Low intermediate risk - judgement call
-	High intermediate/high risk - dose intensive experimental therapy

The preceding description represents what can be achieved using conventional clinical prognostic factors and currently available approaches to therapy. If new approaches to improving both prognosis and treatment are considered, it is important to remember that the identified clinical prognostic features are likely to be surrogate variables that reflect the biologic heterogeneity of large cell lymphomas. The oncologist's ability to make better prognostic predictions and to treat specific risk groups of patients more effectively must inevitably reflect understanding of this biologic heterogeneity.

A variety of features have now been described which relate to the biologic heterogeneity of aggressive non-Hodgkin's lymphoma [24.7]. Some features are clearly associated with known clinical prognostic features: others have independent prognostic significance, suggesting that they reflect heterogeneity that is not identified with currently recognized variables. There are also likely to be features that have clinical significance, but which are not yet well defined.

Features with known significance, which relate to clinical prognostic variables, include the expression of cytokines such as IL-6 and the expression of certain cell surface adhesion molecules. Investigators at the M.D. Anderson Hospital have shown that serum IL-6 levels are significantly higher in patients with aggressive non-Hodgkin's lymphoma than in normal controls [24.8].[3] Furthermore, IL-6 levels are correlated with the presence of B symptoms, elevated serum β2-microglobulin, and poor performance status. Since IL-6 is known to induce cachexia and fevers, this provides a possible explanation for a correlation of elevated IL-6 levels with B symptoms and poor performance status. Furthermore, since performance status is an important component of the International Index, it is not surprising that serum IL-6 levels are very closely correlated with International Index risk groups.

Biological Heterogeneity of Large Cell Lymphoma

-   Features associated with known clinical prognostic factors
    Cytokine expression (IL-6)
    Adhesion molecule expression (CD44s)
    Karyotypic abnormalities (*BCL-2*)
-   Features with independent prognostic significance
    Adhesion molecule expression (CD44 variants)
    Proliferation indices (Ki-67)
    Karyotypic abnormalities (*BCL-6*)
-   Features with probable clinical significance
    Karyotypic abnormalities (p15/p16)
    Immunocompetence

24.8 **IL-6 Levels and Disease Characteristics in Patients with Aggressive NHL**

-   Serum IL-6 levels significantly higher in patients with aggressive NHL than in normal controls (median 4.37 pg/ml vs < 0.35 pg/ml, p < 0.0001).
-   Elevated serum IL-6 levels correlated with the presence of B symptoms, elevated serum β2-microglobulin levels and poor performance status.
-   IL-6 induces cachexia and fevers providing possible explanation for associations with B symptoms and poor performance status.
-   Serum IL-6 levels correlated with International Index (L/LI risk 3.1 pg/ml, HI risk 4.4 pg/ml, H risk 9.9 pg/ml).

Adapted from Seymour *et al.* 1995 [3]

The expression of cell surface adhesion molecules is also likely to have prognostic and therapeutic significance [24.9]. CD44, otherwise known as the lymphocyte homing receptor, mediates cell attachment to extracellular matrix components and to specific cell surface ligands, and binds lymphocytes to the post-capillary venules of lymph nodes, and promotes the extravasation of circulating PBLs into lymphoid organs. This prompted investigation of whether expression of CD44 might also help to promote the dissemination of lymphoma cells [24.9]. Pals and colleagues and other groups have shown this to be the case.[4-6] Patients whose tumors expressed high levels of CD44 were far more likely to present with distant

nodal and extranodal disease. Because stage of disease at presentation has important clinical implications, it is not surprising that patients with high levels of tumor cell CD44 have poor outcomes. This is of particular interest because it provides a potential biologic explanation for the significance of advanced stage disease.

24.9 **Tumor Cell Trafficking - CD44**

-   Mediates cell attachment to extracellular matrix components and specific cell surface ligands (including hyaluronate).
-   Binds lymphocytes to the postcapillary venules of lymph nodes, promoting extravasation of circulating PBL into lymphoid organs.
-   Promotes dissemination of aggressive NHL?
    -   Patients with CD44[hi] tumors more likely to present with distant nodal and extranodal disease.
-   Potential biologic hallmark of advanced stage disease.

Stauder and colleagues [7] have gone on to look more closely at the relationship between the expression of the standard form of CD44 and the International Prognostic Index [24.10]. They found that patients with high levels of cellular CD44 are far more likely to fall into the high risk category of the International Index.

24.10 **CD44 Isoform Expression and the International Index**

Int I	CD44s		CD44v6	
	Neg	Pos	Neg	Pos
L	17	13	20	10
LI	4	4	4	4
HI	1	11	8	4
H	2	9	6	5

Stauder *et al.* 1995 [7]

However, the story is more complicated than originally believed because there are a variety of alternatively spliced forms of CD44 which result from inclusion of extra exons in the membrane-proximal extracellular domain [24.11]. This is of interest because a subset of these isoforms contain the exon 10. The expression of this sequence, both in lymphoid tumors and in epithelial malignancies, seems to confer metastatic potential. This alternatively spliced variant is also expressed transiently on activated B cells, suggesting that it may also participate in the trafficking of normal cells. The author's laboratory and others, including Stauder's group, have demonstrated that these alternatively spliced versions of CD44 are expressed in a subset of aggressive non-Hodgkin's lymphomas, and have independent prognostic significance.[7-9]

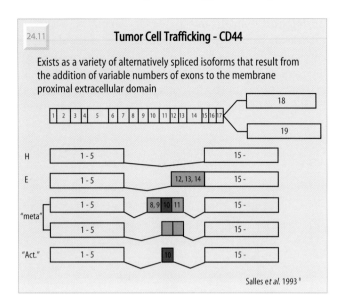

Tumor Cell Trafficking - CD44

Exists as a variety of alternatively spliced isoforms that result from the addition of variable numbers of exons to the membrane proximal extracellular domain

Salles *et al.* 1993 [8]

Other independent factors that have been identified, in addition to the CD44 variants, include proliferation indices, and some karyotypic abnormalities [24.7]. One of the most widely used markers of proliferation is Ki-67, a nuclear protein present in cycling cells that can be used to assess tumor growth fraction. Drs. Miller and Grogan in the Southwest Oncology Group have identified Ki-67 expression as an important prognostic factor in aggressive non-Hodgkin's lymphomas.[10] This enabled them to identify two groups of patients, one with a low proliferative index and one year survival of 82%, and another group with a high proliferative index and a one year survival of only 18%. Of particular interest was the finding that Ki-67 expression has independent prognostic significance, suggesting that it identifies something that is not covered by the clinical variables in the International Index.

One of the most interesting karyotypic abnormalities in aggressive non-Hodgkin's lymphoma is rearrangement of *BCL-6* as a result of chromosomal translocations involving 3q27 [24.12]. *BCL-6* encodes a protein that is homologous with zinc finger transcription factors. When molecular probes became available, *BCL-6* translocations were found in up to a third of large cell lymphomas, and they were shown to be more frequent in the aggressive or large cell B lymphomas than in other lymphoid malignancies.

24.12   *BCL-6* in Large Cell Lymphoma

- Chromosomal translocations affecting band 3q27 observed in 8-12% DLCL by cytogenetics

- *BCL-6* cloned from 3q27 chromosomal translocation

- *BCL-6* protein homologous with zinc finger transcription factors

Ye *et al.* 1993 [11]

Dr. Offit and colleagues at Memorial Sloan Kettering have studied the prognostic significance of *BCL-6* rearrangement in a series of aggressive non-Hodgkin's lymphomas [24.13].[12] One finding was that the great majority of patients with *BCL-6* rearrangement tended to present with extranodal disease. A second feature of interest was that patients with *BCL-6* rearrangement had a much greater freedom from progression than those patients who had germline *BCL-6*. When *BCL-6* rearrangement was assessed in relationship to other clinical features identified by the International Index, it was shown that *BCL-6* rearrangement was an independent prognostic factor.

24.13   Rearrangement of *BCL-6* in Patients with Aggressive NHL

- 23/102 patients with aggressive NHL had *BCL-6* rearrangement by Southern analysis.

- 19/23 patients with *BCL-6* rearrangement had extranodal disease. 2 additional patients had primary splenic lymphoma.

- Freedom from progression (FFP) 82% in patients with *BCL-6* rearrangement vs 56% in patients with germline *BCL-6* (p = 0.009).

- *BCL-6* status an independent prognostic marker of FFP and overall survival.

Offit *et al.* 1994 [12]

There are other karyotypic abnormalities that are also very likely to have prognostic significance, including t(14;18) [24.7]. Overexpression of BCL-2 protein may occur as a result of the 14;18 translocation, but it can also arise through other mechanisms that have yet to be characterized, and it results in the blocking of programmed cell death, or apoptosis, in B cells [24.14]. It is known that *BCL-2* rearrangement plays a major role in follicular lymphomas, but there are also a variety of data, from animal models, clinical trials and *in vitro* studies, to suggest that BCL-2 expression is also likely to be of importance in a subset of the aggressive lymphomas [24.15]. Transgenic mice that have the *BCL-2-Ig* hybrid gene initially develop indolent follicular hyperplasia. However, a subset of these animals subsequently develop immunoblastic lymphoma. There are also data from clinical trials, the largest one of which was performed by the GELA group, suggesting that patients with advanced stage disease are more likely to overexpress BCL-2. BCL-2 overexpression (which was not necessarily dependent on the presence of the (14;18) translocation) was linked to shortened disease-free survival. Other smaller studies have confirmed these initial observations.

BCL-2 in Lymphomas

Mechanism of action

t(14;18)(q32;q21) results in inappropriately elevated levels of the 18q21 gene product, *BCL-2*.

Over-expression of *BCL-2* blocks programmed cell death (apoptosis) in B cells.

Hockenbery *et al.* 1990 [13]

BCL-2 in Aggressive Non-Hodgkin's Lymphoma

Animal model

- Mice expressing a BCL-2/immunoglobulin transgene developed indolent follicular hyperplasia that progressed to immunoblastic lymphoma.

McDonnell *et al.* 1991 [14]

Clinical trials

- Patients with advanced stage disease more likely to have BCL-2 overexpression.
- BCL-2 overexpression linked with shortened disease-free survival.

Hermine *et al.* 1993 [15]

***In vitro* data**

- BCL-2 over-expression correlated with reduced chemosensitivity of murine and human lymphoma cell lines.

Miyashita and Reed, 1993 [16]

In this context, it is of note that Reed and colleagues have demonstrated that over-expression of *BCL-2* in chemosensitive lymphoma cell lines makes them chemoresistant, suggesting a potential mechanism for reduced chemosensitivity.

Similar observations have been made regarding other members of the BCL-2 family, including the long form of BCL-X which functions in a very similar way to BCL-2 [24.16]. Since *BCL-2* and *BCL-X* are both known to protect lymphoid cells from chemotherapy-induced apoptotic cell death, there is the interesting possibility that dysregulated expression of these molecules may contribute to differences in response to high dose therapy. In pilot studies at the author's institution, significant differences in outcome have been seen between patients who quickly achieve complete remission and those who do not.[17]

BCL-2/BCL-X_L and Observed Chemoresistance

- *BCL-2* and *BCL-X_L* protect lymphoid cells from chemotherapy-induced apoptotic cell death
- Dysregulated *BCL-2/BCL-X_L* expression may contribute to observed differences in response to high dose therapy
- In a pilot study of HI- and H-risk patients treated with a high dose induction regimen, patients who achieved CR in 2 cycles are more likely to remain disease-free (91% FFP in CR by 2 cycles vs 11% FFP in no CR by 2 cycles, p 0.0012)

Thus, when thinking about the relationship between biologic and clinical variables, it is necessary to consider not only features that are known to be correlated with previously identified clinical features, but also independent features and no doubt others that remain to be identified [24.17].

24.17 Clinical and Biological Heterogeneity in Large Cell Lymphoma Associated Clinical and Biological Features

Clinical features	Biological features
Stage	CD44s, *BCL-2*
Extranodal disease	*BCL-6, rel*
Performance status	IL-6
LDH	
Independent biological features	
	CD44v
	Ki-67
	BCL-6
Additional features	
	BCL-2/BCL-X_L
	p15/p16
	Immunocompetence

Shipp 1997 [18]

Finally, a commentary may be made about the difference, or lack of difference, between diffuse large cell lymphoma and immunoblastic lymphoma, two entities that have now been combined in the REAL classification [24.18]. Data were derived from the International Index study, based on more than 3,000 patients, and the survival curves for patients with diffuse large cell lymphoma and immunoblastic lymphoma, defined by either Working Formulation or Kiel criteria, are shown in [24.19]. There was a clear difference in outcome between the two categories, and this was statistically significant and of independent prognostic significance following multivariate analysis with other clinical features [24.20]. Therefore, rather than eliminating the distinction between the two entities, pathologists should be encouraged to find criteria which allow them to make the distinction objectively. A grading system like the one that Dr. Harris has proposed for follicular lymphomas (see Chapter 12) might provide one model to follow.

24.18 Aggressive Lymphomas

Working Formulation	REAL Classification	
	B cell neoplasms	T cell neoplasms
Intermediate grade		
G. Diffuse large cell	Diffuse large B cell lymphoma	Peripheral T cell
High grade		
H. Large cell immunoblastic	Diffuse large B cell lymphoma	Peripheral T cell ATL/L Anaplastic large cell

Shipp et al. 1997 [19]

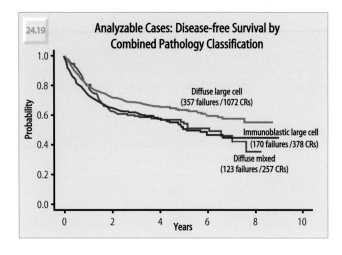

24.19 Analyzable Cases: Disease-free Survival by Combined Pathology Classification

Diffuse large cell (357 failures / 1072 CRs)

Immunoblastic large cell (170 failures / 378 CRs)

Diffuse mixed (123 failures / 257 CRs)

24.20 Combined Pathology Classification and The International Index

Factor	Risk ratio	p-value
Age > 60	1.867	0.0001
Stage	1.495	0.0001
Extranodal sites	1.384	0.0001
Performance	1.711	0.0001
LDH	1.778	0.0001
Diffuse mixed	1.174	0.12
Immunoblastic	1.392	0.0002

ACKNOWLEDGEMENTS

Figures [24.1], [24.10] and [24.11] are reproduced, respectively, from *Blood* 1994; **83**: 1165-73, *Blood* 1995; **85**: 2885-99 and *Blood* 1993; **82**: 3539-47 with copyright permission of W.B. Saunders Company.

Figures [24.2], [24.3], [24.4], [24.5] are reproduced from Shipp MA, Harrington DP, Anderson JR *et al* . (The International Non-Hodgkin's Lymphoma Prognostic Factors Project). A predictive model for aggressive non-Hodgkin's lymphoma. *New Engl J Med* 1993; **329**: 987-94. Copyright ©1993 Massachusetts Medical Society. All rights reserved. Adapted with permission 1998.

Figures [24.7] and [24.17] are reproduced from *Annals of Oncology* 1997; **8** (Suppl): 43-7, Can we improve upon the International Index? Shipp MA. Table 1 © Kluwer Academic Publishers with kind permission from Kluwer Academic Publishers.

Figure [24.18] is reproduced from DeVita VT, Hellman S, Rosenberg SA, eds. *Cancer Principles & Practice of Oncology*. Lippincott-Raven. 1997; Vol 2: 2165-2220, with copyright permission of Lippincott Williams and Wilkins.

REFERENCES

1. Shipp MA. Prognostic factors in aggressive non-Hodgkin's lymphoma: who has "high-risk" disease? *Blood* 1994; **83**:1165-73.

2. Shipp MA, Harrington DP, Anderson JR *et al.* (The International Non-Hodgkin's Lymphoma Prognostic Factors Project). A predictive model for aggressive non-Hodgkin's lymphoma. *New Engl J Med* 1993; **329**: 987-94.

3. Seymour JF, Talpaz M, Cabanillas F, Wetzler M, Kurzrock R. Serum interleukin-6 levels correlate with prognosis in diffuse large-cell lymphoma. *J Clin Oncol* 1995; **13**: 575-82.

4. Pals ST, Horst E, Ossekoppele GJ, Figdor CG, Scheper RJ, Meijer CJ. Expression of lymphocyte homing receptor as a mechanism of dissemination in non-Hodgkin's lymphoma. *Blood* 1989; **73**: 885-8.

5. Jalkanen S, Joensuu H, Klemi P. Prognostic value of lymphocyte homing receptor and S phase fraction in non-Hodgkin's lymphoma. *Blood* 1990; **75**: 1549-56.

6. Horst E, Meijer CJ, Radaszkiewicz T, Ossekoppele GJ, Van Krieken JH, Pals ST. Adhesion molecules in the prognosis of diffuse large-cell lymphoma: expression of a lymphocyte homing receptor (CD44), LFA-1 (CD11a/18), and ICAM-1 (CD54). *Leukemia* 1990; **4**: 595-9.

7. Stauder R, Eisterer W, Thaler J, Gunthert U. CD44 variant isoforms in non-Hodgkin's lymphoma: a new independent prognostic factor. *Blood* 1995; **85**: 2885-99.

8. Salles G, Zain M, Jiang WM, Boussiotis VA, Shipp MA. Alternatively spliced CD44 transcripts in diffuse large-cell lymphomas: characterization and comparison with normal activated B-cells and epithelial malignancies. *Blood* 1993; **82**: 3539-47.

9. Yakushijin Y, Steckel J, Kharbanda S *et al.* A directly spliced exon 10-containing CD44 variant promotes the metastasis and homotypic aggregation of aggressive non-Hodgkin's lymphoma. *Blood* 1998; **91**: 4282-91.

10. Miller TP, Grogan TM, Dahlberg S *et al.* Prognostic significance of the Ki-67-associated proliferative antigen in aggressive non-Hodgkin's lymphomas: a prospective Southwest Oncology Group trial. *Blood* 1994; **83**: 1460-6.

11. Ye BH, Lista F, Lo Coco F *et al.* Alterations of a zinc finger-encoding gene, BCL-6, in diffuse large-cell lymphoma. *Science* 1993; **262**: 747-50.

12. Offit K, Lo Coco F, Louie DC *et al.* Rearrangement of the bcl-6 gene as a prognostic marker in diffuse large-cell lymphoma. *New Engl J Med* 1994; **331**: 74-80.

13. Hockenbery D, Nunez G, Milliman C, Schreiber RD, Korsmeyer SJ. Bcl-2 is an inner mitochondrial membrane protein that blocks programmed cell death. *Nature* 1990; **348**: 334-6.

14. McDonnell TJ; Korsmeyer SJ. Progression from lymphoid hyperplasia to high-grade malignant lymphoma in mice transgenic for the t(14;18). *Nature* 1991; **349**: 254-6.

15. Hermine O, Haioun C, Lepage E *et al.* Bcl-2 protein expression in aggressive non-Hodgkin's lymphoma (NHL). A new adverse prognostic factor? *Fifth International Conference on Malignant Lymphoma* 1993; 28.

16. Miyashita T, Reed JC. Bcl-2 oncoprotein blocks chemotherapy-induced apoptosis in a human leukemia cell line. *Blood* 1993; **81**: 151-7.

17. Janicek M, Kaplan W, Neuberg D, Canellos GP, Shulman LN, Shipp MA. Early restaging gallium scans predict outcome in poor prognosis patients with aggressive non-Hodgkin's lymphoma treated with high-dose CHOP chemotherapy. *J Clin Oncol* 1997; **15**: 1631-7.

18. Shipp MA. Can we improve upon the International Index? *Ann Oncol* 1997; **8** Suppl 1: 43-7.

19. Shipp MA, Harris NL, Mauch PM. Non-Hodgkin's Lymphomas. In: DeVita VT, Hellman S, Rosenberg SA, eds. *Cancer Principles & Practice of Oncology*. Lippincot-Raven. 1997; Vol 2: 2165-2220.

FURTHER READING

Bastion Y, Berger F, Bryon PA, Felman P, Ffrench M, Coiffier B. Follicular lymphomas: assessment of prognostic factors in 127 patients followed for 10 years. *Ann Oncol* 1991; **2** (Suppl 2): 123-9.

Coiffier B, Brousse N, Peuchmaur M *et al.* Peripheral T-cell lymphomas have a worse prognosis than B-cell lymphomas: a prospective study of 361 immunophenotyped patients treated with the LNH-84 regimen. *Ann Oncol* 1990; **1**: 45-50.

Hermans J, Krol AD, van Groningen K *et al.* International Prognostic Index for aggressive non-Hodgkin's lymphoma is valid for all malignancy grades. *Blood* 1995; **86**: 1460-3.

List AF, Spier CM, Miller TP, Grogan TM. Deficient tumor-infiltrating T-lymphocyte response in malignant lymphoma: relationship to HLA expression and host immunocompetence. *Leukemia* 1993; **7**: 398-403.

Minn AJ, Rudin CM, Boise LH, Thompson CB. Expression of bcl-X_L can confer a multidrug resistance phenotype. *Blood* 1995; **86**: 1903-10.

Miyashita T, Reed JC. Bcl-2 gene transfer increases relative resistance of S49.1 and WEHI7.2 lymphoid cells to cell death and DNA fragmentation induced by glucocorticoids and multiple chemotherapeutic drugs. *Cancer Res* 1992; **52**: 5407-11.

Shipp MA. Prognostic factors in aggressive non-Hodgkin's lymphoma: who has "high-risk" disease? *Blood* 1994; **83**: 1165-73.

Swan F Jr, Velasquez WS, Tucker S, Redman JR. A new serologic staging system for large-cell lymphomas based on initial beta 2-microglobulin and lactate dehydrogenase levels. *J Clin Oncol* 1989; **7**: 1518-27.

Yunis JJ, Mayer MG, Arnesen MA, Aeppli DP, Oken MM, Frizzera G. Bcl-2 and other genomic alterations in the prognosis of large-cell lymphoma. *New Engl J Med* 1989; **320**: 1047-54.

Risk-related treatment strategies for diffuse large B cell lymphoma

B Coiffier

Patients with large cell lymphoma have differing prognoses. Even within a single histologic subtype, outcome is influenced by a number of factors (not all of which are recognized), and the optimal treatment differs from one patient to another.

Another lesson of the last 10 years is that patients who are not cured by the first line of treatment will probably never be cured. Shown in [25.1] are the overall survival and progression-free survival of all patients included in the LNH 1984 trial who relapsed or progressed after achieving complete remission. One sees that very few, if any, of them were cured. Consequently if patients are going to be cured, this has to be achieved with the first line treatment.

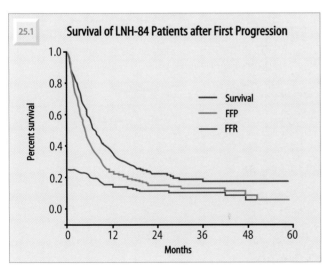

Another clear clinical finding is that, although it is not certain if increasing the dosage of chemotherapy is better for the patient, one can be certain that decreasing the dosage gives worse results. Shown in [25.2] are the results for the GELA group, and similar patterns are found in the literature. When the dose administered was reduced, either by decreasing the dosage or increasing the times between each course, the therapeutic results were clearly worse.

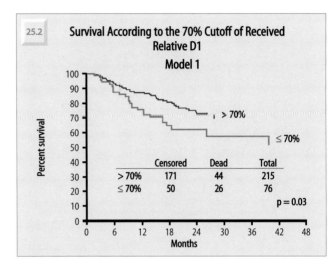

Another lesson is that patients remain at risk of relapse even after 3 or 4 years. Results from the LNH-84 study [25.3] show the number of patients relapsing year by year. Each column represents one year, and the curve indicates the risk of relapse. Although most patients who relapsed did so during the first 2 or 3 years after treatment, nevertheless relapses continued for 8 years, and will probably continue for at least 10 years. In consequence, one must wait for at least 5 or 6 years from initial treatment before talking in terms of a cure.

Another lesson which emerges from the literature is that CHOP is the gold standard for treatment of aggressive lymphomas. Results [25.4 and 25.5] were published by Dr. Fisher more than 10 years ago, and also more recently, concerning different variations of CHOP used in the SWOG studies. It is evident that CHOP is the best treatment available, but also that, during the last ten years, the results obtained with CHOP have not been improved upon with newer regimes, and that 60% of patients are still not cured. A major clinical task is therefore to improve the outlook for the substantial number of patients who are not cured by CHOP or other chemotherapy regimens.

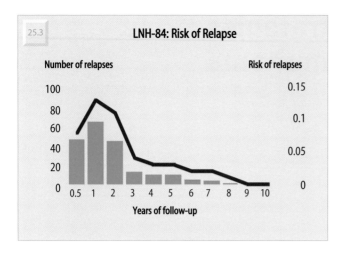

25.3 **LNH-84: Risk of Relapse**

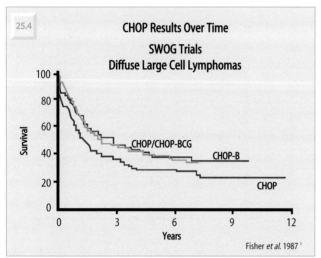

25.4 **CHOP Results Over Time**
SWOG Trials
Diffuse Large Cell Lymphomas

Fisher *et al.* 1987 [1]

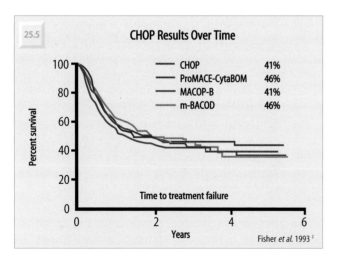

25.5 **CHOP Results Over Time**

Fisher *et al.* 1993 [2]

How may this be achieved? It is clear that prognostic factors enable us to identify different groups of patients, and that patients can be stratified into different treatment groups. In France the LNH-93 protocol has introduced the idea of stratifying patients in a trial according both to age and to adverse prognostic factors [25.6]. The International Index prognostic factors (stage, performance status and LDH) was used so that patients could be treated according to their probable outcome.

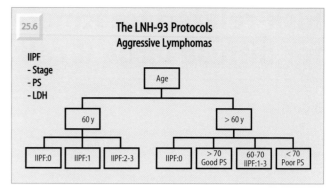

25.6 **The LNH-93 Protocols**
Aggressive Lymphomas

It may be added that, although stage, performance status and LDH are major prognostic factors, β2-microglobulin is also a factor. It was not included in the International Index because at that time β2-microglobulin level was measured at diagnosis in very few patients in America and in Europe. The curves in [25.7] make the point that, for the LNH-84 regimen, the risk of relapse related to the initial LDH level, and that patients with the highest LDH level clearly had the highest risk of relapse. However, β2-microglobulin was also significant, as shown when the survival of patients from the author's center was related to initial LDH and β2-microglobulin levels [25.8]. The patients in whom both were elevated had the worst prognosis, so that it is important to take into account not only the International Index but also β2-microglobulin.

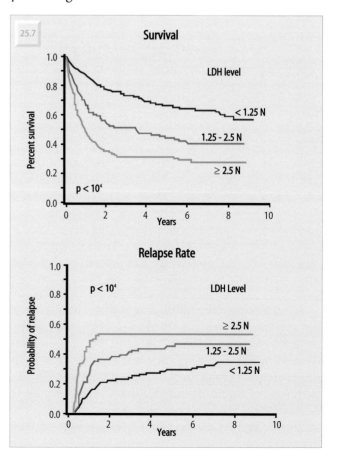

25.7 **Survival**

Relapse Rate

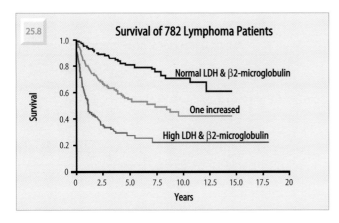

Which drugs should be used for treatment [25.9]? It is now accepted from many trials that there are two major drugs, doxorubicin and cyclophosphamide. Other drugs have a role to play, but they are not valuable if they entail a decrease in the dose of these two major drugs.

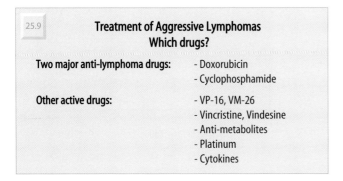

How should we manage patients without any adverse prognostic factors [25.10]? In the author's opinion, one should use a standard chemotherapy regimen. The particular protocol chosen should be the one with which the oncologist is most familiar, for example CHOP or BACOD, provided it can achieve 80% cure. [25.11] shows a trial in which the LNH-84 protocol and m-BACOD were compared, and for low risk patients without any adverse factors, there was no difference in freedom from progression or overall survival. Low-risk patients with localized disease may be treated as well with 3 or 4 courses of CHOP followed by radiation therapy. We are therefore justified in basing our choice on personal preference, although in the author's view CHOP is probably preferable because of its simplicity.

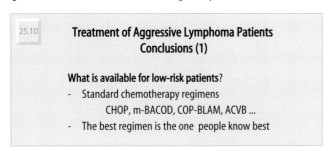

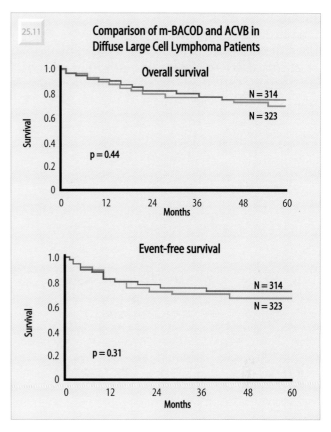

One important point is that for any treatment there is a learning curve, as illustrated in [25.12] for LNH-84. The death rate due to toxicity or treatment failure was greater at the beginning of the trial, when very few patients had been included, but it decreased with time. Every oncologist has to learn how to use a particular treatment regime, and the lesson is not to change the treatment too often.

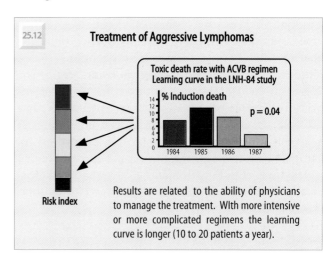

For intermediate risk patients, the combination of high dose cyclophosphamide and high dose doxorubicin is probably among the best [25.13]. It has been in the LNH-84 studies for years, and Dr. Shipp and others have used high dose CHOP or similar regimens under different names. With this type of treatment, one can achieve a ten year survival for intermediate risk patients of around 50% [25.14]. These patients fare better on high dose CHOP than on standard CHOP. We are currently finishing a trial comparing ACVP (high dose CHOP) with CHOP, in which we included 450 patients.

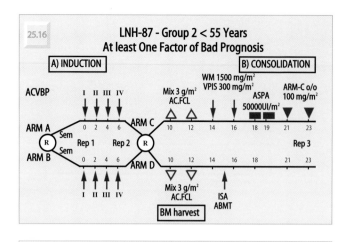

25.16 LNH-87 - Group 2 < 55 Years
At least One Factor of Bad Prognosis

25.13

Treatment of Aggressive Lymphoma Patients
Conclusions (2)

What is available for intermediate-risk patients?
- High-dose combination of cyclophosphamide and doxorubicin LNH-84 regimen is a good candidate
- The role of higher doses with stem cell support is unknown

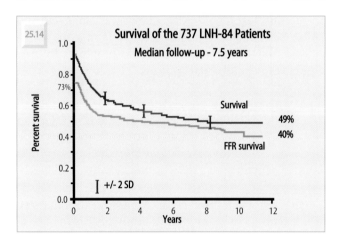

25.14 Survival of the 737 LNH-84 Patients
Median follow-up - 7.5 years

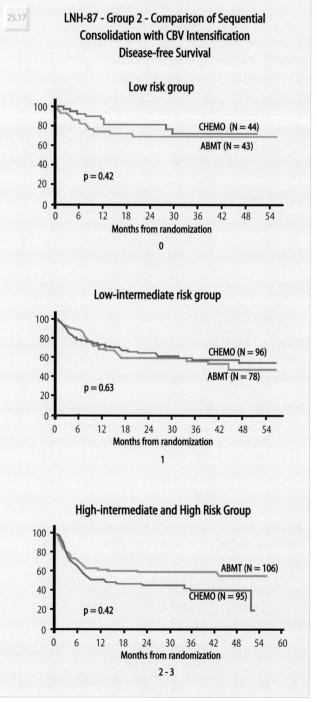

25.17 LNH-87 - Group 2 - Comparison of Sequential Consolidation with CBV Intensification
Disease-free Survival

Low risk group

Low-intermediate risk group

High-intermediate and High Risk Group

What can one offer the high risk patient [25.15]? There is no consensus on this in the literature, but one possibility is to increase the dosage and to combine it with stem cell transplantation. This strategy was adopted in the LNH-87 study for a subgroup of young patients with adverse prognostic factors, who were randomized between a regimen of standard consolidation combined with chemotherapy, versus high dose therapy and bone marrow transplantation [25.16]. The results, published in the *Journal of Clinical Oncology* by Dr. Haioun,[3] showed that for patients with no adverse prognostic factors, or with only one adverse prognostic factor, there was no difference between the two treatments [25.17]. However, for patients with two or three adverse prognostic factors, at the time of publication and subsequently, a statistically significant advantage has emerged for patients transplanted in the first year [25.18].

25.15

Treatment of Aggressive Lymphoma Patients
Conclusions (3)

What is available for low-risk patients?
- No good treatment
- Necessity of prospective randomized studies
  - Intensive chemotherapy regimens
  - Cytokines

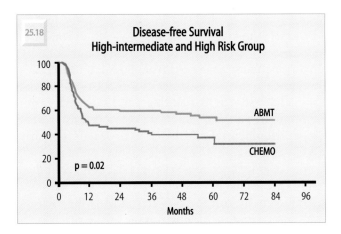

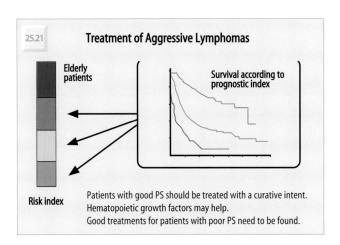

We have tried to improve on this result by giving high dose treatment earlier in the disease, before or just after the patients achieved complete remission [25.19]. Young patients with the same adverse prognostic factors were randomized either to early intensification, accompanied by peripheral blood stem cell transplantation, or to the classical ACVB regimen. We aimed to see if it would be possible in the worst outcome patients to increase the complete remission rate and to decrease relapses.

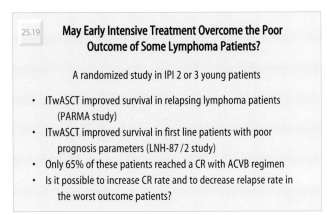

Initially standard CHOP with epirubicin as given [25.20]. Two courses of a higher dosage of epirubicin with a higher dosage of cyclophosphamide were then given, together with G-CSF, to allow harvest of blood stem cells. This was followed by BEAM chemotherapy and auto-transplant.

Unfortunately, this approach was not a success. A total of 300 patients, mainly with diffuse large cell lymphoma, were included, all of whom were aged below 60 and had two or (in 35%) three adverse prognostic factors. When a comparison is made between the standard arm and the intensive arm, the complete remission rate is nearly the same, as is mortality during induction, but the two year event-free survival is worse for the intensive arm, as is the three year survival. The reason is probably that high dose therapy was given too early in the history of the disease.

Any review of the treatment of diffuse large B cell lymphoma should include a consideration of elderly patients since half of the patients are older than 60 years [25.21]. They vary in their prognosis, but those with no or very few adverse prognostic factors should be treated. In this trial the survival of patients older than 70 years was relatively good, even when some adverse prognostic factors are present. These patients will die of their lymphoma, if untreated, within one year, whereas with treatment they may achieve a reasonable survival. For elderly patients, randomized trials have shown that the best outcome was reached with the CHOP regimen too.

In relapsed patients high dose therapy is better than chemotherapy. Shown in [25.22] are the event-free and overall survival curves from the PARMA trial, published by Dr. Philip,[4] showing an improved survival. However, if one looks carefully at the results, one sees that although more than 200 relapsing patients were included in the trial, only a small number, 100 patients, were randomized. The others were not randomized because they did not respond or they progressed. Consequently, there is a need to find a treatment strategy for such patients, since high dose therapy in relapse is not the final answer. It is useful only for those patients who respond to a salvage regimen and who do not relapse subsequently. However, salvage chemotherapy followed by high-dose therapy and autotransplant is currently considered the standard regimen for relapsing aggressive patients.

In conclusion, what can we hope for in the feature in the treatment of lymphoma [25.23]? We need to find new drugs to add to cyclophosphamide and doxorubicin, for example taxol. So far, however, this strategy has not been successful, and Dr. Fisher and others have shown that adding a third drug does not increase the survival rate.[1,2] We also need to prevent the development of resistance to drugs, particularly taking into account the MDR or other phenotypes. Some trials are currently in progress, but no definitive results are available, and it is not clear if this will offer a solution in the future. For some patients, the solution may come from increasing dosage of the drugs with the help of growth factors. Another approach, that may be feasible, is to exploit biological factors, using, for example, immunotherapy. We may also in the future prevent relapse by attacking minimal residual disease, using agents such as interferon and cytokines.

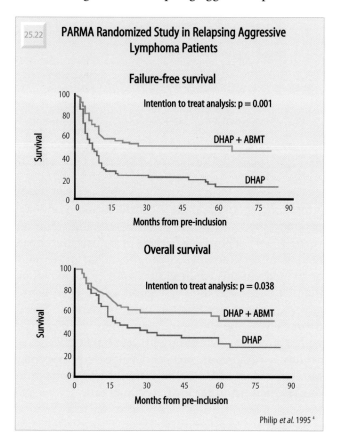

25.22

PARMA Randomized Study in Relapsing Aggressive Lymphoma Patients

Failure-free survival

Intention to treat analysis: p = 0.001

DHAP + ABMT

DHAP

Survival

Months from pre-inclusion

Overall survival

Intention to treat analysis: p = 0.038

DHAP + ABMT

DHAP

Survival

Months from pre-inclusion

Philip *et al.* 1995 [4]

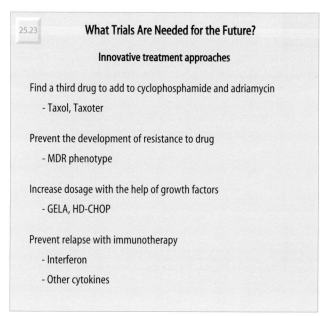

25.23

What Trials Are Needed for the Future?

Innovative treatment approaches

Find a third drug to add to cyclophosphamide and adriamycin

- Taxol, Taxoter

Prevent the development of resistance to drug

- MDR phenotype

Increase dosage with the help of growth factors

- GELA, HD-CHOP

Prevent relapse with immunotherapy

- Interferon

- Other cytokines

REFERENCES

1. Fisher RI, Miller TP, Dana BW, Jones SE, Dahlberg S, Coltman CA Jr. Southwest oncology group clinical trials for intermediate and high-grade non-Hodgkin's lymphomas. *Semin Hematol* 1987; **24** (2 Suppl 1): 21-5.

2. Fisher RI, Gaynor ER, Dahlberg S *et al*. Comparison of a standard regimen (CHOP) with three intensive chemotherapy regimens for advanced non-Hodgkin's lymphoma. *N Engl J Med* 1993; **328**: 1002-6.

3. Haioun C, Lepage E, Gisselbrecht C *et al*. Comparison of autologous bone marrow transplantation with sequential chemotherapy for intermediate-grade and high-grade non-Hodgkin's lymphoma in first complete remission: a study of 464 patients. Groupe d'Etude des Lymphomes de l'Adulte. *J Clin Oncol* 1994; **12**: 2543-51.

4. Philip T, Guglielmi C, Hagenbeek A *et al*. Autologous bone marrow transplantation as compared with salvage chemotherapy in relapses of chemotherapy-sensitive non-Hodgkin's lymphoma. *N Engl J Med* 1995; **333**: 1540-5.

FURTHER READING

Diviné M, Lepage E, Brière J *et al*. Is the small non-cleaved-cell lymphoma histologic subtype a poor prognostic factor in adult patients? A case-controlled analysis. Groupe d'Etude des Lymphomes de l'Adulte. *J Clin Oncol* 1996; **14**: 240-8.

Haioun C, Lepage E, Gisselbrecht C *et al*. Benefit of autologous bone marrow transplantation over sequential chemotherapy in poor-risk aggressive non-Hodgkin's lymphoma: updated results of the prospective study LNH87-2. Groupe d'Etude des Lymphomes de l'Adulte. *J Clin Oncol* 1997; **15**: 1131-7.

Miller TP, Dahlberg S, Cassady JR *et al*. Chemotherapy alone compared with chemotherapy plus radiotherapy for localized intermediate- and high-grade non-Hodgkin's lymphoma. *N Engl J Med* 1998; **339**: 21-6.

The International Non-Hodgkin's Lymphoma Prognostic Factors Project. A predictive model for aggressive non-Hodgkin's lymphoma. *N Engl J Med* 1993; **329**: 987-94.

The Non-Hodgkin's Lymphoma Classification Project. A clinical evaluation of the International Lymphoma Study Group classification of non-Hodgkin's lymphoma. *Blood* 1997; **89**: 3909-18.

The Non-Hodgkin's Lymphoma Classification Project. Effect of age on the characteristics and clinical behavior of non-Hodgkin's lymphoma patients. *Ann Oncol* 1997; **8**: 973-0.

Tilly H, Gaulard P, Lepage E *et al*. Primary anaplastic large-cell lymphoma in adults: clinical presentation, immuno-phenotype, and outcome. *Blood* 1997; **90**: 3727-34.

Treatment of early stage diffuse large B cell lymphoma, including mediastinal large cell lymphoma

P M Mauch

In the 1970s the standard treatment for Stage I and II diffuse large cell lymphoma was involved field, regional field or extended field radiation. However, a number of published studies showed a high recurrence rate with radiation therapy alone [26.1]. The best results were seen in patients with limited Stage I disease, who achieved about a 50% freedom from recurrence, and in Stage II patients, who showed about 20% freedom from recurrence. About 15-20% were "in field" recurrences, but the majority were extranodal. Early randomized trials, published in the early 1980s, compared involved field or regional radiation to radiation followed by chemotherapy (initially CVP, and then BACOP or other regimens). It was demonstrated that disease-free and overall survival results were superior for patients receiving combined radiation and chemotherapy, versus radiation alone.

26.1

Stage I - II DLCL
Early Studies

High recurrence rates with regional radiotherapy alone:
50% freedom from recurrence for Stage I patients

Chen et al. 1979 [1]

20% freedom from recurrence for Stage II patients

Reddy et al. 1977 [2]

Early randomized trials of radiotherapy vs radiotherapy + chemotherapy demonstrated freedom from recurrence and survival advantages for combined therapy in the early 1980s.

Monfardini et al. 1980; [3] Nissen et al. 1983 [4]

Several studies have reported more favorable results with radiation therapy alone, and they fall into two categories. One of these [26.2] was a study from the Princess Margaret Hospital of carefully selected patients with minimal disease, which reported favorable results with radiation alone in patients with early stage disease and a recurrence rate of only about 25%. To be included, the patients had to be young, to have minimal nodal disease (less than 2.5 cm in size), and to be Stage I or Stage II, with two contiguous groups of involved nodes.

26.2

Stage I - II DLCL
Favorable Results with RT

PMH experience; favorable results with RT alone in patients with early stage disease (23% recurrence rates)

Age < 60
Nodes < 2.5 cm
Stage I or Stage II (contiguous groups)

Stage I experience with extensive staging and treatment

Gospodarowicz et al. 1984; [5] Sutcliffe et al. 1985 [6]

There is also experience with more extensive staging and treatment. An approach involving surgical staging (laparotomy) and wide-field irradiation was pioneered at the Universities of Minnesota, Chicago and Stanford [26.3]. All three institutions used staging laparotomy to exclude patients with abdominal involvement. The minimum field of radiation would be a mantle field, treating all the nodes above the diaphragm, and often the abdominal and/or pelvic nodes would also be treated. In these studies, the survival figures achieved in patients with disease limited to a single node site were 70-75%. The results were substantially poorer, even in this very extensively staged and treated group, for patients with Stage II disease, whose survival was only 35-50%.

26.3

Stage I - II DLCL
Surgically Staged - TR Alone

Institution	Treatment	Stage	Survival
U. of Minn [7]	STLI, TLI (11)	I	75% (10 year)
U. of Chicago [8]	M, MPA (36)	I	91% (10 year)
		II	35% (10 year)
Stanford U. [9]	STLI, TLI (32)	I	73% (5 year)
		II	56% (5 year)

The advent of effective combination chemotherapy regimens led to studies based on the use of chemotherapy alone in limited stage large cell lymphoma. Two studies [26.4], one from the MD Anderson Hospital and the other from the University of Arizona, reported relapse-free survival rates in the 75-85% range for Stage I, and a little lower for Stage II.

26.4	Stage I - II DLCL Chemotherapy Alone				
Institution	Treatment	Stage	RNS	Survival
MDAH [10]	CHOP (30)	I	83%	100%
		II	65%	63%
U. of Arizona [11]	CHOP (28)	I - II	75%	80%

There have been larger studies of combined modality therapy, building on the initial randomized trials, with follow-up of 5 to 6 years [26.5]. At Stanford University, standard chemotherapy with the CHOP regimen mixed with extended field radiation gave disease-free survivals in a total of 48 Stage I and II patients of 90 and 70% respectively. At the University of Arizona, using more limited radiation fields after CHOP, an 85-90% disease-free survival was achieved for Stage I and II disease.

26.5	Stage I - II DLCL Combined Modality Therapy (5-6 year)				
Study	Treatment	Stage	RFS	Survival
Standard chemotherapy				
Stanford U. [9]	CHOP - EFRT (48)	I	90%	80%
		II	70%	68%
U. of Arizona [11]	CHOP - IFRT (17)	I - II	87%	93%
Reduced chemotherapy				
Vancouver [12]	CHOPx3 - IFRT (78)	I - II (78)	84%	85%
NCI [13]	ProMace-MOPP x 4 - IFRT (47)	I	100%	96%

Several institutions have proposed that involved field radiation could be combined with a reduction in either the number of cycles or the total dose of chemotherapy. In the Vancouver study, limited doses of standard CHOP for three cycles were followed by involved field radiation, and in the NCI study, a 75% dose of the ProMace-MOPP regimen was used for four cycles, followed by involved field irradiation. Both studies, which comprised about 130 patients in total, showed very good results with a combination of reduced chemotherapy and limited radiation therapy.

The effectiveness of combination chemotherapy means that there has been much discussion about the role of radiation in early stage large cell lymphoma, and in this context a randomized trial from the Eastern Co-operative Oncology Group for Stage I and

II patients is relevant [26.6].[14] Patients had bulky or extranodal Stage I disease or Stage II disease, and all patients received CHOP for eight cycles. There were 365 patients in the study, and patients who achieved complete remission were randomized to receive radiation (at 3,000 cGy) or no further treatment, and patients in partial remission received radiation at somewhat higher dose. In this study 32% of patients were Stage I and 68% Stage II. The median age was 59, and about a third of the patients had bulky disease. For patients who achieved complete remission, the addition of involved field radiation to the CHOP regimen brought a significant advantage in terms of disease-free survival and freedom from recurrence, and also an advantage, of borderline significance, in terms of overall survival [26.6]. The SWOG trial randomized patients (Stage I and II) to 3 cycles CHOP and involved field RT vs 8 cycles of CHOP alone. CHOP + RT had a significantly better progression-free survival (p = 0.03) and overall survival (p = 0.02) compared to CHOP alone.[15]

26.6	ECOG Stage I - II Randomized Trial		
Design			
Bulky or extranodal Stage I patients; Stage II patients			
All patients received CHOP x 8			
Patients in CR were randomized to receive			
RT (3,000 cGy) or			
No further treatment			
Patients in PR received RT (4,000 cGy)			
Results of Patients in CR			
Results	CHOP + RT	CHOP alone	p
DFS	73%	58%	0.03
FFR	73%	58%	0.04
OS	84%	70%	0.06
			Glick *et al.* 1995 [14]

Despite these excellent results, there is a group of patients with Stage I or Stage II disease who have a poor prognosis. Three different institutions have studied Stage I - II patients for prognostic factors. Cause-specific survival data from the author's institution on 144 patients who were treated with chemotherapy, with or without radiation is shown in [26.7].[16] The upper curve, giving an 82% survival at ten years, represents patients with Stage I or Stage II disease limited to two contiguous sites. The lower curve, with a 54% survival, represents patients with bulky abdominal disease, bulky thoracic disease or more than two sites of involvement.

Similar data have been reported from other institutions. In a study published in 1988 from Stanford, 94 patients were given combined chemotherapy and radiation [26.8].[17] The three most important factors, in terms of predicting a poor prognosis, were elevated LDH, tumor bulk greater than 10 cm, and whether or not patients had been treated by the "sandwich" technique. Patients who received a combination of radiation and chemotherapy, but with the radiation being given in the middle as opposed to initially or at the end, had a somewhat better prognosis.

also a frustrating area in terms of giving adjuvant radiation, because of the very extensive involvement of the heart and lung in many of these patients. The CT scan shown in [26.10] shows very extensive anterior mediastinal involvement in a patient with diffuse large cell lymphoma.

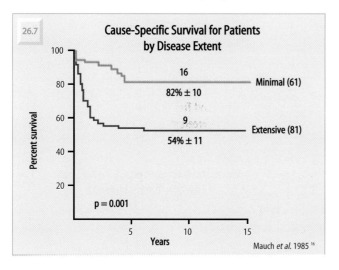

Cause-Specific Survival for Patients by Disease Extent

Mauch *et al.* 1985 [16]

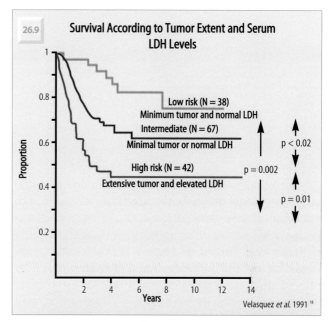

Survival According to Tumor Extent and Serum LDH Levels

Velasquez *et al.* 1991 [18]

26.8 — Results Univariate Analysis of Presentation and Treatment Variables for Correlation with Freedom from Relapse (FFR) and Survival

Covariate	p-value for FFR	p-value for survival
LDH (≤ 200 U/L vs > 200 U/L)	< 0.0001	< 0.001
Histology (immunoblastic vs other)	0.005	0.005
Therapy sequence ("sandwich" vs other)	0.007	0.011
Chemotherapy cycles (≤ 6 vs > 6)	0.026	0.018
Tumor bulk (≤ 10 cm vs > 10 cm)	0.045	0.014

Prestidge *et al.* 1988 [17]

The curves in [26.9] are from the MD Anderson Hospital. The top curve shows patients who did not have extensive disease or an elevated LDH, the middle group are patients that had either extensive disease or an elevated LDH, and the bottom group shows patients that had both extensive involvement and an elevated LDH. Extensive involvement was defined as either an abnormal chest radiograph or tumor bulk greater than 7 cm.

Some comments may be made on patients who have localized primary mediastinal involvement. This is often a difficult group to manage because of the very extensive involvement within the chest, often with invasion of tissues such as the chest wall. This is

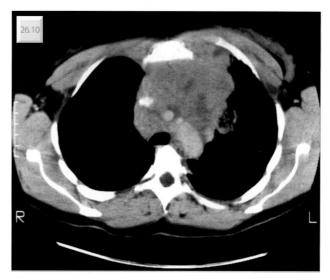

A series of such patients was published in the *Journal of Clinical Oncology* by Dr. Kirn,[19] who was working with Dr. Shulman at the Brigham and Women's Hospital, and with a number of collaborators at the Dana Farber Institute in Boston [26.11]. He reviewed 57 patients, comprising 60% diffuse large cell lymphomas and 40% immunoblastic lymphomas. The median age was 31 years, and the median follow-up was about two and a half years. About 75% of patients had bulky disease, defined as greater than 10 cm in size, and a third of the patients had B symptoms. The chemotherapy regimens varied [26.11], but most patients received either BACOD or CHOP.

26.11

Mediastinal Lymphoma

57 patients
Large cell or immunoblastic lymphoma
(lymphoblastic lymphoma excluded)
M:F 30:27
Median age = 31 years
Median follow-up = 30 months

Chemotherapy regimen
M/m-BACOD 37 pts (65%)
CHOP 7 pts (19%)
Other 6 pts (16%)

Relapse rate
M/m-BACOD 18/37 (49%)
CHOP 5/7 (71%)
(p = 0.25 Fisher's)

26.13

Prognostic Factors for Relapse and Survival

Variable	Significance (p)	
	Relapse	Survival
Pleural effusion	0.015	0.001
Positive post therapy ^{67}Ga scan	0.01	0.027
Number of extranodal sites (≤ 1 vs ≥ 2)	< 0.01	0.022
Response to primary therapy	0.02	0.27
LDH ratio (> 3 vs < 3)	0.04	0.33
Age	0.95	0.95
Sex	0.99	0.99
B symptoms	0.45	0.55
Radiation therapy	0.10	0.57
Bulk disease	0.33	0.45

Kirn *et al.* 1993[19]

When the freedom from progression and survival in this group of patients are reviewed [26.12], plateaux of approximately 50% are seen. These patients are therefore at higher risk than are routine patients with Stage I or Stage II disease. The prognostic factors that appeared to be most important for relapse and survival were the presence of pleural effusions, positive post-therapy gallium scans, and the number of initial extranodal sites of involvement [26.13]. In terms of relapse-free survival, an elevated LDH and the response to primary treatment were also prognostically significant. Patients who had positive gallium scans, either half way through chemotherapy or at the end of chemotherapy, all recurred, whereas there was about a 60% freedom from progression in patients who had negative scans [26.14]. In terms of pleural effusions and tumor bulk, the most favorable group of patients were those who did not have an effusion, and who had less than 10 cm disease: their disease-free survival was very similar to that of patients with more favorable diffuse large cell lymphoma [26.15]. Again, one adverse feature in this group was large bulky disease, giving a disease-free survival of about 50%. If a pleural effusion was present, the prognosis was also poor.

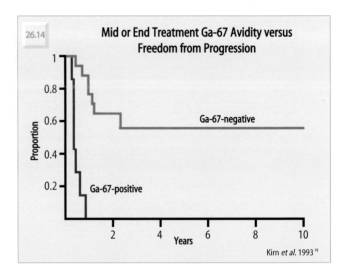

26.14

Mid or End Treatment Ga-67 Avidity versus Freedom from Progression

Kirn *et al.* 1993[19]

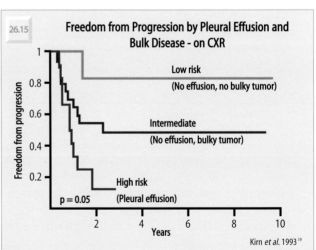

26.15

Freedom from Progression by Pleural Effusion and Bulk Disease - on CXR

Kirn *et al.* 1993[19]

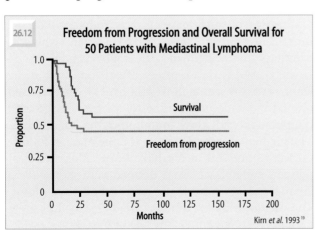

26.12

Freedom from Progression and Overall Survival for 50 Patients with Mediastinal Lymphoma

Kirn *et al.* 1993[19]

In summary [26.16], it is evident that there is still a lot to learn about prognostic categories among these different groups of patients. Some of the biologic factors that are discussed elsewhere by Dr. Shipp for advanced disease (Chapter 24) may also help in the treatment of early stage patients. However, for patients with minimal disease, Stage I or limited Stage II disease, cure rates approaching 90% can be achieved with modified chemotherapy (three to four cycles of CHOP for example) and involved field radiation (i.e. radiation limited to the initial nodal group of involvement). There are also patients who can respond well to larger numbers of cycles of chemotherapy, especially patients with very minimal initial disease. There is also a subgroup of patients who fare well with radiation alone, but patients need to be carefully selected for both of these alternative treatments. There is evidence from the ECOG and SWOG trials for Stage I and for Stage II patients, that the addition of involved field radiation to standard dose CHOP adds significantly to disease-free survival.

Finally, there is the group of Stage II patients with poor prognostic features. These are largely patients with bulky thoracic disease, although patients with abdominal disease fall into the same category, and they are very difficult to treat. One option is to use higher dose chemotherapy, such as the high dose

CHOP and G-CSF approach which Dr. Shipp and the CALGB are studying. The role for radiation therapy in high-risk CS I - II patients remains unanswered because of the extent of the disease and the large radiation fields that are often needed.

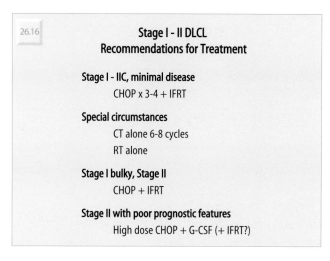

26.16

**Stage I - II DLCL
Recommendations for Treatment**

Stage I - IIC, minimal disease
CHOP x 3-4 + IFRT

Special circumstances
CT alone 6-8 cycles
RT alone

Stage I bulky, Stage II
CHOP + IFRT

Stage II with poor prognostic features
High dose CHOP + G-CSF (+ IFRT?)

REFERENCES

1. Chen MG, Prosnitz LR, Gonzalez-Serva A, Fischer DB. Results of radiotherapy in control of stage I and II non-Hodgkin's lymphoma. *Cancer* 1979; **43**: 1245-54.

2. Reddy S, Saxena VS, Pellettiere EV, Hendrickson FR. Early nodal and extra-nodal non-Hodgkin's lymphomas. *Cancer* 1977; **40**: 98-104.

3. Monfardini S, Banfi A, Bonadonna G *et al*. Improved five year survival after combined radiotherapy-chemotherapy for stage I-II non-Hodgkin's lymphoma. *Int J Radiat Oncol Biol Phys* 1980; **6**: 125-34.

4. Nissen NI, Ersboll J, Hansen HS *et al*. A randomized study of radiotherapy versus radiotherapy plus chemotherapy in stage I-II non-Hodgkin's lymphomas. *Cancer* 1983; **52**: 1-7.

5. Gospodarowicz MK, Bush RS, Brown TC. Role of radiation in treatment of patients with localized intermediate and high-grade non-Hodgkin's lymphoma. *Proc Amer Soc Clin Onc* 1984a; **3**: C-922 (abstr).

6. Sutcliffe SB, Gospodarowicz MK, Bush RS *et al*. Role of radiation therapy in localized non-Hodgkin's lymphoma. *Radiother Oncol* 1985; **4**: 211-23.

7. Levitt SH, Lee CK, Bloomfield CD, Frizzera G. The role of radiation therapy in the treatment of early stage large cell lymphoma. *Hematol Oncol* 1985; **3**: 33-7.

8. Hallahan DE, Farah R, Vokes EE *et al*. The patterns of failure in patients with pathological stage I and II diffuse histiocytic lymphoma treated with radiation therapy alone. *Int J Radiat Oncol Biol Phys* 1989; **17**: 767-71.

9. Hoppe RT. The role of radiation therapy in the management of the non-Hodgkin's lymphomas. *Cancer* 1985; **55** (Suppl): 2176-83.

10. Cabanillas F, Bodey GP, Freireich EJ. Management with chemotherapy only of stage I and II malignant lymphoma of aggressive histologic types. *Cancer* 1980; **46**: 2356-9.

11. Miller TP, Jones SE. Initial chemotherapy for clinically localized lymphomas of unfavorable histology. *Blood* 1983; **62**: 413-8.

12. Connors JM, Klimo P, Fairey RN, Voss N. Brief chemotherapy and involved field radiation therapy for limited-stage, histologically aggressive lymphoma. *Ann Intern Med* 1987; **107**: 25-30.

13. Longo DL, Glatstein E, Duffey PL *et al*. Treatment of localized aggressive lymphomas with combination chemotherapy followed by involved-field radiation therapy. *J Clin Oncol* 1989; **7**: 1295-302.

14. Glick J, Kim K, Earle J, O'Connell M. An ECOG randomized phase III trial of CHOP vs. CHOP + radiotherapy for inter-mediate grade early stage non-Hodgkin's lymphoma. *Proc Amer Soc Clin Oncol* 1995; **14**: 391a.

15. Miller TP, Dahlberg S, Cassady JR *et al*. Chemotherapy alone compared with chemotherapy plus radiotherapy for localized intermediate- and high-grade non-Hodgkin's lymphoma. *N Engl J Med* 1998; 339: 21-6.

16. Mauch P, Leonard R, Skarin A *et al*. Improved survival following combined radiation therapy and chemotherapy for un-favorable prognosis stage I-II non-Hodgkin's lymphomas. *J Clin Oncol* 1985; **3**: 1301-8.

17. Prestidge BR, Horning SJ, Hoppe RT. Combined modality therapy for stage I-II large cell lymphoma. *Int J Radiat Oncol Biol Phys* 1988; **15**: 633-9.

18. Velasquez WS, Fuller LM, Jagannath S *et al*. Stages I and II diffuse large cell lymphomas: prognostic factors and long-term results with CHOP-bleo and radiotherapy. *Blood* 1991; **77**: 942-7.

19. Kirn D, Mauch P, Shaffer K *et al*. Large-cell and immunoblastic lymphoma of the mediastinum: prognostic features and treatment outcome in 57 patients. *J Clin Oncol* 1993; **11**: 1336-43.

FURTHER READING

Jones SE, Miller TP, Connors JM. Long-term follow-up and analysis for prognostic factors for patients with limited-stage diffuse large-cell lymphoma treated with initial chemotherapy with or without adjuvant radiotherapy. *J Clin Oncol* 1989; **7**: 1186-91.

Morphologic, immunologic and genetic features of peripheral T cell lymphomas (unspecified category)

E S Jaffe

It is widely agreed, even by its strongest supporters, that the Working Formulation did not deal very successfully with T cell lymphomas [27.1]. No specific category of T cell lymphoma is recognized, with the exception of mycosis fungoides, which was included in the "miscellaneous" group. The T cell lymphomas that we diagnose today would fall into a number of different Working Formulation categories. These are principally the diffuse small cleaved, diffuse mixed, and large cell immunoblastic groups, although a few T cell neoplasms would probably be categorized as diffuse large cell lymphomas.

27.1 NCI Working Formulation of Non-Hodgkin's Lymphomas for Clinical Use

Low grade
- A. Small lymphocytic
- B. Follicular, predominantly small cleaved cell
- C. Follicular, mixed small cleaved and large cell

Intermediate grade
- D. Follicular, predominantly large cell
- E. Diffuse, small cleaved cell
- F. Diffuse, mixed small cleaved and large cell
- G. Diffuse, large cell

High grade
- H. Large cell, immunoblastic
- I. Lymphoblastic
- J. Small non-cleaved cell

Miscellaneous
- Composite
- Mycosis fungoides
- Histiocytic
- Extramedullary plasmacytoma
- Unclassifiable, other

Cancer, 1982 [1]

The Kiel classification [27.2] represented an improvement in dealing with T cell lymphomas. It recognized a large number of cytologic entities and divided them into low grade and high grade categories.

However, it was a cytologically based classification, which did not take clinical data into account, and it focused primarily on nodal lymphomas.

27.2 Post-thymic T Cell Lymphomas in the Kiel Scheme

Low grade
- Chronic lymphocytic leukemia & prolymphocytic leukemia
- Small cerebriform cell (MF/SS)
- Lymphoepithelioid cell (Lennert's lymphoma)
- Angioimmunoblastic
- T-zone lymphoma
- Pleomorphic small cell (HTLV-1 +/-)

High grade
- Pleomorphic medium and large cell (HTLV-1 +/-)
- Immunoblastic (HTLV-1 +/-)
- Large cell anaplastic lymphoma (Ki1+)

Cytologically based classification which does not rely on clinical data. Intended for nodal lymphomas.

The International Lymphoma Study Group felt that this was not a satisfactory way to approach T cell lymphomas, and, for several reasons, decided to modify the classification of T cell lymphomas when they formulated the REAL scheme [27.3]. First, several studies, mainly from Europe, had shown that the categories of node-based T cell lymphomas in the Kiel classification could not be identified reliably by pathologists, and furthermore that they did not seem to have clinical relevance. In addition, because the Kiel classification was concerned primarily with nodal lymphomas, the distinctive features of different types of extranodal T cell lymphoma were not recognized. Finally, the Kiel classification did not recognize adult T cell leukemia/lymphoma as a distinct disease entity, whereas the ILSG felt that this was a disease which should be separated out. It is true that we cannot recognize all cases purely on morphologic grounds, but certainly ample clinical and biologic data exist to indicate that it is a separate entity.

27.3   **Rationale for Not Adopting Kiel Classification of Post-thymic T Cell Lymphomas**

Categories of node-based T cell lymphomas are not reliably distinguished histologically or clinically (Noordyun *et al.* 1990; [2] Hastrup *et al.* 1991 [3])

Distinctive features of extranodal PTL not recognized, e.g.

-   nasal angiocentric lymphoma

-   enteropathy-associated PTL

-   hepatosplenic γδ lymphoma, subcutaneous

ATL/L (HTLV-1+ lymphoma/leukemia) is a distinct disease entity, and should be distinguished from other PTL

The ILSG therefore proposed a more logical classification of T cell malignancies [27.4]. They can be divided into several groups for the purposes of discussion. The first three entities present with leukemia or systemic disease. The next three are primarily lymph node based. And finally there are extranodal T cell lymphomas, and anaplastic large cell lymphoma.

27.4   **Post-thymic T Cell & NK Cell Neoplasms in the REAL Scheme**

T cell CLL/PLL

Large granular lymphocyte leukemia: T & NK

Mycosis fungoides/Sézary syndrome

Peripheral T cell lymphoma, unspecified

Angioimmunoblastic T cell lymphoma (AILD-like)

Adult T cell leukemia/lymphoma (HTLV-1+)

Angiocentric T/NK cell lymphoma

Intestinal T cell lymphoma

Subcutaneous panniculitis-like T cell lymphoma

Hepatosplenic γδ T cell lymphoma

Anaplastic large cell lymphoma (T and null cell)

This chapter is concerned with "peripheral T cell lymphoma, unspecified", which includes most nodal PTL not conforming to a specific category [27.5]. This is really a diagnosis of exclusion, and it encompasses as many as five separate categories in the Kiel classification. Its establishment in the REAL scheme therefore represents a significant simplification. Furthermore, these five Kiel categories included both low grade and high grade subtypes. It should be added that the REAL scheme refers to various provisional cytologic subtypes. However, these represent descriptive terms (medium, mixed + large cell, large cell + lymphoepithelioid) rather than distinct disease entities .

27.5   **Comparison of REAL and Kiel Classifications for Nodal Peripheral T Cell Lymphomas**

Peripheral TCL, unspecified *	Kiel categories
Medium sized cell **	Pleomorphic, small cell (HTLV +/-) T zone lymphoma
Lymphoepithelioid cell	Lymphoepithelioid cell
Mixed medium and large **	Pleomorphic medium and large (HTLV +/-)
Large cell **	Immunoblastic (HTLV +/-)

* Excludes ATL/L, AILD and other specific PTL entities
** Cytologic subtypes are provisional, not entities

Kiel entities are divided between low and high grade categories

The problems that arise when using the Kiel scheme to categorize T cell neoplasms are summarized in more detail in [27.6]. As already noted, pathologists have found practical difficulties in identifying some of the Kiel subtypes reproducibly. However, there are also problems over Kiel categories such as T zone lymphoma. Is this a distinct disease, or does it simply represent a stage in the development of the lymphoma when the node is only partially involved? The category of Lennert's lymphoma also poses problems. Epithelioid histiocytes are very characteristic of Lennert's lymphoma but can in practice be found in many subtypes of peripheral T cell lymphoma. How many epithelioid cells are needed to justify a diagnosis of Lennert's lymphoma? The clinical relevance of the Kiel classification has also been questioned. For example, a study from the Netherlands found that stage was a better indicator of clinical outcome than cytologic subtype.

27.6   **Difficulties in Use of Kiel Subtypes of Peripheral T Cell Lymphomas**

-   Subclassification is difficult and not reproducible
    (Noordyun *et al.* 1990; [2] Hastrup *et al.* 1991 [3])

-   Problem areas in classification
    Is T-zone lymphoma a disease, or a phase of involvement?
    Epithelioid histiocytes are seen in many subtypes of PTL.
    When is a lymphoma with epithelioid cells, a "Lennert's lymphoma"?

-   Stage is a more important predictor of clinical outcome than cytologic subtype, or low grade vs high grade [1]

For these reasons the members of the ILSG felt that they were justified in creating the "T cell lymphoma, unspecified" category, and in saying that any cytologic sub-categorization was purely provisional [27.7]

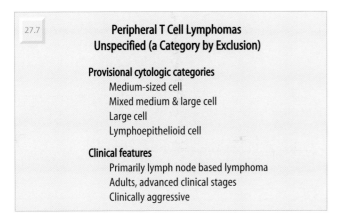

27.7

**Peripheral T Cell Lymphomas
Unspecified (a Category by Exclusion)**

Provisional cytologic categories
Medium-sized cell
Mixed medium & large cell
Large cell
Lymphoepithelioid cell

Clinical features
Primarily lymph node based lymphoma
Adults, advanced clinical stages
Clinically aggressive

Peripheral T cell lymphoma is primarily a disease of adults, is lymph node based, and is clinically aggressive. It also shows considerable histologic diversity. [27.8] would be classified in the Kiel classification as being of medium-sized cell type, and in the Working Formulation one might call this a diffuse small cleaved cell lymphoma. The cells are relatively small, irregular and they frequently show mitotic figures.

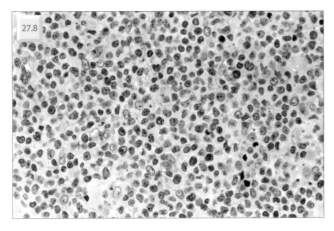

Seen in [27.9] is a peripheral T cell lymphoma composed of a mixture of medium-sized and larger cells. There is an inflammatory background containing eosinophils and scattered epithelioid histiocytes, although these are not so numerous that one would call this a lymphoepithelioid cell lymphoma.

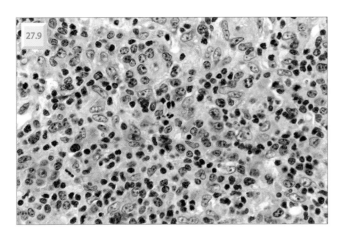

The tumor in [27.10] is composed of a mixture of small atypical and larger lymphoid cells, again with an inflammatory background. Many of the large cells have immunoblastic features and might evoke the differential diagnosis of Hodgkin's disease.

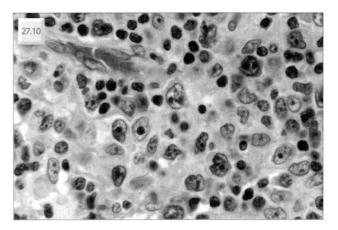

At the far end of the spectrum T cell tumors are sometimes encountered which are composed predominantly of large cells. These can show considerable pleomorphism and multilobation (as in the two examples in [27.11]) or they can be relatively monomorphic in appearance (as shown in the case in [27.12] in which the cells are large, mostly with a round nuclear outline).

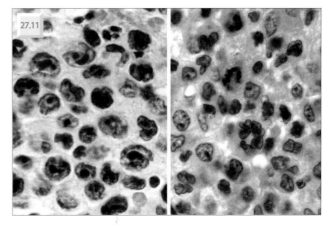

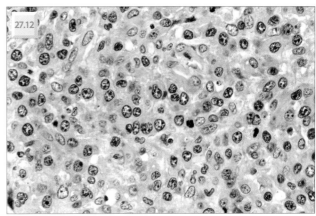

Epithelioid histiocytes can be numerous in some T cell lymphomas, and a case like [27.13], containing clusters of epithelioid histiocytes throughout the lymph node, fulfills the criteria for a lympho-epithelioid cell lymphoma. This is a distinct entity in the Kiel classification, but only a provisional subtype in the REAL scheme. The malignant cells are of course the intervening medium and occasional large lymphoid cells [27.14]. Often the epithelioid cell component is not a constant feature of the tumor and is lost with time, providing further evidence that this Kiel subtype is not a distinct biologic or clinical entity.

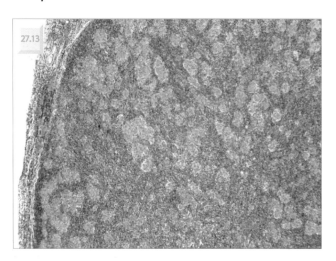

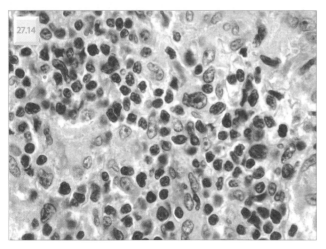

Although one may suspect a T cell lymphoma on histologic grounds, the need for immunophenotypic confirmation of the diagnosis is universally accepted [27.15]. This has become easier in recent years with a panel of antibodies that can be used on paraffin sections, and immunophenotypic characterization is within the reach of every practising pathologist. The most reliable T cell marker that can be detected in paraffin sections is CD3. CD45RO and CD43 are not completely specific T-associated markers, but they can give valuable information when used in a panel of monoclonal antibodies.

27.15	**Monoclonal Antibodies for Paraffin Section Immunohistochemistry of Lymph Node Lesions**
B cell:	CD20 (L26), CD79a (mb-1), CD43 (Leu22, MT-1), κ/λ
T cell:	CD3, CD45RO, CD43, CD8, CD4, TIA-1
Hodgkin's:	CD30+, CD15+ (Leu M1), CD45-
Histiocytic:	CD68 (KP1/PGM1), lysozyme
Granulocytic:	Lysozyme, myeloperoxidase, CD68
Misc:	BCL-2, MIB1 (Ki-67), EMA, TDT

Although a T cell lymphoma can now be detected using paraffin sections, much more insight into its immunophenotype can be obtained using fresh tissue, which can be studied by frozen section immunohistochemistry or flow cytometry, using a wider panel of markers. This reveals that most peripheral T cell lymphomas express either CD4 or CD8 [27.16]. In addition, we often find that T cell lymphomas have an aberrant T cell phenotype. Antigens are frequently lost, most commonly CD7 [27.17]. A number of years ago Picker et al. reported that about 80% of peripheral T cell lymphomas have an abnormal phenotype [27.18].[4] Although in most instances this was manifested by loss of one or more pan-T cell antigens, in a sizeable proportion of cases there was also abnormal expression of subset antigens, either absence of both CD4 and CD8 or dual expression of these two markers.

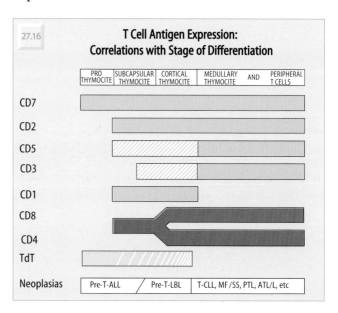

The use of antigenic markers can give a hint that the proliferation is neoplastic, but they cannot provide direct evidence of clonality. The only way to prove that a T cell proliferation is clonal is by molecular techniques, a procedure which has become easier in recent years. In the past, Southern blotting of DNA extracted from fresh tissue was the only way to show T cell gene rearrangement, but now, even with paraffin-embedded tissue, one can use polymerase chain reaction (PCR) methods to demonstrate re-arrangement of the T cell receptor γ chain gene [27.19].[4]

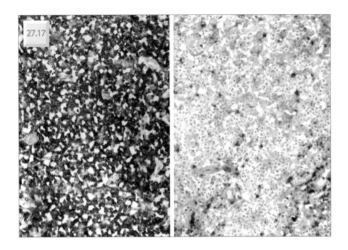

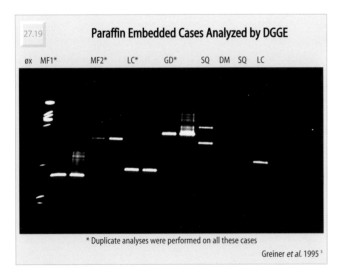

27.18	Incidence of "Abnormal" T-Lineage Phenotype
	Peripheral T cell lymphomas (excluding mycosis fungoides) (N = 88)
Pan-T antigen lost (1 or more antigens)	67 (76%)
"Abnormal" subset antigen expression (Leu-2-/3- or 2+/3+)	16 (18%)
Leu-6 T lineage	0
Total "abnormal"	70 (80%)

Picker *et al.* 1987 [4]

Paraffin Embedded Cases Analyzed by DGGE

øx MF1*   MF2*   LC*   GD*   SQ DM SQ LC

* Duplicate analyses were performed on all these cases

Greiner *et al.* 1995 [5]

From a clinical point of view, peripheral T cell lymphomas are frequently aggressive, and most patients present with generalized lymphadenopathy and often have hepatosplenomegaly. There is a high incidence of skin involvement, and in three studies, from the NCI, Nebraska and Japan, its frequency ranged from 20 to 50% [27.20].[1,6,7]

27.20	Clinical Features of Peripheral T Cell Lymphomas (Based on series from NCI, Nebraska, & Nagoya, Japan [1,6,7])	
Generalized lymphadenopathy		50-75%
Skin Involvement		20-50%
Hepatosplenomegaly		25-20%
Liver involvement		10-25%
Bone marrow involvement		25-35%
Hypergammaglobulinemia		25-50%
Stage III/IV		75%
"B" Symptoms		50-60%

When one sees skin involvement, it tends to be "top heavy" in contradistinction to B cell lymphomas, which tend to be "bottom heavy". Also, as shown in [27.21], there is an absence of the type of epidermal infiltration seen in mycosis fungoides or Sézary syndrome.

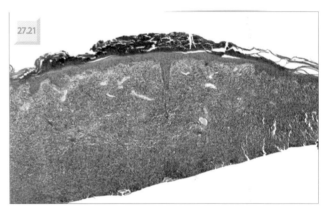

This group of "peripheral T cell lymphomas, unspecified" is the largest group of T cell lymphomas in the REAL classification, and the question still remains as to whether they can meaningfully be subclassified. A large study from Japan reported that the low grade groups in the Kiel classification had a better prognosis than the high grade groups [27.22]. Noticeably, large cell anaplastic lymphomas had the best prognosis. However, as noted already, the Kiel classification subdivides low grade T cell lymphoma into several different histopathologic sub-types, and it is significant that in this study there were no significant survival differences between these proposed subcategories [27.23]. Furthermore, although differences were reported between the low grade and high grade groups, it was not clear that this was independent of Stage since the high grade peripheral T cell lymphomas tended to be more advanced clinically. T cell receptor gene rearrangement was also analyzed, in particular in the low grade T cell lymphomas, and it was possible to identify clonality in only 62% of the cases. This was ascribed to a low percentage of tumor cells in some biopsies, but it raises the possibility that some of the so-called low grade peripheral T cell lymphomas may have been examples of benign atypical lymphoid hyperplasia.

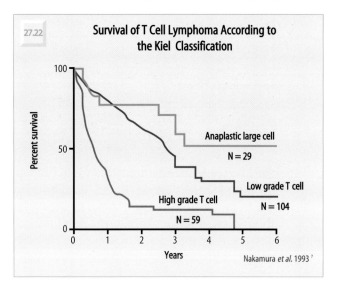

27.22   Survival of T Cell Lymphoma According to the Kiel Classification

Percent survival

Anaplastic large cell
N = 29

Low grade T cell
N = 104

High grade T cell
N = 59

Years

Nakamura *et al.* 1993 [7]

27.23   Clinical Relevance of Classification of PTL

- No significant survival differences among low grade Kiel categories of PTL

- Statistic differences in survival between low grade, high grade, and ALCL groups

- High grade PTL are more often of high clinical stage

- Clonal TCR β gene rearrangement seen in only 62% of low grade PTL:

      19/29 (66%) AILD

      8/14 (57%) T-zone lymphoma

      5/9 (56%) lymphoepithelioid lymphoma

May be secondary to low % of tumor cells (or ? benign)

Nakamura *et al.* 1993; [7]   Takagi *et al.* 1992 [8]

Cytogenetics has been very important in identifying distinctive biologic and clinical entities among other lymphoid neoplasms, so the question arises as to whether this approach can be used to identify distinct entities within the broad group of peripheral T cell lymphomas. The largest cytogenetic study published to date is that of Schlegelberger *et al.*[9] based on the Kiel classification, and they found considerable overlap in the cytogenetic findings among the low grade T cell lymphoma categories [27.24]. However, T cell CLL, prolymphocytic leukemia and mycosis fungoides were different from nodal T cell neoplasms, supporting the notion that these entities should be considered separately. They found a much higher

frequency of clonal cytogenetic abnormalities in the high grade T cell lymphomas than in the low grade lymphomas, and the high grade lymphomas had more complex cytogenetic findings. The only recurrent cytogenetic abnormality in this series was the (2;5) translocation, characteristic of anaplastic large cell lymphoma.

27.24   Is There Biological Evidence for Kiel Subclassification of PTL? Cytogenetic Findings in PTL

- There is considerable overlap in cytogenetic findings in low grade PTL (AILD, T-zone lymphoma, and lymphoepithelioid lymphoma)

- T-CLL, T-PLL, and MF/SS differ in their cytogenetic features from nodal PTL

- Aberrant clones found in 69% low grade PTL vs 95% high grade PTL

- High grade PTL (pleomorphic, immunoblastic) have more complex cytogenetic findings than low grade PTL

- t(2;5) in ALCL was the only specific abnormality detected

Schlegelberger *et al.* 1994 [9]

Thus, there were no recurrent cytogenetic lesions which allow, at least for the moment, subtypes of low grade nodal peripheral T cell lymphomas to be distinguished [27.25]. The findings in high grade T cell lymphomas are consistent with histologic progression, but they do not necessarily indicate a different entity. Furthermore, the differential diagnosis between atypical hyperplasia and low grade peripheral T cell lymphoma can still be a diagnostic problem. Finally, specific entities cannot be delineated within the broad group of "peripheral T cell lymphoma, unspecified".

27.25   Cytogenetic Findings in PTL : Conclusions

- Subtypes of low grade nodal PTL cannot be distinguished

- Findings in high grade PTL are consistent with histologic progression

- Differential diagnosis of atypical hyperplasia vs. low grade PTL may still be a diagnostic problem

- Specific entities are not identified in the "PTL, unspecified" category of REAL

Finally, [27.26] summarizes in a single figure the salient features of this lymphoma category.

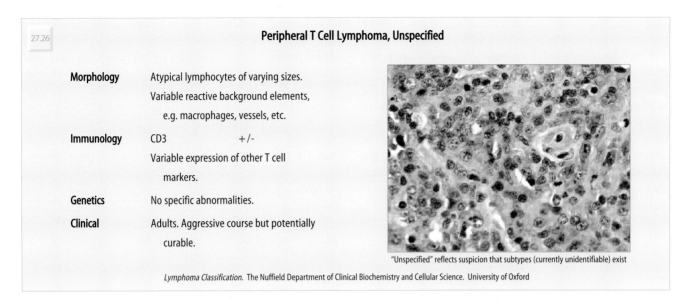

27.26

Peripheral T Cell Lymphoma, Unspecified

Morphology	Atypical lymphocytes of varying sizes.
	Variable reactive background elements,
	e.g. macrophages, vessels, etc.
Immunology	CD3 +/-
	Variable expression of other T cell
	markers.
Genetics	No specific abnormalities.
Clinical	Adults. Aggressive course but potentially
	curable.

"Unspecified" reflects suspicion that subtypes (currently unidentifiable) exist

Lymphoma Classification. The Nuffield Department of Clinical Biochemistry and Cellular Science. University of Oxford

ACKNOWLEDGEMENT

This chapter is based on U.S. government work. There are no restrictions on its use.

REFERENCES

1. National Cancer Institute sponsored study of classifications of non-Hodgkin's lymphomas: summary and description of a working formulation for clinical usage. The Non-Hodgkin's Lymphoma Pathologic Classification Project. *Cancer* 1982; **49**: 2112-35.

2. Noorduyn LA, van der Valk P, van Heerde P *et al*. Stage is a better prognostic indicator than morphologic subtype in primary noncutaneous T-cell lymphoma. *Am J Clin Pathol* 1990; **93**: 49-57.

3. Hastrup N, Hamilton-Dutoit S, Ralfkiaer E, Pallesen G. Peripheral T-cell lymphomas: an evaluation of reproducibility of the updated Kiel classification. *Histopathology* 1991; **18**: 99-105.

4. Picker L, Weiss L, Medeiros L, Wood G, Warnke R. Immunophenotypic criteria for the diagnosis of non-Hodgkin's lymphoma. *Am J Pathol* 1987; **128**: 181-201.

5. Greiner TC, Raffeld M, Lutz C, Dick F, Jaffe ES. Analysis of T cell receptor-gamma gene rearrangements by denaturing gradient gel electrophoresis of GC-clamped polymerase chain reaction products. Correlation with tumor-specific sequences. *Am J Pathol* 1995; **146**: 46-55.

6. Armitage J, Greer J, Levine A *et al*. Peripheral T-cell lymphoma. *Cancer* 1989; **63**: 158-63.

7. Nakamura S, Suchi T, Koshikawa T *et al*. Clinicopathologic study of 212 cases of peripheral T-cell lymphoma among the Japanese. *Cancer* 1993 ; **72**: 1762-72.

8. Takagi N, Nakamura S, Ueda R *et al*. A phenotypic and genotypic study of three node-based, low-grade peripheral T-cell lymphomas: angioimmunoblastic lymphoma, T-zone lymphoma, and lymphoepithelioid lymphoma. *Cancer* 1992; **69**: 2571-82.

9. Schlegelberger B, Himmler A, Godde E, Grote W, Feller AC, Lennert K. Cytogenetic findings in peripheral T-cell lymphomas as a basis for distinguishing low-grade and high-grade lymphomas. *Blood* 1994; **83**: 505-11.

FURTHER READING

Coiffier B, Brousse N, Peuchmaur M *et al*. Peripheral T-cell lymphomas have a worse prognosis than B-cell lymphomas: a prospective study of 361 immunophenotyped patients treated with the LNH-84 regimen. *Ann Oncol* 1990; **1**: 45-50.

Kim H, Jacobs C, Warnke R, Dorfman R. Malignant lymphoma with a high content of epithelioid histiocytes: a distinct clinicopathologic entity and a form of so-called "Lennert's lymphoma". *Cancer* 1978; **41**: 620-35.

Lippman S, Miller T, Spier C, Slymen D, Grogan T. The prognostic significance of the immunotype in diffuse large-cell lymphoma: a comparative study of the T-cell and B-cell phenotype. *Blood* 1988; **72**: 436-41.

Patsouris E, Noel H, Lennert K. Histological and immunohistological findings in lymphoepithelioid cell lymphoma (Lennert's lymphoma). *Am J Surg Pathol* 1988; **12**: 341-50.

Suchi T, Lennert K, Tu L-Y. Histopathology and immunohistochemistry of peripheral T-cell lymphomas: a proposal for their classification. *J Clin Pathol* 1987; **40**: 995-1015.

POST-SCRIPT

The International Lymphoma Classification Project conducted by Armitage and colleagues[10] confirmed the importance of distinguishing PTL, unspecified, from anaplastic large cell lymphomas of T and null cell types. ALCL has an excellent prognosis, whereas nearly all other PTL have an aggressive clinical course. Within PTL, unspecified, cytologic subclassification is not likely to be clinically significant.

REFERENCES

10. The Non-Hodgkin's Lymphoma Classification Project. A clinical evaluation of the International Lymphoma Study Group classification of non-Hodgkin's lymphoma. *Blood* 1997; **89**: 3909-18.

Do lymphomas in the peripheral T cell (unspecified) category differ clinically from B cell lymphomas?

F Cabanillas

This chapter presents some background information on peripheral T cell lymphomas and also some data that we have generated at our institution.

There are several controversies in the area of T cell lymphoma [28.1]. The first is whether post-thymic (otherwise known as "peripheral") T cell non-Hodgkin's lymphomas have a worse prognosis because they present with more advanced disease, or whether a T cell phenotype by itself is an independent prognostic factor? This question has not been answered clearly, and it is necessary to study peripheral T cell lymphoma patients with poor prognostic features, and compare them with B cell non-Hodgkin's lymphomas with similar prognostic features. Data presented below aimed to make exactly that comparison.

It is made up of many different subtypes and, within this heterogeneous collection of entities, there may be some that have a better prognosis than others.

There are two problems in answering these questions [28.2]. Firstly, only 10 - 15% of all aggressive non-Hodgkin's lymphomas are of peripheral T cell type. The other problem, which has not been widely appreciated, is that many of the published series probably contain a significant number of "T cell-rich B cell lymphomas". This entity was described some time ago by Dr. Jaffe but there was little awareness of it until recently, so that earlier series of peripheral T cell lymphoma may have been contaminated with such cases. Hodgkin's disease of mixed cellularity type is also not uncommonly confused with peripheral T cell lymphoma.

28.1 **Controversies Regarding Aggressive Post-thymic T Cell NHL**

- Is poor outcome described for post-thymic T cell NHL entirely due to their more advanced presentation?

or

- Is T cell phenotype an independent adverse prognostic feature?
- Is the prognosis of post-thymic T cell NHL really different from that of aggressive B cell NHL?
- Is the prognosis of T cell DLCL different from other T cell histologic types?

28.2 **Problems in Comparing Aggressive Post-thymic T Cell with Aggressive B Cell NHL**

- Only 10-15% of aggressive NHL are of T cell origin
- Published series probably contain significant numbers of "T cell-rich B cell NHL" and Hodgkin's mixed cellularity incorrectly diagnosed as PTCL
- More heterogeneous in histologic subtypes than B cell lymphomas

---

Most studies that have asked the question of whether the prognosis of post-thymic or peripheral T cell non-Hodgkin's lymphoma is really different from that of aggressive B cell non-Hodgkin's lymphoma have concluded that peripheral T cell lymphomas do indeed fare worse than B cell lymphomas. However, they have not addressed the important question of whether the prognosis of T cell diffuse large cell lymphoma is different from other T cell types. Peripheral T cell lymphoma is not really a homogeneous entity.

To complicate things even more, there are many proposed histologic subtypes within peripheral T cell lymphomas, so that it is difficult to gather meaningful numbers of patients in many of these different subtypes. Thus, not only are peripheral T cell lymphomas rare, but the numbers of cases within the different subtypes is even smaller.

In our own institution, we have gone back ten years and reviewed all the patients who had been included in our studies of aggressive non-Hodgkin's lymphoma. This series consisted of 560 patients, after exclusion of cases which had not been adequately phenotyped [28.3]. Of these, 85% had a B cell phenotype and 15% a T cell phenotype. However, the finding of a T cell phenotype did not necessarily mean that they were peripheral T cell lymphomas, and we identified 16 T cell-rich B cell lymphomas. We were then left with a relatively small number of cases that fulfilled the criteria for T cell lymphoma. However, when our pathologist, Dr. Pugh, reviewed these cases, the number fell even further because in reality two were cases of Hodgkin's disease, one was an atypical Sézary syndrome and one could not be classified. So finally we were left with 68 patients, or 12% of the original group, who met the criteria for post-thymic/peripheral T cell lymphoma.

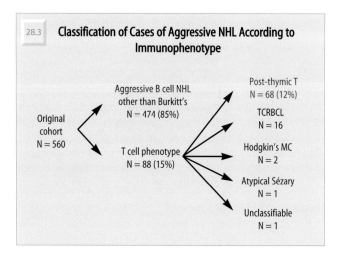

28.3   Classification of Cases of Aggressive NHL According to Immunophenotype

When Dr. Pugh subdivided them down into different subtypes, it was evident that, as expected, the largest group corresponded to the "peripheral T cell lymphoma, unspecified" REAL category [28.4]. An effort was made to split them further into different histologic categories, and diffuse large cell lymphoma was the commonest type, followed closely by the diffuse mixed subtype. There were two cases of lympho-epithelioid lymphoma, and seven could not be classified further.

28.4   Histologic Types of Post-thymic T Cell Lymphoma

MD Anderson Cancer Center Service

Histology	N	%
Peripheral T cell (unspecified)	45	66
- DLCL	19	28
- DMxL	17	25
- Lymphoepithelioid	2	3
- Unclassified	7	10
Anaplastic Ki-1+	10	15
AILD	8	12
Angiocentric	5	7
TOTAL	**68**	**100**

In addition to the "peripheral T cell lymphoma, unspecified" cases, there were cases of anaplastic large cell lymphoma, angioimmunoblastic T cell lymphoma, and angiocentric lymphoma. The angiocentric cases, even though they frequently presented with localized disease, did extremely poorly. In contrast, as expected, anaplastic large cell lymphomas did better than other T cell lymphomas.

When we compared the clinical characteristics of these patients with those of the B cell lymphomas, we found that 78% of the cases presented with advanced disease (stages III or IV), compared to only 49% of the B cell neoplasms [28.5]. There were other significant differences, such as a two-fold greater frequency of constitutional symptoms. β2-microglobulin levels were also higher, and LDH somewhat higher. When we applied the MD Anderson Tumor Score, which is our way of assessing prognosis, patients with PTCL presented with a Tumor Score of 3 more frequently than did the B cell type, and this achieved borderline statistical significance.

28.5   Comparison of Characteristics of Aggressive B Cell and Post-thymic T Cell NHL

MD Anderson Series

Feature	B cell N = 492	PTCL N = 68	p
Ann Arbor stage 3-4	49%	78%	< 0.0001
"B" symptoms	28%	54%	< 0.0001
β2-m ≥ 3.0	26%	44%	0.002
High LDH	44%	57%	0.03
MDA Tumor Score ≥ 3	44%	56%	0.08
Performance status ≥ 2	15%	22%	0.14
International Index ≥ 3	28%	31%	0.3
Age (median)	57	54	0.3

The complete response rate in this group of patients was lower in the peripheral T cell lymphomas [28.6]. Furthermore, the five year failure-free survival was significantly different, as well as the five year survival. However, this did not address the question of whether this difference was because the peripheral T cell lymphomas presented with more advanced disease.

28.6   Comparison of Characteristics of Aggressive B Cell and Post-thymic T Cell NHL

MD Anderson Series

Result	B cell (N = 492)	PTCL (N = 68)	p
CR rate	76%	65%	0.04
5-year FFS	56%	38%	0.0006
5-year survival	63%	39%	0.0006

Consequently, we stratified the patients according to the International Index, and then compared the failure-free survival of the T and B cell cases [28.7]. We found that the 23 good prognosis T cell lymphoma patients (with an International Index of 0 to 1) did significantly worse than B cell lymphoma patients in the same prognostic groups. However, they still had a relatively good outcome, in keeping with the fact that they were within the most favorable category in the International Index.

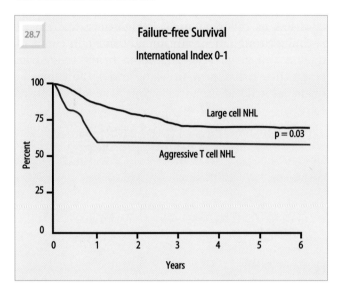

Most of our cases of T cell lymphoma, however, had an International Index of 2 to 5, and for these patients there is a clear-cut separation between the failure-free survival for T and B cell lymphomas [28.8]. The values were even more significant than for the good prognosis cases, because of the larger number of patients.

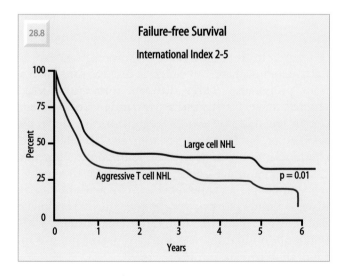

We can conclude from these studies that a diagnosis of peripheral T cell lymphoma is a prognostic factor which is independent of the fact that the patients tend to present with more advanced disease.

Data from the literature is summarized in [28.9], and it is evident from the last column that the five year survival ranges from very poor to suboptimal, i.e. from less than 10% to 45%. The only exception is the series from Stanford. However, if one analyzes that report in more detail, it is evident that the cases were very different from the other patients. For example, their median age was less than 50 and only 18% presented with advanced stage III to IV disease, versus 70 80% in the other series. Very few had constitutional symptoms, and the great majority of them achieved complete remission. So there was something atypical about this group of patients from Stanford, perhaps because only diffuse large cell lymphoma were included, many of which were anaplastic large cell lymphomas.

28.9	Literature Series Post-thymic T Cell Lymphomas					
Institution	N	Median age	% Stage 3-4	% BSI	% CR	5-year survival
Vanderbilt U.	33	64	79	67	24	< 10
U. Arizona	20	59	80	60	50	10
Netherlands	20	57	60	NA	NA	27
Stanford	21	< 50	18	29	95	78
Austria	38	54	NA	NA	37	< 40
U. Nebraska	80	57	72	57	50	40
Franco	108	NA	77	58	72	45
MD Anderson	68	54	74	56	65	39

Finally, it is relevant to add a comment on T cell-rich B cell lymphoma. In the author's opinion this is just a large B cell lymphoma that happens to contain many T cells, rather than a separate entity [28.10]. Our criteria for T cell-rich B cell lymphoma include a diffuse architecture, a minor population of atypical large cells, and a preponderance of cytologically mature small T lymphocytes. More than 50% of the neoplastic cells are T lymphocytes, and the atypical large cells stain positively for pan-B markers and are negative for T cell markers. A report from our institution [28.11], published in *Blood* a few years ago,[1] compared 23 cases with 495 cases of aggressive B cell lymphoma. No significant differences from the B cell cases were observed, including clinical Stage constitutional symptoms, β2-microglobulin, and age. The only possible difference is that we found splenomegaly in 35% of patients. Data on this feature for our B cell lymphomas are not available, but it is a high figure. A group from Vanderbilt University have also published data to indicate that splenomegaly is frequent in these patients. It is conceivable that this phenomenon represents an immune reaction associated with the high number of T cells.

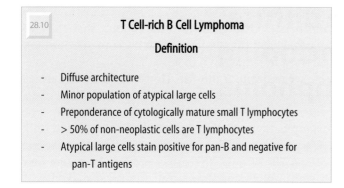

28.10   T Cell-rich B Cell Lymphoma

Definition

- Diffuse architecture
- Minor population of atypical large cells
- Preponderance of cytologically mature small T lymphocytes
- > 50% of non-neoplastic cells are T lymphocytes
- Atypical large cells stain positive for pan-B and negative for pan-T antigens

28.11   Comparison of Characteristics of T Cell-rich B Cell Lymphoma vs Aggressive B Cell

MD Anderson Series

Feature	B cells N = 495	TCRBCL N = 23	p
Ann Arbor stage 3-4	49%	57%	0.4
"B" symptoms	28%	26%	0.5
β2-m ≥ 3.0	26%	60% (N = 10)	0.3
High LDH	44%	42%	0.5
Splenomegaly	n.a.	35%	-
Age (median)	57	59	0.5

Rodriguez *et al.* 1993 [1]

The single most important point about the T cell-rich B cell lymphomas is summarized in [28.12] . It lists the diagnoses that were made before these patients were referred to the MD Anderson Hospital, and reveals that six of them were misdiagnosed as Hodgkin's disease, four were called diffuse mixed non-Hodgkin's lymphoma, two were incorrectly called peripheral T cell lymphoma, and two were called diffuse large cell lymphoma. One was even called mantle cell lymphoma. Therefore the important point is not that these patients are essentially identical to other large cell lymphomas, but that an inexperienced pathologist may make a misdiagnosis. This can lead to a B cell large cell lymphoma being treated as Hodgkin's disease, with very undesirable consequences.

28.12   How Were Cases of T Cell-rich B Cell Lymphoma Diagnosed Before Referral to MDACC

Diagnosis	N
Hodgkin's Disease	6
Diffuse Mixed Cell NHL	4
Peripheral T cell NHL	2
Diffuse Large cell NHL	2
Mantle Cell NHL	1

REFERENCES

1. Rodriguez J, Pugh WC, Cabanillas F. T-cell-rich B-cell lymphoma. *Blood* 1993; **82:** 1586-9.

Optimal treatment strategies for peripheral T cell lymphoma (unspecified category)

B Coiffier

This review combines peripheral "T cell lymphoma, unspecified", whatever the cell morphology and the specific variants described in the REAL classification [29.1]. If one is going to identify clinical differences between the subtypes, one requires a very large number of patients. We have therefore amalgamated all subtypes together for the purposes of our study [29.2].

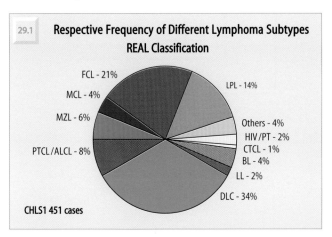

29.1 Respective Frequency of Different Lymphoma Subtypes REAL Classification

FCL - 21%
MCL - 4%
MZL - 6%
PTCL/ALCL - 8%
LPL - 14%
Others - 4%
HIV/PT - 2%
CTCL - 1%
BL - 4%
LL - 2%
DLC - 34%
CHLS1 451 cases

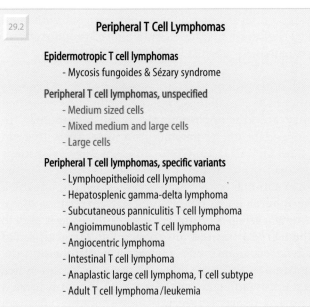

29.2 Peripheral T Cell Lymphomas

Epidermotropic T cell lymphomas
- Mycosis fungoides & Sézary syndrome

Peripheral T cell lymphomas, unspecified
- Medium sized cells
- Mixed medium and large cells
- Large cells

Peripheral T cell lymphomas, specific variants
- Lymphoepithelioid cell lymphoma
- Hepatosplenic gamma-delta lymphoma
- Subcutaneous panniculitis T cell lymphoma
- Angioimmunoblastic T cell lymphoma
- Angiocentric lymphoma
- Intestinal T cell lymphoma
- Anaplastic large cell lymphoma, T cell subtype
- Adult T cell lymphoma/leukemia

Some years ago we introduced the LNH-84 regimen and presented in the first issue of the *Annals of Oncology* a comparative study of B and T cell lymphoma [29.3].[1] The study was performed on 361 phenotyped patients who had been treated with the LNH-84 regime. Patients with indolent subtypes, mostly B cell lymphoma, are excluded from this update.

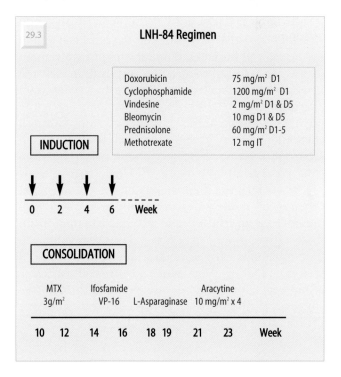

29.3 LNH-84 Regimen

Doxorubicin	75 mg/m^2 D1
Cyclophosphamide	1200 mg/m^2 D1
Vindesine	2 mg/m^2 D1 & D5
Bleomycin	10 mg D1 & D5
Prednisolone	60 mg/m^2 D1-5
Methotrexate	12 mg IT

INDUCTION

0   2   4   6   Week

CONSOLIDATION

| MTX 3g/m^2 | Ifosfamide VP-16 | L-Asparaginase | Aracytine 10 mg/m^2 x 4 |

10   12   14   16   18 19   21   23   Week

The frequency of patients with T cell lymphoma was approximately 12%. When the clinical features were reviewed [29.4] there were very few differences between B and T cell neoplasms. The numbers of patients with disseminated disease were similar. There were slightly more T cell lymphoma patients with B symptoms, with weight loss, with a large number of extranodal sites, and with spleen and skin involvement. The B cell lymphoma patients more frequently had bulky tumors or gastrointestinal involvement and high LDH levels.

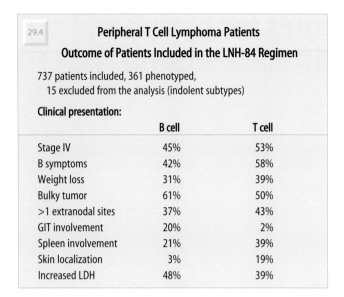

Peripheral T Cell Lymphoma Patients

Outcome of Patients Included in the LNH-84 Regimen

737 patients included, 361 phenotyped,
15 excluded from the analysis (indolent subtypes)

Clinical presentation:

	B cell	T cell
Stage IV	45%	53%
B symptoms	42%	58%
Weight loss	31%	39%
Bulky tumor	61%	50%
>1 extranodal sites	37%	43%
GIT involvement	20%	2%
Spleen involvement	21%	39%
Skin localization	3%	19%
Increased LDH	48%	39%

The survival curves reported at that time [29.5] showed a short recurrence-free survival for T cell lymphoma, which was statistically different from the B cell curve. At that time a multivariate analysis of all prognostic factors was performed, and only the phenotype correlated significantly with the duration of complete remission [29.6].

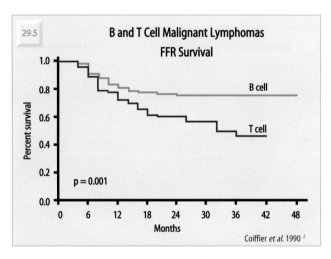

B and T Cell Malignant Lymphomas

FFR Survival

p = 0.001

B cell

T cell

Coiffier *et al.* 1990 [2]

Prognostic Factors for Duration of CR

	B cell	T cell	All	Cox regression
Histologic subtypes	-	-	0.001	-
Phenotype			0.002	0.04
PS ≥ 2	0.001	-	-	-
Weight loss > 10%	-	-	-	-
Spleen	-	-	-	-
Bone marrow +	0.001	-	0.0002	-
Stage	0.001	-	0.0009	-
B symptoms	0.0005	-	-	-
No of sites ≥ 2	0.02	-	0.05	-
Bulky tumor	-	-	-	-
Increased LDH	$<10^{-4}$	-	0.01	-
Serum albumin ≤ 30g/l	-	-	-	-

Subsequently some data have emerged to indicate why T cell lymphoma patients may have a worse prognosis. Many studies have shown that neoplastic cells in T cell lymphoma can secrete cytokines, and this may explain why these patients have a poorer prognosis and a shorter survival than B cell lymphoma cases. Shown in [29.7] is one such study, but similar results have been shown for many factors, including IL-10, TNF and cytokine receptors.

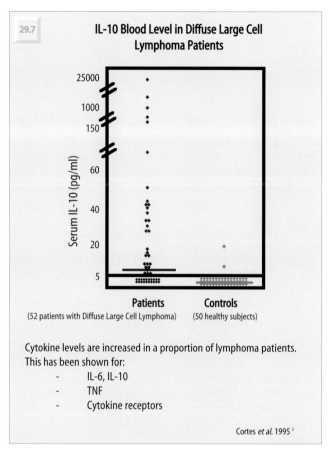

IL-10 Blood Level in Diffuse Large Cell Lymphoma Patients

Serum IL-10 (pg/ml)

Patients
(52 patients with Diffuse Large Cell Lymphoma)

Controls
(50 healthy subjects)

Cytokine levels are increased in a proportion of lymphoma patients. This has been shown for:
- IL-6, IL-10
- TNF
- Cytokine receptors

Cortes *et al.* 1995 [2]

In our centre, we have measured TNF and TNF-receptor levels, and shown that patients with high levels of these markers have a poorer prognosis than patients with normal levels [29.8].

If other prognostic factors are evaluated, for example high LDH and high β2-microglobulin, it is clear that they are also applicable for T cell lymphoma. In [29.9] data for 74 patients from our centre in Lyon show the separation into different survival groups according to these prognostic factors. If the International Index is applied, however, to these peripheral T cell lymphomas, the correlation is not strong. When survival curves [29.10] for patients in the LNH-84 regimen are analyzed, the large group of low/intermediate and high/intermediate risk categories are not separable, and the only group which separates out is the high risk group, in which there is clearly a poorer survival.

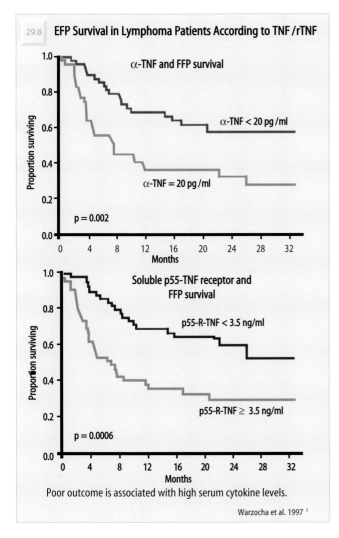

29.8 **EFP Survival in Lymphoma Patients According to TNF /rTNF**

α-TNF and FFP survival

α-TNF < 20 pg /ml

α-TNF = 20 pg /ml

p = 0.002

Soluble p55-TNF receptor and FFP survival

p55-R-TNF < 3.5 ng/ml

p55-R-TNF ≥ 3.5 ng/ml

p = 0.0006

Poor outcome is associated with high serum cytokine levels.

Warzocha et al. 1997 [3]

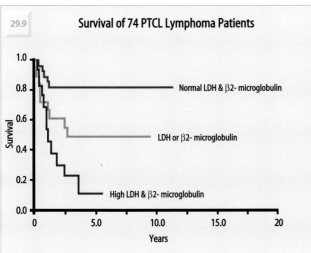

29.9 **Survival of 74 PTCL Lymphoma Patients**

Normal LDH & β2- microglobulin

LDH or β2- microglobulin

High LDH & β2- microglobulin

categories. There is a large difference in survival between B cell and T cell lymphomas for good risk patients, but the poor risk T cell cases had the same poor survival as the good risk T cell patients. The only significant difference between the two risk categories is for B cell lymphomas. Thus it is mostly in low risk patients that there is a difference between B and T cell lymphomas.

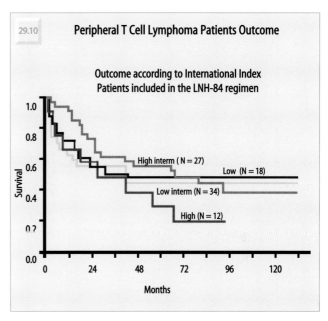

29.10 **Peripheral T Cell Lymphoma Patients Outcome**

Outcome according to International Index Patients included in the LNH-84 regimen

High interm (N = 27)

Low (N = 18)

Low interm (N = 34)

High (N = 12)

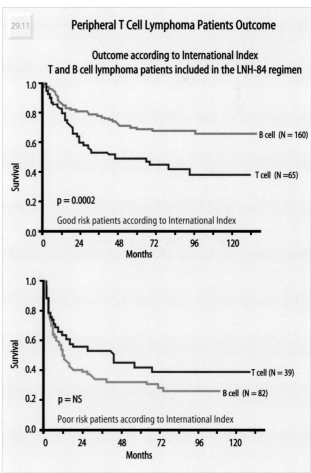

29.11 **Peripheral T Cell Lymphoma Patients Outcome**

Outcome according to International Index T and B cell lymphoma patients included in the LNH-84 regimen

B cell (N = 160)

T cell (N =65)

p = 0.0002

Good risk patients according to International Index

T cell (N = 39)

B cell (N = 82)

p = NS

Poor risk patients according to International Index

Since that time an update of the LNH-84 study has been performed by Dr. Gisselbrecht, based on patients included in the more recent LNH-87 protocol.[4]

An updated LNH-84 trial [29.11] shows a five year follow-up. The patients are classified according to the International Index into good and poor risk

When the data are analyzed for all LNH-84 patients [29.12], including both B cell and T cell lymphomas, the difference described several years ago still persists, and the two phenotypes differ in both event-free survival and overall survival.

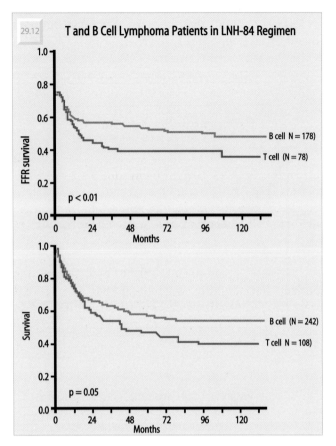

In the LNH-87 protocol [29.13] a regimen was introduced in which patients were stratified at diagnosis into four groups, according to prognostic factors. In each group patients received either the standard arm, which is ACVB (the LNH-84-like regimen), ACVB with second-shot consolidation, or an experimental protocol. All of the 3,500 patients in this protocol have been analyzed in terms of phenotype. More than 1,800 patients with diffuse mixed or diffuse large cell morphology could be reviewed, and 15% were T cell lymphomas. They were subdivided using the Kiel classification into different subcategories, such as T-zone, pleomorphic large cell, etc [29.14].

The clinical differences between T cell and B cell lymphomas are shown in [29.15], and the pattern is essentially what was found for the LNH-84 patients [29.4]. Disseminated disease, B symptoms, skin and bone marrow involvement, and elevated β2-microglobulin levels all tended to be more frequent among the T cell lymphomas. B cell lymphomas more frequently had bulky tumors and gastrointestinal involvement, but the LDH levels were not different between the two groups.

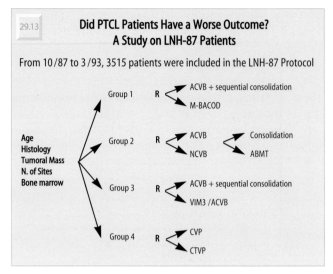

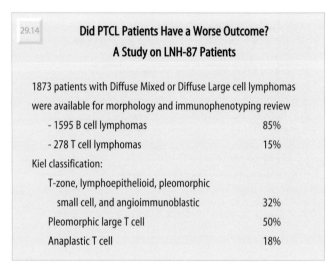

29.14

Did PTCL Patients Have a Worse Outcome?

A Study on LNH-87 Patients

1873 patients with Diffuse Mixed or Diffuse Large cell lymphomas were available for morphology and immunophenotyping review

- 1595 B cell lymphomas	85%
- 278 T cell lymphomas	15%

Kiel classification:

T-zone, lymphoepithelioid, pleomorphic small cell, and angioimmunoblastic	32%
Pleomorphic large T cell	50%
Anaplastic T cell	18%

29.15

Did PTCL Patients Have a Worse Outcome

A Study on LNH-87 Patients

	T cell	B cell
Disseminated stage	64%	47%
B symptoms	60%	40%
Bulky tumor	25%	40%
BM involvement	35%	27%
Skin involvement	20%	4%
GIT involvement	15%	29%
Increased LDH	51%	49%
Increased β2-m	45%	32%

When the five year survival and the event-free survival are considered, T cell lymphomas had a significant poorer prognosis [29.16]. If the analysis is restricted to patients with T cell lymphoma of large cell type, i.e. pleomorphic or anaplastic large cell cases, the poorer prognosis for T cell lymphomas is still evident [29.16].

29.16	**Did PTCL Patients have a Worse Outcome? A Study on LNH-87 Patients**			
		T cell	B cell	p-value
All patients:				
5-year Survival		42%	52%	< 0.001
5-year Event-free survival		33%	45%	< 0.0001
Large cell lymphomas only				
(140 T cell and 1387 B cell):				
5-year Survival		45%	52%	< 0.0001
5-year Event-free survival		28%	35%	< 0.0001

- Comparison according to the score of International Prognostic Index
- In each score, overall survival of PTCL patients was inferior to the survival of diffuse large B cell lymphoma patients. However, it did not reach statistical significance
- PTCL patients have a poorer outcome than diffuse large B cell lymphoma patients
- This poorer outcome is mainly related to the presence of adverse prognostic parameters at diagnosis
- Pleomorphic large T cell lymphomas have a worse outcome independently of other parameters

Cox multivariate analysis of survival

For all patients
- Age > 60 years   < 0.0001
- Increased LDH level   < 0.0001
- Poor performance status   < 0.0001
- BM involvement   < 0.0001
- Disseminated stage   = 0.054
- T phenotype   = 0.088

For large cell lymphoma patients:
Age, LDH level, PS, BM involvement remained.
T cell phenotype was independent (p = 0.003)

For each category in the International Index, large cell T cell lymphomas had a poorer prognosis than B cell lymphomas, but this did not reach statistical significance [29.16]. A statistically significant poorer survival for T versus B cell tumors was seen when the whole group was analyzed, but, when each International Index category was analyzed, this disappeared, probably because the number of patients was not sufficient. A Cox multivariate analysis for these patients showed a trend towards a poorer prognosis for T cell lymphomas [29.16], and if only the large cell T cell lymphomas are analyzed, the difference is still statistically significant.

Thus, T cell lymphomas have a worse prognosis on the whole, but this is probably due to their poor prognostic factors. The poorer prognosis is, however, attributable to adverse factors for the small and intermediate cell categories, but to both adverse factors and phenotype for the large cell group.

In conclusion, peripheral T cell lymphoma patients have a poorer outcome than diffuse large B cell lymphoma patients. This poor outcome is mainly related to the presence of adverse prognostic factors, except for polymorphic large cell T cell lymphoma [29.16].

REFERENCES

1. Coiffier B, Brousse N, Peuchmaur M, Berger F, Gisselbrecht C, Bryon PA, Diebold J. Peripheral T-cell lymphomas have a worse prognosis than B-cell lymphomas: a prospective study of 361 immunophenotyped patients treated with the LNH-84 regimen. The GELA (Groupe d'Etude des Lymphomes Agressives). *Ann Oncol* 1990; **1**: 45-50.

2. Cortes JE, Talpaz M, Cabanillas F, Seymour JF, Kurzrock R. Serum levels of interleukin-10 in patients with diffuse large cell lymphoma: lack of correlation with prognosis. *Blood* 1995; **85**: 2516-20.

3. Warzocha K, Salles G, Bienvenu J *et al*. Tumor necrosis factor ligand-receptor system can predict treatment outcome in lymphoma patients. *J Clin Oncol* 1997; **15**: 499-508.

4. Gisselbrecht C, Gaulard P, Lepage E *et al*. Prognostic significance of T-cell phenotype in aggressive non-Hodgkin's lymphomas. Groupe d'Etude des Lymphomes de l'Adulte (GELA). *Blood* 1998; **92**: 76-82.

FURTHER READING

Tilly H, Gaulard P, Lepage E *et al*. Primary anaplastic large-cell lymphoma in adults: clinical presentation, immunophenotype, and outcome. *Blood* 1997; **90**: 3727-34.

Morphologic, immunologic and genetic features of angioimmunoblastic T cell lymphoma (AILD)

R A Warnke

This review of angioimmunoblastic T cell lymphoma can be begun by relating this entity to the categories of the Working Formulation. A number of the cases correspond to the diffuse large cell or large cell immunoblastic categories [30.1]. However, many of the cases in the Working Formulation study would have been categorized as lymphomas of diffuse mixed small and large cell type [30.1].

30.1	Working Formulation	REAL Classification
		T cell neoplasms
	Diffuse large cell	Peripheral T cell, unspecified
	Large cell immunoblastic	Angioimmunoblastic T cell
		Angiocentric T cell
		Intestinal T cell
		Adult T cell lymphoma / leukemia
		Anaplastic large cell
	Diffuse mixed small and large cell	Peripheral T cell, unspecified
		Angioimmunoblastic T cell
		Angiocentric T cell
		Intestinal T cell
		Adult T cell lymphoma / leukemia

T cell neoplasms account for about 13% of the adult non-Hodgkin's lymphomas at Stanford [30.2], and this is virtually identical to the percentages seen in series from France and Houston. Of these cases, a little over half are in the "unspecified" category, and a quarter are anaplastic large cell lymphomas. Of the remaining T cell neoplasms, angioimmunoblastic T cell lymphoma, lymphoblastic lymphoma and mycosis fungoides each represent about a third. However, more mycosis fungoides patients are probably seen at Stanford than in some other centers.

Shown in [30.3] is the definition of the disease in the REAL scheme. The morphology is fairly distinctive [30.4]. It is a diffuse lymphoma, but abnormal follicles can be present, and it is not uncommon for sinuses to be preserved. The neoplastic cell nuclei tend to be heterogeneous in size and shape, and the cytoplasm, especially in the cases that are clearly diagnosable as lymphoma, is often clear. The cellular composition varies greatly - one often sees a mixture of eosinophils and plasma cells, and in some cases large numbers of epithelioid histiocytes are present. The high endothelial venules provide a hallmark of the disease, since they increase in number and have an arborizing pattern. Another feature, that was emphasized even in the earliest reports in the mid 1970s, is the presence of amorphous interstitial material, which is eosinophilic and PAS-positive.

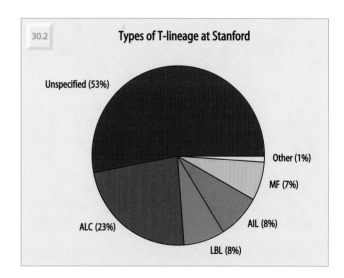

30.2 **Types of T-lineage at Stanford**

Unspecified (53%)
Other (1%)
MF (7%)
AIL (8%)
LBL (8%)
ALC (23%)

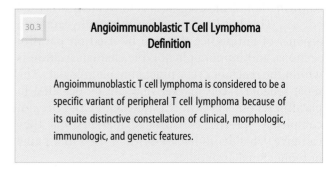

30.3 **Angioimmunoblastic T Cell Lymphoma Definition**

Angioimmunoblastic T cell lymphoma is considered to be a specific variant of peripheral T cell lymphoma because of its quite distinctive constellation of clinical, morphologic, immunologic, and genetic features.

Angioimmunoblastic T Cell Lymphoma Morphology

30.4

Diffuse pattern with abnormal follicles and preserved sinuses
Nuclei of variable size and shape
Cytoplasm often clear
Mixed and variable cellular composition
Increased and arborizing high endothelial venules
Eosinophilic amorphous interstitial material (PAS+)

The morphology of the disease can be illustrated by showing two cases: one at the benign end of the morphologic spectrum and the other at the opposite, malignant, extreme.

The low power view of the benign case in [30.5] shows a typical feature, which is that the lymph node looks less cellular than normal. One can see patent medullary sinuses and a diffuse pattern of involvement.

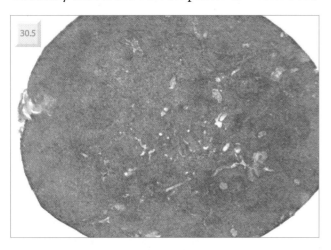

Clusters of cells with very abundant eosinophilic cytoplasm are seen in [30.6]. These were initially thought to be granulomas, but over time it has become clear that these are usually B cell follicles which have undergone regression [30.7]. They are composed mainly of dendritic reticulum cells, the antigen-presenting cell characteristic of B cell follicles. In [30.7] one can also see the admixture of small lymphocytes with some eosinophils and plasma cells.

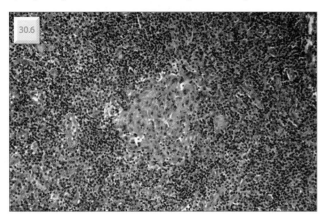

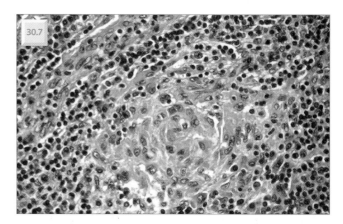

The hypervascularity characteristic of this condition can be highlighted with a PAS stain, which shows the large number of vessels and also their arborizing pattern [30.8]. The amorphous eosinophilic interstitial material [30.9] is also highlighted by a PAS stain [30.10]. In early reports it was said to have some features of fibrin. In some areas in this case [30.11] large cells are prominent, a feature which accounts for the name "immunoblastic lymphadenopathy".

The second case, from the malignant end of the spectrum, still shows some patent subcapsular sinuses, but the lymph node is more cellular and the infiltrate extends into the surrounding soft tissue [30.12]. Another kind of abnormal B cell follicle, lacking a mantle zone, can be found in this condition and is seen in [30.13]. Essentially, all cases contain EBV-positive B cells, and these abnormal follicles are one of the sites where they can be found. Shown in [30.14] is quite striking vascularity, which is even more prominent at higher magnification [30.15]. In addition to these high endothelial venules, one sees large cells with abundant clear cytoplasm. In consequence, a number of these cases have been designated "clear cell immunoblastic" lymphoma in the past [30.16]. In a case such as this [30.17], in which the nuclei are highly irregular and there is abundant clear cytoplasm, it is easy to make a diagnosis of T cell lymphoma.

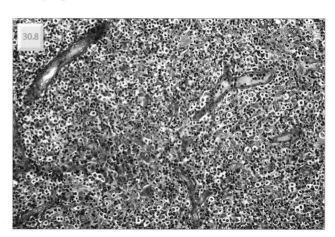

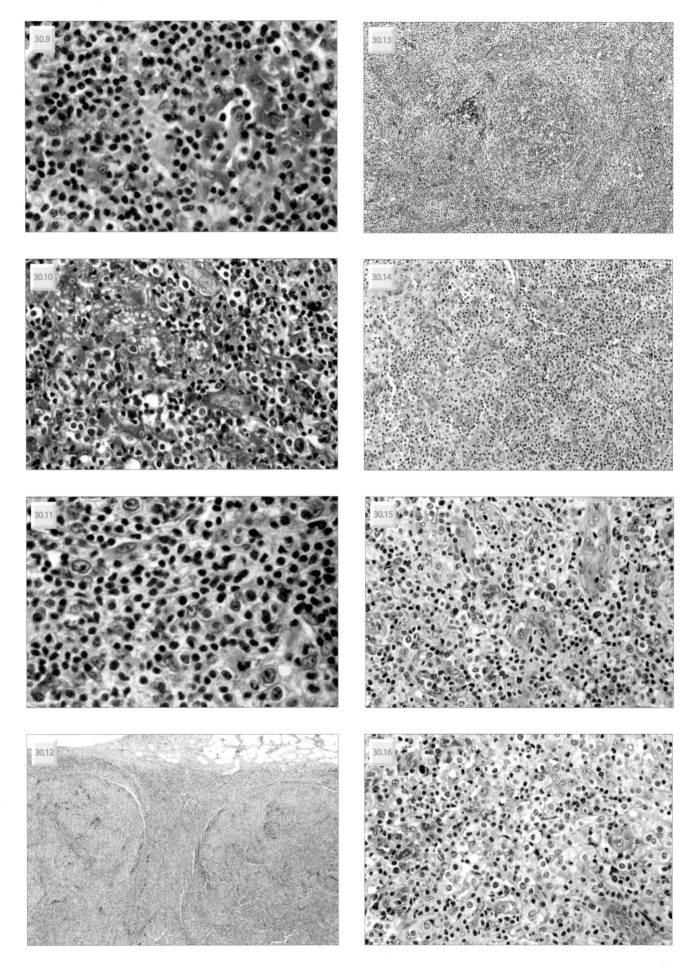

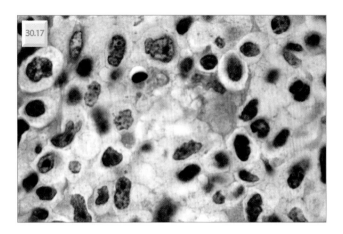

Turning to the immunologic features [30.18], these cases lack TdT, as one would expect, being post-thymic peripheral T cell lymphomas. Most cases in the literature are CD4-positive, and a couple of studies have suggested that this may be true even in cases which appear CD8-positive, since double-labelling shows that the proliferating cells are CD4-positive. Furthermore, when multiple biopsies are taken over time, cases that initially have a predominance of CD8-positive cells may develop a predominance of CD4-positive cells. Another feature revealed by immunohistologic staining, seen in more than half of all cases, is the presence of clusters of follicular dendritic cells around the high endothelial venules.

30.18	Angioimmunoblastic T Cell Lymphoma Immunology	
TdT		-
CD4+		+/-
FDC clusters around HEV		+/-

There are no specific karyotypic abnormalities, but it is of interest that those cytogenetic features that are present may vary over time, or even among different sites. This had been reported in some of the Japanese studies, and it appears that cytogenetic abnormalities may arise and then disappear [30.19].

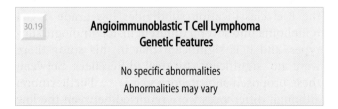

30.19	Angioimmunoblastic T Cell Lymphoma Genetic Features
	No specific abnormalities
	Abnormalities may vary

Highlighted in [30.20] are a number of the special problems encountered in diagnosing and under-standing this category of T cell lymphoma. Firstly, the morphology may not appear diagnostic of

lymphoma, and one may have difficulties in differentiating it from atypical diffuse hyperplasia. This is especially true at the benign end of the spectrum and in younger patients. If immunologic studies are performed, no specific abnormalities are found in the majority of cases, so one often gets little support for a diagnosis of lymphoma from this approach. Consequently, in many of these problem cases, we proceed straight to molecular biological studies.

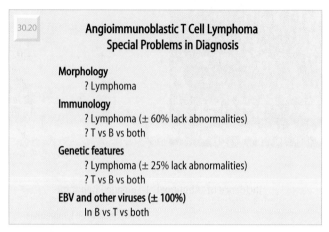

30.20	Angioimmunoblastic T Cell Lymphoma Special Problems in Diagnosis
Morphology	
	? Lymphoma
Immunology	
	? Lymphoma (± 60% lack abnormalities)
	? T vs B vs both
Genetic features	
	? Lymphoma (± 25% lack abnormalities)
	? T vs B vs both
EBV and other viruses (± 100%)	
	In B vs T vs both

Another problem is that the immunologic findings may be discordant. One may think, on morphologic grounds, that the lesion is a T cell lymphoma, but immunologic studies reveal numerous large B cells, and this raises the possibility of a B cell lymphoma. These B cells are often infected with EB virus, and the proliferations may be analogous to the immunodeficiency lymphomas, except that in this instance they are associated with T cell neoplasia.

The genetic features can also cause problems. About three quarters of the cases show evidence of clonal gene rearrangement. One Japanese study suggested that this depends on how many tumor cells are present in the infiltrate, because double-labelling studies indicate that the likelihood of picking up a clone by gene rearrangement analysis is dependent on the number of proliferating CD4-positive cells.

A further confusion arising from molecular biological studies is that they may reveal both B cell and T cell clones. As already noted, virtually all cases contain increased numbers of EBV-infected cells. In several studies these were shown predominantly to be B cells, but in one study, a number of the neoplastic T cells were found to be infected. In some samples the number of EBV-infected cells is low, suggesting that EBV plays no major role in those particular cases. However, if one looks at more than one biopsy in the same patient one may find differing numbers of EBV-infected cells.

FURTHER READING

Anagnostopoulos I, Hummel M, Finn T *et al*. Heterogeneous Epstein-Barr virus infection patterns in peripheral T-cell lymphoma of angioimmunoblastic lymphadenopathy type. *Blood* 1992; **80**: 1804-12.

Feller AC, Griesser H, Schilling CV *et al*. Clonal gene rearrangement patterns correlate with immunophenotype and clinical parameters in patients with angioimmunoblastic lymphadenopathy. *Am J Pathol* 1988; **133**: 549-56.

Frizzera G, Moran E, Rappaport H. Angio-immunoblastic lymphadenopathy with dysproteinemia. *Lancet* 1974; **i**: 1070-3.

Jaffe E. Post-thymic lymphoid neoplasia. In: Jaffe E, ed. *Surgical pathology of the lymph nodes and related organs*. Philadelphia, PA: W. B. Saunders, 1985; **16**: 218-48.

Namikawa R, Suchi T, Ueda R *et al*. Phenotyping of proliferating lymphocytes in angioimmunoblastic lymphadenopathy and related lesions by the double immunoenzymatic staining technique. *Am J Pathol* 1987; **127**: 279-87.

Ohshima K, Takeo H, Kikuchi M *et al*. Heterogeneity of Epstein-Barr virus infection in angioimmunoblastic lymphadenopathy type T-cell lymphoma. *Histopathology* 1994; **25**: 569-79.

Patsouris D, Noel H, Lennert K. AILD type of T-cell lymphoma with a high content of epithelioid cells. Histopathology and comparison with lymphoepithelioid cell lymphoma. *Am J Surg Pathol* 1989; **13**: 161-75.

Schlegelberger B, Feller A, Godde W, Lennert K. Stepwise development of chromosomal abnormalities in angio-immunoblastic lymphadenopathy. *Cancer Genet Cytogenet* 1990; **50**: 15-29.

Weiss L, Strickler J, Dorfman R, Horning S, Warnke R, Sklar J. Clonal T-cell populations in angioimmunoblastic lymphadenopathy and angioimmunoblastic lymphadenopathy-like lymphoma. *Am J Pathol* 1986; **122**: 392-7.

Weiss LM, Jaffe ES, Liu XF, Chen YY, Shibata D, Medeiros LJ. Detection and localization of Epstein-Barr viral genomes in angioimmunoblastic lymphadenopathy and angio-immunoblastic lymphadenopathy-like lymphomas. *Blood* 1992; **79**: 1789-95.

POST-SCRIPT

Angioimmunoblastic T cell lymphomas continue to pose difficult problems in diagnosis. A significant number of these lymphomas are complicated by an EBV-associated lymphoproliferative disorder. Thus, a pathologist may favor a diagnosis of angio-immunoblastic T cell lymphoma based on morphologic findings but be perplexed when most of the large cells label as B cells (suggesting a T cell-rich B cell lymphoma). If stains for kappa and lambda light chains are performed, they will typically show an admixture of kappa and lambda stained large cells. Molecular studies to investigate the clonality of the T cells and B cells as well as *in situ* hybridization studies for EBV are essential in clarifying the nature of these lymphomas and the associated B cell proliferations.

Clinical aspects and treatment of angio-immunoblastic T cell lymphoma (AILD)

W H Wilson

The entity, known as angioimmunoblastic lymphadenopathy with dysproteinemia, or AILD, was described for the first time more than twenty years ago. Since that time, several syndromes have been named which overlap with AILD as originally described, and a variety of different names have been used [31.1].

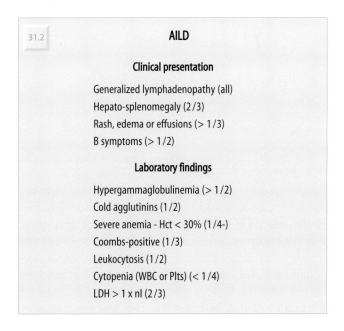

31.1	AILD Synonyms
	Histopathology
	Immunoblastic lymphadenopathy (IBL)
	Angioimmunoblastic lymphadenopathy (AIL)
	Lymphogranulomatosis X (LgX)

A classical finding in AILD, as described in Chapter 30, is effacement of the lymph node architecture. One sees infiltrating lymphocytes, lymphoblasts, immunoblasts, plasma cells and histiocytes, and typically arborizing post-capillary venules. The infiltrating cells are usually T cells and, more commonly than not, express CD4, although one can also find CD8 positivity. Recent studies of T cell receptor rearrangement have found evidence of clonality in up to 75% of cases, and the EBV genome is frequently detectable.

For these reasons, most cases of AILD can be considered to be T cell non-Hodgkin's lymphomas. The histopathologic findings suggest a low-grade lymphoma, but from the clinical point of view most cases behave in a way that is far from low grade.

In up to 25% of cases one cannot find evidence of T cell receptor rearrangement, and it is not clear at present whether these patients have a different disease or whether the clone cannot be identified because of normal infiltrating cells. One of the clinical hallmarks of this disorder, and one presumes that this

is induced by an abnormal T cell clone, is a general immune dysregulation, associated with B cell proliferation.

When one looks at the clinical characteristics, there appears to be no clear sex predilection. It tends to be a disease of older people, with the median age in the seventh decade, although one does see some younger cases, even in their thirties. All patients present with generalized lymphadenopathy, usually involving cervical, axillary, mediastinal and abdominal nodes [31.2]. The nodes tend to be in the 2-3 cm size range, are not matted and are freely mobile. They may or may not be tender, and frequently patients will report that lymph nodes have enlarged very abruptly.

31.2	AILD
	Clinical presentation
	Generalized lymphadenopathy (all)
	Hepato-splenomegaly (2/3)
	Rash, edema or effusions (> 1/3)
	B symptoms (> 1/2)
	Laboratory findings
	Hypergammaglobulinemia (> 1/2)
	Cold agglutinins (1/2)
	Severe anemia - Hct < 30% (1/4-)
	Coombs-positive (1/3)
	Leukocytosis (1/2)
	Cytopenia (WBC or Plts) (< 1/4)
	LDH > 1 x nl (2/3)

More than half of the patients will have severe constitutional symptoms, notably high fevers, severe malaise, anorexia and weight loss, and this may be coincidental with the appearance of the nodes or may pre-date it by several weeks. On physical examination, the spleen and liver is moderately enlarged in up to two thirds of patients, and these organs tend not to be tender. An interesting observation is that around 25% of patients present with rashes, which may be coincidental with the lymphadenopathy or may precede it by one to three months. Furthermore, in about 25% of cases, one can elicit an antecedent history of a drug reaction or a viral infection, and this has led to the hypothesis that AILD may be a hyper-immune reaction to an allergic process. One also sees edema and effusions in up to a third of patients.

The laboratory findings [31.3], show evidence of a hyperimmune process. Hypergammaglobulinemia is present in over half of the patients, with elevations of IgG, IgA and IgM. Monoclonal spikes are sometimes found, and occasionally these presage the emergence of a B cell non-Hodgkin's lymphoma. Late in the course of the disease process, the patient will some-times develop hypogammaglobulinemia, and this may be related to the process burning itself out. Other evidence of a hyper- or auto-immune process is found in the high frequency of cold agglutinins. Moderate to severe anemia is found in over half of the patients, and, in a third of patients, it is a Coombs-positive hemolytic anemia. From 30 to 40% of patients will have circulating immune complexes, rheumatoid factor and smooth muscle antibodies.

AILD
Treatment Approaches
Prednisone +/- Cytoxan
Combination chemotherapy
Interferon
High-dose chemotherapy with BMT

31.3

Up to half of the patients will have a leukocytosis, but about 50% of patients will also have an absolute lymphopenia. A quarter of the patients will have an overall leucopenia, and occasionally thrombocytopenia is also seen. Elevation of LDH is seen in up to two thirds of patients.

The optimal treatment for this disease is unclear [31.3]. In part, this may be because there have been no good randomized studies, and also because the disease is heterogeneous in terms of clinical presentation. Some studies have evaluated prednisone plus or minus cyclophosphamide. Other studies have investigated the value of combination chemotherapy, either as primary therapy, or following the failure of prednisone. There have now been some limited

claims of the transient efficacy of interferon, and anecdotal reports of the use of high dose chemotherapy with bone marrow transplant.

The report from Siegert et al. published in 1995 [31.4][1] was a retrospective evaluation, rather than a randomized study, and it was based on 62 patients. Patients either received prednisone, to which chemotherapy was added if they failed on this initial treatment, or they received primary chemotherapy up front. It is interesting that patients who received primary chemotherapy tended to have a higher complete and partial remission rate than those who received prednisone followed by chemotherapy. However, if the complete remission rates after four years are reviewed, there was no difference, with survival rates in both groups of about 36 per cent.

AILD			
Clinical outcome			
Therapy	CR	PR	Continuous CR at 4 years
Prednisone / chemotherapy	41%	24%	24%
Primary chemotherapy	52%	40%	20%
Prognostic factors			
Variable	4-year survival (%)		p2
Age < 64	43%		0.032
> 64	28%		
Stage I/II	83%		
III	43%		0.037
IV	15%		
B-symptoms +	65%		0.007
–	22%		
LDH > 274	16%		0.0007
< 274	63%		

31.4

Study based on 62 patients

Siegert et al. 1995 [1]

Since this study was a retrospective one, there may have been some bias in patient selection. For example, patients with less severe presentations, who may also have a somewhat better prognosis, would tend to receive steroids first, rather than chemotherapy. Nevertheless, the overall results suggest that there is no argument for starting patients on chemotherapy as primary treatment.

These authors analyzed prognostic factors which might predict outcome [31.4]. As one might expect, younger patients tended to have a better four year survival, and patients with more limited stage disease also fared better than those with advanced stage disease. Survival was better in patients without constitutional symptoms, as it was in those with a low LDH. However, as already noted, patients in this better prognosis group represent a small minority.

There is also some limited experience with interferon treatment. In one study of twelve patients, half of whom received interferon as primary therapy, and half of whom received interferon after having received prednisone and/or chemotherapy, four complete and four partial remissions were observed. However, the median duration of responses was four months, and only one patient remained in complete remission beyond seven months. Although interferon deserves further study, at least in this limited study, there were no long-standing remissions.

How do these patients fare from a clinical point of view [31.5]? There are essentially three clinical patterns. In about a quarter of patients there is an indolent course and one can even see spontaneous remissions and relapses without therapy. Others are very responsive to prednisone and enter complete remission, but those patients frequently suffer multiple relapses. About a quarter of patients with more aggressive presentations can be very responsive to chemotherapy, and can achieve long-term durable complete remissions. Consequently, it is the author's view that one should consider combination chemotherapy early in the disease, because a subset of these patients may indeed be curable. Finally, there is a group of patients whose disease runs a very aggressive course, and who tend to respond very poorly to combination chemotherapy and die fairly rapidly.

AILD

Clinical Outcome

Usually runs an aggressive course

Less than 25% of patients may have indolent course

Up to one third of patients may develop an aggressive T cell lymphoma or occasionally a B cell NHL

31.5

Why do patients die with this disease? Up to one third of patients will develop an aggressive large T cell neoplasm, although occasionally B cell lymphomas are seen. The development of an aggressive

T cell lymphoma has been likened to the histologic transformation of a low grade lymphoma, but, as noted previously, there is little justification to call the disease, except in a small minority of patients, a low grade process.

One of the interesting observations in this disease is that it is associated with immunodeficiency, and this seems to be secondary to T cell abnormalities. When peripheral blood is analyzed by flow cytometry, these patients have decreased numbers of both CD4 and CD8 cells. Over time, however, a further and more profound immunodeficiency state tends to develop, so that up to 40% of patients who die from this disorder do so from infections. The most common of these are opportunistic infections, including Pneumocystis, Mycobacteria, Pseudomonas, fungi, and a variety of viruses such as CMV, HSV and EBV.

In conclusion [31.6], on the basis of our current understanding, we can view this disease as a lymphoproliferative disorder, in which there is usually both a clonal expansion of T cells and a polyclonal expansion of B cells that are, at least in cell culture, being stimulated by these clonal T cells. Hence a combined T- and B-cell immune dysregulation occurs. There is evidence that this is a clonal disease in most patients since T cell gene rearrangements can be found, and EBV appears to play some etiologic role, because it is very commonly present.

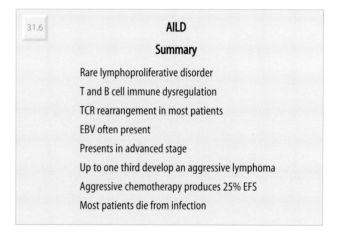

AILD

Summary

Rare lymphoproliferative disorder

T and B cell immune dysregulation

TCR rearrangement in most patients

EBV often present

Presents in advanced stage

Up to one third develop an aggressive lymphoma

Aggressive chemotherapy produces 25% EFS

Most patients die from infection

31.6

Most patients present with advanced stage. Up to a third develop an aggressive lymphoma, but, with aggressive chemotherapy, up to 25% may enjoy an extended event-free survival. Finally, the majority of patients will die from an opportunistic infection, presumably due to profound T cell dysfunction.

REFERENCES

1. Siegert W, Nerl C, Agthe A *et al*. Angioimmunoblastic lymphadenopathy (AILD)-type T-cell lymphoma: Prognostic impact of clinical observations and laboratory findings at presentation. The Kiel Lymphoma Study Group. *Ann Oncol* 1995; **6**: 659-64.

FURTHER READING

Frizzera G, Moran EM, Rappaport H. Angio-immunoblastic lymphadenopathy - diagnosis and clinical course. *Am J Med* 1975; **59**: 803-18.

Jaffe ES. Angioimmunoblastic T-cell lymphoma: New insights, but the clinical challenge remains. *Ann Oncol* 1995; **6**: 631-2.

Siegert W, Agthe A, Griesser H *et al*. Treatment of angioimmunoblastic lymphadenopathy (AILD)-type T-cell lymphoma using prednisone with or without the COP-BLAM / IMVP-16 regimen. *Ann Intern Med* 1992; **117**: 364-70.

Siegert W, Nerl C, Meuthen I *et al*. Recombinant human interferon-alpha in the treatment of angioimmunoblastic lymphadenopathy: Results in 12 patients. *Leukemia* 1991; **5**: 892-5.

Steinberg AD, Seldin MF, Jaffe ES *et al*. Angioimmunoblastic lymphadenopathy with dysproteinemia (NIH Conference). *Ann Intern Med* 1988; **108**: 575-84.

Nasal/nasal type NK/T cell lymphoma (angiocentric lymphoma) and lymphomatoid granulomatosis

E S Jaffe

The REAL classification differs from prior classifications, such as the Working Formulation or the Kiel classification, in that it integrates clinical information into the diagnosis of distinctive entities. In contrast, both the Kiel classification and the Working Formulation were based purely on cell morphology and phenotype. While this information is important, the clinical pattern is often essential to accurate diagnosis. This is particularly true for angiocentric lymphoma, which is a distinct clinicopathologic entity among the T cell lymphomas in the REAL classification [32.1].

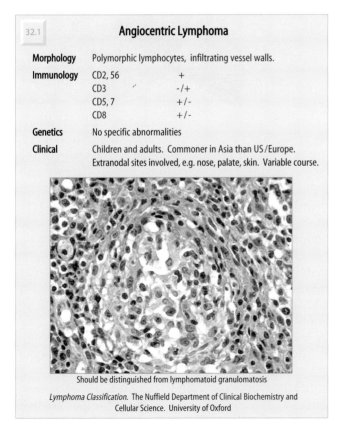

32.1 Angiocentric Lymphoma

Morphology	Polymorphic lymphocytes, infiltrating vessel walls.
Immunology	CD2, 56 +
	CD3 -/+
	CD5, 7 +/-
	CD8 +/-
Genetics	No specific abnormalities
Clinical	Children and adults. Commoner in Asia than US/Europe. Extranodal sites involved, e.g. nose, palate, skin. Variable course.

Should be distinguished from lymphomatoid granulomatosis

Lymphoma Classification. The Nuffield Department of Clinical Biochemistry and Cellular Science. University of Oxford

This disease commonly presents in the nasal area and palate, often with the syndrome of lethal midline granuloma. It tends to spread to other extranodal sites of disease [32.2], such as the gastrointestinal tract, subcutaneous tissue and testis, and its initial presentation can occasionally be at one of these other extranodal sites as well. Lymph node involvement, on the other hand, is conspicuous by its absence.

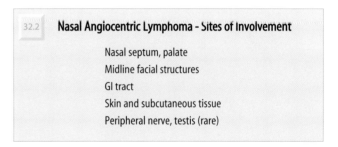

32.2 Nasal Angiocentric Lymphoma - Sites of Involvement

Nasal septum, palate

Midline facial structures

GI tract

Skin and subcutaneous tissue

Peripheral nerve, testis (rare)

The term "angiocentric lymphoma" was coined because extensive tissue necrosis with vascular invasion is a common feature [32.3]. However, vascular invasion is not seen in all cases. This may be due to variation in sampling, since many of the nasal biopsies are small, or it could be that the necrosis is due to other factors. Release of chemokines contribute to the vascular damage. Nevertheless, extensive tissue necrosis suggesting vascular impairment is very characteristic.

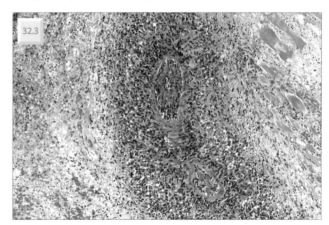

The cytologic composition is quite variable. At one end of the spectrum, as in the case from the Philippines shown in [32.4] in which vascular invasion

is very evident, the neoplastic cells are rather small, with minimal cytologic atypia, and are associated with a reactive background of plasma cells and occasional histiocytes. One is often uncertain that a case such as this is indeed a lymphoma. At the other end of the spectrum are tumors composed of large pleomorphic cells. The aggressive and lymphomatous nature of this form of the disease is obvious in [32.5].

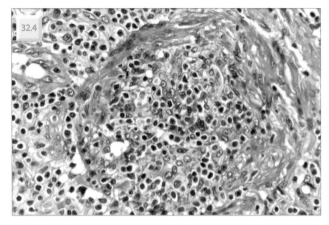

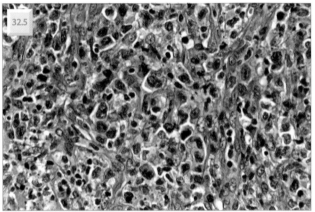

In virtually all cases of this disease one can find Epstein-Barr virus in the neoplastic cells [32.6], and in situ hybridization for EBV using the EBER1 probe is particularly helpful in distinguishing low grade lesions from an atypical inflammatory process. The EBV is in the neoplastic cells, as shown in [32.7] by double staining for EBV and the T cell associated antigen CD43.

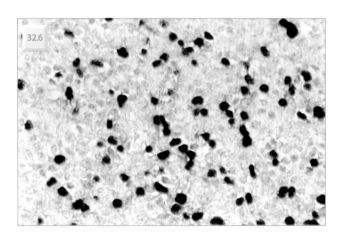

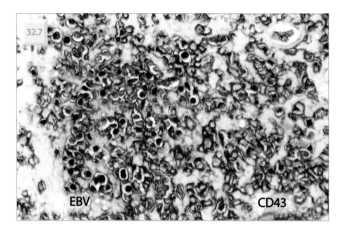

We know that the nasopharynx is frequently a reservoir for EBV, where it is associated with undifferentiated carcinomas, but in the case illustrated in [32.8], by combining *in situ* hybridization with staining for cytokeratin, it is evident that the epithelial cells are EBV-negative.

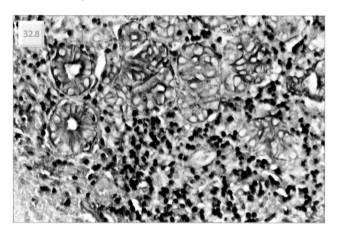

This disease has very interesting epidemiologic features. It is rare in North America and in Europe, but is common in Asian countries, and many of the largest series are from Hong Kong,[1] Taiwan and Japan. It is also seen on the American continent, mainly in Central and South America, where it seems to be especially prevalent among native Americans.[2] Shown in [32.9] is a patient from Peru presenting with nasal angiocentric lymphoma. The geographic distribution pattern suggests that racial factors may predispose to the disease, and certainly there is laboratory evidence to suggest that different ethnic populations handle EBV differently.

The disease has a distinctive immunophenotype [32.10]. It was originally categorized as a T cell lymphoma, because many T cell associated antigens, such as CD2, are present, but other T cell associated markers, such as surface CD3, are usually lacking. T cell arrangement is also generally absent, and a study published by Emile *et al.*[3] provided evidence for the NK-cell origin of this tumor. These tumors contain cytoplasmic CD3, which is a feature of NK cells. Another NK-associated molecule, found in virtually all cases, is CD56. In contrast, CD16 and CD57, which are often found in NK cells, are generally absent.

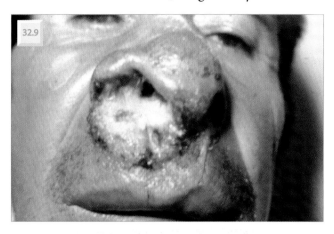

32.10 Phenotypic and Genotypic Features of Nasal and Nasal-type Angiocentric T/NK Cell Lymphomas

Usually pos:	CD2, CD56, cCD3, CD45RO, CD43, EBER 1/2 (EBV by *in situ* hybridization)
Occasionally pos:	CD7, CD4, CD8, LMP-1
Usually neg:	sCD3, βF1, TCRd, CD5, TCR rearr., CD57, CD16, B-cell ag, Ig gene rearr.

We can therefore conclude that angiocentric lymphoma, as defined in the REAL classification, is a distinct sub-type of lymphoma, probably of NK-cell origin, which contains Epstein-Barr viral genome and lacks T cell receptor gene rearrangement [32.11].

32.11

"Angiocentric lymphoma" occurring in the nose and other sites is a distinct type of "T-cell lymphoma" containing **EBV viral genomes**, and **lacking T cell rearrangement**.

The cells express markers of both **T & NK cells**.

It has provisionally been designated as: **Nasal and nasal-type T/NK cell lymphoma**.

The other topic covered in this Chapter is lymphomatoid granulomatosis, a lesion which exhibits similarities in morphology and clinical presentation, but which is a quite different entity [32.12]. Initially we and others had thought that lymphomatoid granulomatosis and nasal angiocentric lymphoma, or "polymorphic reticulosis", were part of a single clinicopathologic entity, but more recent data indicate that lymphomatoid granulomatosis is a clearly different disease.

32.12 Angiocentric Immunoproliferative Lesions

Lymphocytic vasculitis
Lymphomatoid granulomatosis
Polymorphic reticulosis
Midline malignant reticulosis
Angiocentric lymphomas

In common with nasal angiocentric lymphoma, it tends to present at extranodal sites, but it differs in that it most frequently involves the lung, with kidney, liver and central nervous system as other frequent sites. It shares with nasal angiocentric lymphoma a tendency to spread to skin and sub-cutaneous tissue and also to the gastrointestinal tract [32.13].

32.13 Lymphomatoid Granulomatosis Sites of Involvement

Lung and upper respiratory tract
Skin & subcutaneous tissue
Kidney
Liver
Central nervous system
GI tract (uncommon)

In [32.14] one sees a lung in which large tumor nodules with extensive necrosis are present, and a similar picture is seen in the kidney in [32.15].

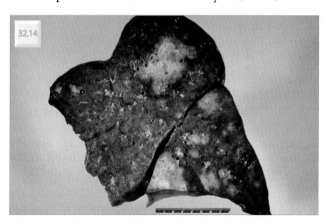

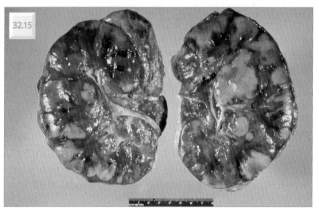

The disease also tends to exhibit a spectrum in histologic grade. In the case illustrated in [32.16], at the low grade end of the spectrum, one sees predominantly small cells with an inflammatory background. At the opposite end of the spectrum [32.17] a tumor in the brain is composed predominantly of large cells, which are much more monomorphic in appearance. Tissue necrosis is seen at the edge of the lesion.

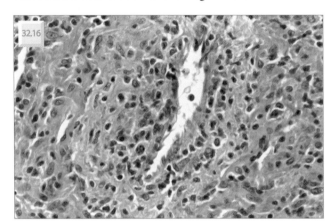

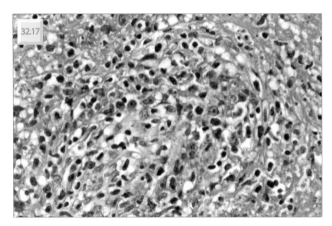

This disease is also associated with EBV. In situ hybridization for EBV on the brain lesion illustrated in [32.18] reveals numerous EBV-positive cells within a vessel. However, the EBV is localized to B cells, as shown in [32.19] by double staining with anti-CD20. Moreover, when Guinee *et al.*[4] [32.20] analyzed a number of cases for evidence of clonal immunoglobulin gene rearrangement by the V-J PCR technique, most cases were positive. This suggests that the EBV-positive B cells are clonal, and represent the neoplastic component. In contrast, when we and others have studied lymphomatoid granulomatosis for T cell gene rearrangement, the results were nearly always negative.

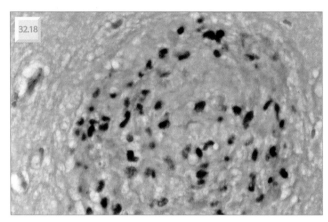

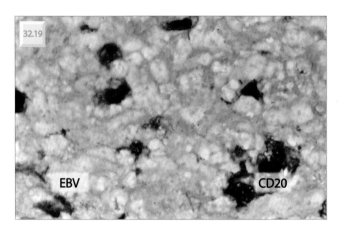

32.20	**Summary of Combined Immunocytochemistry / *In Situ* Hybridization for EBV, PCR for IgH Chain Gene Rearrangements, and Grade**				
Patient N	**Combined IHC for UCHL-1 and ISH for EBV**	**Combined IHC for L26 and ISH for EBV**	**PCR for IgH Chain gene rearrangement**	**EBV + cells/hpf**	**Grade**
1	Negative	Positive in rare immunoblastic cells	Insufficient tissue for analysis	< 1	I
2	Negative	Positive in large atypical cells	Clonal	11	II
3	Negative	Positive in large atypical cells	Clonal	10	II
4	Negative	Positive in large atypical cells	Non reactive	25	III
5	Negative	Positive in large atypical cells	Clonal	40	III
6	Negative	Positive in large atypical cells	Non reactive	59	III
7	Negative	Positive in large atypical cells	Clonal	17	III
8	Negative	Positive in large atypical cells	Indeterminant	28	III
9	Negative	Positive in large atypical cells	Clonal	51	III
10	Negative	Negative	Clonal	62	III

Key: IHC = immunohistochemistry; ISH = *in situ* hybridization; hpf = high power field; EBV = Epstein-Barr virus

Guinee *et al.* 1994[4]

These findings suggest that lymphomatoid granulomatosis is an EBV-associated B cell lymphoproliferative disorder associated with an exuberant T cell response [32.21]. In fact, a number of observations in the past had linked lymphomatoid granulomatosis to EBV-associated lymphoproliferative disease [32.22]. It was shown a number of years ago in a study by Sordillo *et al.* that patients with lymphomatoid granulomatosis frequently had underlying defects in cell mediated immunity.[7] Furthermore, histologic similarities had been noted between lymphomatoid granulomatosis and post-transplant lymphoproliferative disease. Finally, lymphomatoid granulomatosis has frequently been reported in the post-transplant setting, as well as in other immunodeficiency states such as Wiskott-Aldrich syndrome, AIDS and other congenital and acquired immunodeficiencies.

It is perhaps not surprising that in the past we linked nasal angiocentric lymphomas and lymphomatoid granulomatosis, because they do share a number of common features, namely a propensity for extranodal disease, the presence of coagulative necrosis with a vasculitic component, a polymorphous cellular infiltrate with variations in cytologic grade, and a predominance of cells which exhibit a T cell phenotype [32.23]. It is worth noting that in both of these disorders, which were each thought to be T cell lymphomas, clonal T cell gene rearrangement is absent. Interestingly, both disorders are also associated with an increased risk of a hemophagocytic syndrome, probably secondary to the presence of EBV.

32.21 · Molecular Features of LYG

Sporadic LYG is a "T cell" LPD that contains EBV viral genomes but lacks TCR rearrangements

Katzenstein & Peiper 1990 [5] – PCR detects EBV sequences in LYG

Medeiros *et al.* 1991 [6] – Grade III AIL contains clonal EBV, but no Ig or TCR clones

The EBV can be localized to B cells, which represent the minority of cells present.

Clonal Ig rearrangements may be shown in some cases by PCR

Guinee *et al.* 1994 [4]

Conclusion: LYG is a form of EBV-associated B-cell LPD with an exuberant T-cell response

By Contrast: Nasal angiocentric lymphoma is an EBV+ "T/NK-cell" lymphoma lacking T-cell receptor rearrangements

---

32.22 · Relationship of LYG to EBV+ Lymphoproliferative Disease

1. Patients with LYG have underlying defects in cell mediated immunity

2. There are histologic similarities between LYG and Post Tx-LPD

3. LYG has been reported in the post-transplant setting

4. LYG occurs in congenital and acquired immunodeficiency, where it has been linked to EBV;

   — and the vascular lesions may contain a predominance of T cells

---

32.23 · Common Features of Nasal /Nasal-type Angiocentric Lymphomas and LYG

- Propensity for extranodal disease
- Coagulative necrosis with "vasculitic" component
- Polymorphous cellular infiltrate with variations in "cytologic grade"
- Predominant cell exhibits a "T cell" phenotype
- Paradoxic absence of clonal T cell gene R
- Increased risk of hemophagocytic syndrome
- Associated with EBV which is clonal in abnormal cells

However, despite these similarities it now seems clear that nasal angiocentric lymphoma and lymphomatoid granulomatosis are indeed different disorders [32.24], arising respectively from NK cells and B cells.

32.24 · Comparison of Nasal Angiocentric Lymphomas / Lymphomatoid Granulomatosis

	Nasal T /NK lymphoma	LYG
Site	Nasal, palate, URT, GI, skin, testis	Lung, kidney, GI, brain, skin, URT
Necrosis	Yes	Yes
Phenotype	T/NK	B (with reac. T)
TCR	Neg	Neg
Ig R	Neg	Pos (PCR)
EBV	Pos (T/NK)	Pos (B)
HPS	Yes	Yes

ACKNOWLEDGEMENT

This chapter is based on U.S. government work. There are no restrictions on its use.

REFERENCES

1. Chan J, Ng C, Lau W, Ho S. Most nasal/nasopharyngeal lymphomas are peripheral T cell neoplasms. *Am J Surg Pathol* 1987; **11**: 418-29.

2. Arber DA, Weiss LM, Albujar PF, Chen YY, Jaffe ES. Nasal lymphomas in Peru. High incidence of T-cell immuno-phenotype and Epstein-Barr virus infection. *Am J Surg Pathol* 1993; **17**: 392-9.

3. Emile J-F, Boulland M-L, Haioun C *et al*. CD5– CD56+ T-cell receptor silent peripheral T-cell lymphomas are natural killer cell lymphomas. *Blood* 1996; **87**: 1466-73.

4. Guinee DJ, Jaffe E, Kingma D *et al*. Pulmonary lymphomatoid granulomatosis. Evidence for a proliferation of Epstein-Barr virus infected B-lymphocytes with a prominent T-cell component and vasculitis. *Am J Surg Pathol* 1994; **18**: 753-64.

5. Katzenstein ALA, Peiper SC. Detection of Epstein-Barr virus genomes in lymphomatoid granulomatosis: Analysis of 29 cases by the polymerase chain reaction technique. *Mod Pathol* 1990; **3**: 435-41.

6. Medeiros LJ, Peiper SC, Elwood L, Yano T, Raffeld M, Jaffe ES. Angiocentric immunoproliferative lesions: a molecular analysis of eight cases. *Hum Pathol* 1991; **22**: 1150-7.

7. Sordillo PP, Epremian B, Koziner B, Lacher M, Lieberman P. Lymphomatoid granulomatosis: an analysis of clinical and immunologic characteristics. *Cancer* 1982; **49**: 2070-6.

FURTHER READING

Dictor M, Cervin A, Kalm O, Rambech E. Sinonasal T-cell lymphoma in the differential diagnosis of lethal midline granuloma using in situ hybridization for Epstein-Barr virus RNA. *Mod Pathol* 1996; **9**: 7-14.

Ferry JA, Sklar J, Zukerberg LR, Harris NL. Nasal lymphoma. A clinicopathologic study with immuno-phenotypic and genotypic analysis. *Am J Surg Pathol* 1991; **15**: 268-79.

Ho F, Choy D, Loke S *et al*. Polymorphic reticulosis and conventional lymphomas of the nose and upper aerodigestive tract - a clinicopathologic study of 70 cases, and immunophenotypic studies of 16 cases. *Hum Pathol* 1990; **21**: 1041-50.

Ho F, Srivastava G, Loke S *et al*. Presence of Epstein-barr virus DNA in nasal lymphomas of B and T cell type. *Hematol Oncol* 1990; **8**: 271-81.

Imamura N, Kusunoki Y, Kawa-Ha K *et al*. Aggressive natural killer cell leukemia/lymphoma: report of four cases and review of the literature. Possible existence of a new clinical entity originating from the third lineage of lymphoid cells. *Br J Haematol* 1990; **75**: 49-59.

Jaffe ES. Classification of natural killer (NK)-cell and NK-like T-cell malignancies. *Blood* 1996; **87**: 1207-10.

Jaffe ES. Post-thymic T-cell lymphomas. In: Jaffe ES, ed. *Surgical pathology of the lymph nodes and related organs, major problems in pathology* (ed 2nd). Philadelphia: W.B. Saunders, 1995: 344-89.

Jaffe ES, Chan JKC, Su IJ *et al*. Report of the workshop on nasal and related extranodal angiocentric T/NK cell lymphomas: definitions, differential diagnosis, and epidemiology. *Am J Surg Pathol* 1996; **20**: 103-11.

Jaffe ES, Costa J, Fauci AS, Cossman J, Tsokos M. Malignant lymphoma and erythrophagocytosis simulating malignant histiocytosis. *Am J Med* 1983; **75**: 741-9.

Lipford EH, Margolich JB, Longo DL, Fauci AS, Jaffe ES. Angiocentric immunoproliferative lesions: a clinico-pathologic spectrum of post-thymic T cell proliferations. *Blood* 1988; **5**: 1674-81.

Medeiros LJ, Peiper SC, Elwood L, Yano T, Raffeld M, Jaffe ES. Angiocentric immunoproliferative lesions: a molecular analysis of eight cases. *Hum Pathol* 1991; **22**: 1150-7.

Teruya-Feldstein J, Jaffe ES, Burd PR *et al*. The role if Mig, the monokine induced by interferon-gamma, and IP-10, the interferon-gamma-inducible protein-10, in tissue necrosis and vascular damage associated with Epstein-Barr virus-positive lymphoproliferative disease. *Blood* 1997; **90**: 4099-105.

Tsang WY, Chan JK, Yip TT *et al*. In situ localization of Epstein-Barr virus encoded RNA in non-nasal/nasopharyngeal CD56-positive and CD56-negative T-cell lymphomas. *Hum Pathol* 1994; **25**: 758-65.

POST-SCRIPT

Nasal angiocentric lymphoma has an aggressive clinical course. Localized Stage I nasal lesions show a good response to radiation therapy, but there is a high relapse rate. This neoplasm generally shows a poor response to chemotherapy. LYG, especially if low grade, may respond to interferon alpha 2b.[8]

REFERENCES

8. Wilson WH, Kingma DW, Raffeld M *et al*. Association of lymphomatoid granulomatosis with Epstein-Barr viral infection of B lymphocytes and response to interferon-alpha 2b. *Blood* 1996; **87**: 4531-7.

Clinical aspects and treatment options in nasal/nasal type lymphoma (angiocentric lymphoma) and lymphomatoid granulomatosis

33

W H Wilson

This chapter is concerned with the treatment of nasal angiocentric (T/NK) lymphomas (NAL) and lymphomatoid granulomatosis. Nasal T/NK lymphomas are characterized histologically by a mixture of small to large atypical cells and an angiocentric distribution causing obliteration of vessels and necrosis. The disorder was known in the past as "lethal midline granuloma lymphoma". For a long time the cell of origin was unclear, but it is now clear that the cells are mostly of NK phenotype and occasionally of T-CPLL phenotype, often expressing CD2 and CD56. Many of the abnormal cells are positive for EBER1 and therefore contain EBV. They generally do not show T cell receptor rearrangement, so they do not appear to be classical T cells, and they normally lack CD16 or CD57.

Turning to their clinical characteristics, nasal T/NK lymphomas are rare, but they constitute the largest single group of lymphomas which present primarily in the nasal cavity. They have a male predilection, and a peak incidence in the sixth decade. At presentation, more than 70% are early stage lesions, and less than 20% of patients have constitutional symptoms. They are uncommon tumors in the West, but are far from rare in Asia, and in a recent report from a large center in Hong Kong, they constituted 10.7% of their cases of non-Hodgkin's lymphomas.[1]

Patients usually present with a midline facial lesion, and often complain of nasal obstruction due to a destructive mass. Extranasal presentations are rare, and include the upper aerodigestive tract, gastrointestinal tract and the testis. There may be secondary spread to the skin, and occasionally there is pulmonary involvement. However, in one large series, these sites were involved in less than 5% of patients, emphasizing the relative infrequency of extranasal involvement.[2]

Therapy has not been well studied in randomized trials, but radiation, with or without chemotherapy, is commonly used on an empirical basis for Stage I and II disease, and chemotherapy, with or without radiation, for Stage III and IV disease.

A retrospective analysis of 100 patients was published in 1995 from Hong Kong [33.1].[2] Most of the cases, as judged by the histologic criteria given in the paper, seemed to fit fully the characteristics of nasal T/NK lymphomas. If the results are reviewed in terms of clinical Stage, the complete remission rate was high (85%) in patients who had limited disease, and the overall five year survival was also quite good, at 66%. In patients with Stage II disease, the complete remission rate fell by half, as did the five year survival rate, and for the patients with advanced disease, Stages III and IV, the survival rate was quite low (30%) and the five year survival was less than 10% [33.1].

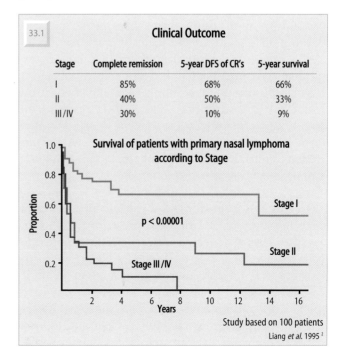

In this study the patients with Stage I and II disease were treated with radiation with or without chemotherapy, but the patients who received chemotherapy fared only slightly better than those who received radiation therapy alone. These data are not based on a randomized study, and the treatment regime varied from patient to patient, but at least they give us a hint that chemotherapy may be of limited value. Combination chemotherapy, often combined with radiation therapy, was used for all patients with Stage III and IV disease, and these patients did not have very good long term outlook. When prognostic factors were assessed in a univariate analysis, younger age and the absence of B symptoms were two favorable prognostic findings, but in a multivariate analysis Stage was the only significant variable.

In summary, this tumor has a T/NK phenotype, without T cell receptor rearrangement. Most cases are EBV-positive, and clonal integration of the virus can be found in these tumors. They are usually angiocentric, are rare in the West, but are the most common lymphoma type to present in the nasal region. Given our current state of knowledge, it appears that Stage I and II disease should receive combined modality therapy, using an intermediate grade lymphoma regimen followed by involved field radiation. With regard to patients who have advanced disease, chemotherapy is obviously the mainstay of therapy, but local failure, particularly in a site like the nasal cavity, poses a very real problem, so that local radiation is indicated in that setting.

The other topic of this chapter, lymphomatoid granulomatosis (LYG), was felt in the past to be a different manifestation of T/NK lymphoma, usually presenting with pulmonary disease. This was because LYG is histopathologically very similar to NAL, containing a mixture of small lymphocytes, plasma cells, histiocytes and variable numbers of large atypical cells. In addition, LYG tends to have an angiocentric distribution, like T NAL, resulting in angiodestruction and necrosis. For this reason, the term "angioimmunoproliferative lesion" (AIL) was coined to include both lymphomatoid granulomatosis and nasal angiocentric lymphomas.

A grading scheme for LYG was developed based on both the number of large cells present in the lesion and the amount of necrosis. Grade I lesions tended to have few scattered large cells and very little necrosis, and grade II had an intermediate number of large cells and more necrosis. Grade III lesions contained many large cells, frequently forming sheets, and were felt at that time, and would still be seen in that light today, to represent an aggressive large cell lymphoma.

When the phenotype is considered, the large cells are usually EBV-positive by *in situ* hybridization, and double staining for CD20 shows that they are also B cells. However, the small cells have a normal T cell phenotype and appear to be infiltrating reactive T cells. We have investigated four patients for evidence that the large cells are monoclonal, and have not found a consistent pattern. Some patients had multiple clones whereas others had single clones, and we do not know the significance of these findings at present.

If the patient characteristics [33.2] are compared to those of nasal T/NK lymphomas, both diseases have a male predilection. However, lymphomatoid granulomatosis tends to present earlier. Nasal lymphomas have a T/NK phenotype whereas lymphomatoid granulomatosis are of B cell phenotype. Early stage disease is common in nasal T/NK lymphomas, whereas lymphomatoid granulomatosis tends to be of advanced stage, with over 50% of patients having disease outside the lung. There is also now evidence that patients with lymphomatoid granulomatosis have some type of T cell defect and are in fact immunocompromised.

33.2	**Patient Characteristics**	
Nasal T /NK lymphomas	**Lymphomatoid granulomatosis**
Male predilection	Male predilection
Presents in 6th decade	Presents in 4th-5th decade
T/NK phenotype	B cell phenotype
Early stage (Nasal) > 70%	Advanced Stage (> 50%)
B symptoms < 20%	B symptoms > 60%
	Immunocompromised

If the clinical presentations are compared [33.3], lymphomatoid granulomatosis almost always presents with pulmonary disease, while nasal lymphoma presents with nasopharyngeal disease. Whereas involvement of the upper aerodigestive and gastrointestinal tracts and the skin is rare in nasal lymphoma, one sees skin, kidney and liver involvement in 30-40% of lymphomatoid granulomatosis patients. One also finds CNS or peripheral nerve involvement in up to 30% of patients with LYG.

33.3	**Presentation**	
Nasal T /NK lymphomas	**Lymphomatoid granulomatosis**
Facial disease	Pulmonary nodules
Upper aerodigestive tract	Frequent skin, kidney,
May involve GI tract and testis	liver involvement
Secondary spread to skin	Occasional CNS disease
Rare pulmonary involvement	

Therapy options for LYG have been very variable and have included antibiotics, prednisone and/or cyclophosphamide, and also combination chemotherapy. However, this is a very rare disorder, so that there are few large studies. In the largest single retrospective series in the literature, from Katzenstein and colleagues in 1979 [33.4], a variety of treatments was used, but the death rate and the number of patients alive and well or alive with disease were all essentially identical for the four treatment groups.[3]

33.4	Clinical Outcome			
Therapy	N	Deaths	Alive / well	Alive / disease
Steroids +/− Chemo	134	64%	24%	12%
Steroids + Chemo	42	64%	24%	12%
Chemotherapy	26	69%	1%	0%
Antibiotics / Observe	21	62%	27%	11%
Median follow-up approximately 24 months				
				Katzenstein et al. 1979[3]

A more recent study from Dr. Fauci at the NIH in the mid-1980s reported 15 patients treated with prednisone and cyclophosphamide over a three year period, and a follow-up of approximately two years.[4] He noted that six patients were in continuing complete remission, so there may be some merit to that therapy. However, a disturbing finding was that seven of these patients went on to develop grade III lymphomatoid granulomatosis, or an aggressive large cell lymphoma.

Since this is a disorder involving B cells infected with EBV, we reasoned that it may well be an EBV-driven B cell lymphoproliferative disorder. We have therefore treated four patients with interferon [33.5]. The only patient who had received previous treatment was the first subject, a 21 year old man who had failed CHOP chemotherapy, and presented with lung and liver disease two months after completing chemotherapy.

33.5	Clinical Summary			
Case history	Interferon therapy	Response	Survival	
1. Man, 21, failed CHOP lung, hepatic	40 months	Complete	DFS 60 months	
2. Woman, 53, with fevers lung, renal, hepatic	24 months	Complete	DFS 43 months	
3. Man, 16, with fevers lung, skin, CNS	16 months	Partial	PD 18 months	
4. Man, 28, with fevers lung, skin, CNS	36 months	Complete	DFS 36 months	

We found EBV-positive B cells in patients Nos. 1, 3 and 4. We were unable to find evidence of a clonal process by immunoglobulin gene rearrangement in patient No. 1, but a single clone was found in patient No. 2 and we found two different clones in patient No. 4.

We treated these patients with interferon, at 10-30 x 10^6 units three times a week, for periods ranging from 16 to 40 months. We achieved complete remission in patients Nos. 1, 2 and 4, and these patients are now all disease-free three to five years later. The only patient who did not enter complete remission was non-compliant with his medication and stopped treatment, and four months later he developed a large cell lymphoma. When his tumor was analyzed, three different clones of EBV-positive B cells could be found.

It was also of interest to look for evidence of immunodeficiency in these patients, because all four of our patients were anergic when tested with skin panels of allergens, and one patient had a history of oral thrush. We found that, although there was variable reduction of both CD4 cells and B cells, all four patients had a decrease in CD8 cells. We did not have pre-therapy values for these patients, but our working hypothesis is that these patients have some type of CD8 or cytotoxic T cell deficit that prevents them from handling EBV infections normally [33.6].

33.6	Lymphomatoid Granulomatosis Lymphocyte Subset Analysis		
Case Nos.	CD4 cells / mm³	CD8 cells / mm³	Total B cells CD19 /mm³
1. Post-therapy	416	147	139
2. Post-therapy	837	198	599
3. During therapy	383	145	ND
Post-therapy	1151	451	ND
4. Pre-therapy	273	48	26
Normal ranges	700-1100	500-900	200-400

To summarize, the large cells in LYG are clearly EBV-positive B cells, and we have seen evidence of a monoclonal, oligoclonal and polyclonal immunoglobulin gene rearrangement. It appears to be associated with immunodeficiency, and in fact one can find evidence of lymphomatoid granulomatosis in patients who are infected with HIV or have other known immunodeficiency states.

Clinically LYG usually presents in the lungs. There is no agreed therapy for grade I and II disease, although consideration should be given to prednisone or cyclophosphamide. It would be hard to disagree if a physician chose to try combination chemotherapy up front. There is too little evidence with interferon for it to be recommended as standard therapy at the present time but our preliminary results are promising. Finally, grade III lesions, which are in effect aggressive lymphomas, should be treated with aggressive combination chemotherapy.[5]

REFERENCES

1. Cheung MM, Chan JK, Lau WH *et al.* Primary non-Hodgkin's lymphoma of the nose and nasopharynx: clinical features, tumor immunophenotype, and treatment outcome in 113 patients. *J Clin Oncol* 1998; **16**: 70-77.

2. Liang R, Todd D, Chan TK *et al.* Treatment outcome and prognostic factors for primary nasal lymphoma. *J Clin Oncol* 1995; **13**: 666-70.

3. Katzenstein AL, Carrington CB, Liebow AA. Lymphomatoid granulomatosis: A clinicopathologic study of 152 cases. *Cancer* 1979; **43**: 360-73.

4. Fauci AS, Haynes BF, Costa J, Katz P, Wolff SM. Lymphomatoid granulomatosis; Prospective clinical and therapeutic experience over 10 years. *N Engl J Med* 1982; **306**: 68-74.

5. Jaffe ES, Wilson WH. Lymphomatoid granulomatosis: pathogenesis, pathology and clinical implications. In Wotherspoon AC (ed). Imperial Cancer Research Fund. *Cancer Surveys* 30. Cold Spring Harbor Laboratory Press 1997.

FURTHER READING

Guinee D Jr, Jaffe E, Kingma D *et al.* Pulmonary lymphomatoid granulomatosis; evidence for a proliferation of Epstein-Barr virus infected B-lymphocytes with a prominent T-cell component and vasculitis. *Am J Surg Pathol* 1994; **18**: 753-64.

Jaffe ES, Chan JK, Su IJ *et al.* Report of the workshop on nasal and related extranodal angiocentric T / Natural Killer-cell lymphomas: Definitions, differential diagnosis, and epidemiology. *Am J Surg Pathol* 1996; **20**: 103-11.

Liebow AA, Carrington CRB, Friedman PJ. Lymphomatoid granulomatosis. *Hum Pathol* 1972; **3**: 457-558.

Wilson WH, Kingma DW, Raffeld M, Wittes RE, Jaffe ES. Association of lymphomatoid granulomatosis with Epstein-Barr viral infection of B lymphocytes and response to interferon-alpha 2b. *Blood* 1996; **87**: 4531-7.

Subcutaneous panniculitis-like T cell lymphoma

E S Jaffe

Although the classification of T cell lymphomas in the REAL scheme is complex, there are sufficient data to warrant separating some of these disorders into separate entities, both because of their unique clinical presentations and because of the complications to which these patients often succumb. This is certainly also true of subcutaneous panniculitic cell lymphoma, or if one prefers, subcutaneous panniculitis-like T cell lymphoma [34.1].

The striking histopathologic appearance is seen in [34.2]. The disease is usually remarkably confined to the subcutaneous adipose tissue, with minimal involvement of the overlying dermis and epidermis. There is a lace-like infiltrate of atypical lymphoid cells throughout the subcutaneous tissue [34.3]. Frequently there is associated fat necrosis and karyorrhexis, and necrosis can be extensive [34.4].

34.1	Subcutaneous Panniculitis-like T Cell Lymphoma

Presents with subcutaneous nodules 1 to 12 cm in size - primarily affecting extremities

Age range: 19-54 years   Males = Females

Reminiscent of panniculitis histologically - with varying degrees of cytologic atypia

Referral diagnosis was benign in 5/8 cases

Progression over time with greater cytologic atypia

Follow-up: 3/8 alive in remission (5-26 months)

       5/8 dead at 6- 60 months with both lymphoma and HPS

Median survival : 27 months

Gonzalez *et al.* 1991 [1]

It is a disease seen primarily in adults, and it has an equal male : female ratio. The patients typically present with subcutaneous nodules, primarily affecting the extremities. Histologically these lesions are often reminiscent of panniculitis, and some of the cases that we have seen were diagnosed as benign lesions by the contributing pathologist.

Early on in the course of the disease there may be only minimal degrees of cytologic atypia. However, it tends to progress histologically, acquiring greater cytologic atypia, and the diagnosis of lymphoma then becomes obvious. It is an aggressive disease, with a median survival of only about two years, and many patients succumb to a hemophagocytic syndrome.

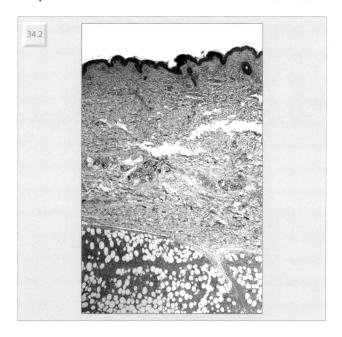

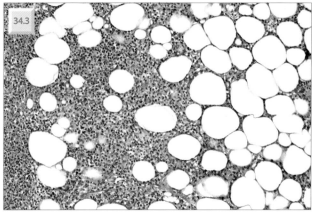

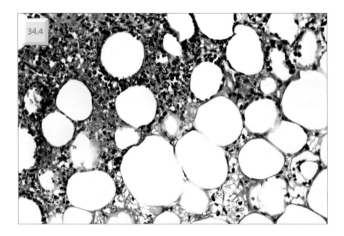

In some cases the cells are predominantly small, but in others, as in this case shown in [34.5], cytologic atypia is obvious and large lymphoid cells are present, with frequent mitotic figures.

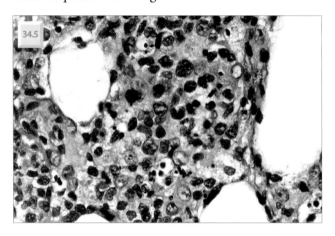

The differential diagnosis of this condition includes angiocentric T cell lymphoma, which can also involve the skin [34.6]. As discussed elsewhere (Chapter 32), the latter disorder usually lacks T cell gene rearrangement and is associated with Epstein-Barr virus. We therefore studied our cases of sub-cutaneous panniculitic T cell lymphoma for the presence of EBV and T cell gene rearrangement. All of the cases investigated for EBV were negative by *in situ* hybridization, which is quite different from angiocentric T cell lymphoma. In most cases with amplifiable DNA which could be studied by the PCR technique, we were able to show clonal rearrangement of the T cell receptor γ chain gene. These findings suggest that this process is distinct from angiocentric lymphoma involving the skin.

An important feature of this disorder is a hemo-phagocytic syndrome [34.7]. Three patients in our initial series had a hemophagocytic syndrome at presentation, and another three developed this complication at some point during their clinical course. Furthermore, the hemophagocytic syndrome was responsible for the patient's death in most cases.

One patient presented with a hemophagocytic syndrome, and this resolved when chemotherapy for the lymphoma was instituted. However, in the other patients this was a fatal complication, causing profound pancytopenia and infectious complications.

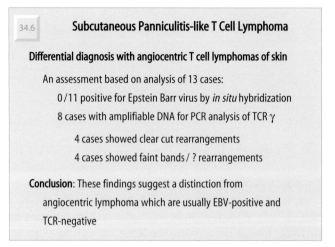

34.6   **Subcutaneous Panniculitis-like T Cell Lymphoma**

Differential diagnosis with angiocentric T cell lymphomas of skin

An assessment based on analysis of 13 cases:

     0/11 positive for Epstein Barr virus by *in situ* hybridization

     8 cases with amplifiable DNA for PCR analysis of TCR γ

         4 cases showed clear cut rearrangements

         4 cases showed faint bands / ? rearrangements

Conclusion: These findings suggest a distinction from angiocentric lymphoma which are usually EBV-positive and TCR-negative

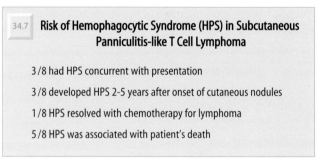

34.7   **Risk of Hemophagocytic Syndrome (HPS) in Subcutaneous Panniculitis-like T Cell Lymphoma**

     3/8 had HPS concurrent with presentation

     3/8 developed HPS 2-5 years after onset of cutaneous nodules

     1/8 HPS resolved with chemotherapy for lymphoma

     5/8 HPS was associated with patient's death

In the bone marrow of patients with a hemo-phagocytic syndrome one sees histiocytes containing numerous red cells [34.8]. These histiocytes are cytologically benign, and one would not suspect malignant involvement of the marrow. Indeed, we have no evidence that the malignant cells are present in the marrow. In bone marrow aspirates one can identify histiocytes which are phagocytosing not only red cells, but also neutrophils and frequently platelets [34.9].

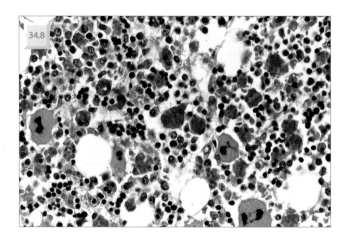

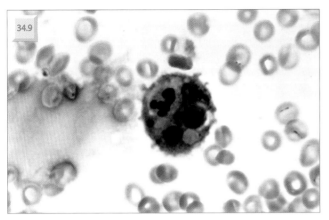

34.9

The mechanism of the hemophagocytic syndrome in this condition is still not clear [34.10]. One possibility is that this is a consequence of cytokine production by the neoplastic cells, or perhaps by bystander cells. We have previously found *in vitro* evidence for the production of cytokines in angiocentric lymphomas, and this is also a possibility in this disorder. In a study by Burg *et al.* of a patient with subcutaneous lymphoma of γδ phenotype who developed a hemophagocytic syndrome, it was shown that T cell clones produced *in vitro* large amounts of interferon-γ and GM-CSF.[3]

Another intriguing possibility is that lipid is the cause of histiocyte activation, and there have been reports of patients undergoing hyperalimentation with intravenous fat emulsions who develop activation of monocytes and histiocytes, and clinical thrombocytopenia. Hyperlipidemia has also been seen in the hemophagocytic syndrome in familial erythrophagocytic lymphohistiocytosis. There may also be a component of direct suppression of hemopoiesis by the neoplastic T cells, as has been shown for certain types of T cell lymphomas.

If one reviews published reports of subcutaneous T cell lymphomas with panniculitis, one finds that hemophagocytic syndrome is common [34.11]. Furthermore, most cases in the literature which have been studied for EBV have been negative, with the exception of a single report. These disorders have a T cell phenotype and in most cases clonal T cell gene rearrangement can be demonstrated. This process is probably identical to what was called in the past "histiocytic cytophagic panniculitis" by Winkelmann.[9,10] This was thought to be malignant histiocytic proliferation, but it is almost certainly a manifestation of subcutaneous T cell lymphoma with panniculitis.

34.10

Possible Mechanisms of HPS in Subcutaneous Panniculitis-like TCL

- Cytokine production by neoplastic or bystander cells
    - in vitro production of cytokines in "AIL"   (Simrell *et al.* 1985 [2])
    - interferon γ & GM-CSF produced by T cell clones from subcutaneous lymphoma   (Burg *et al.* 1991 [3])
- Intravenous lipid as a cause of histiocyte activation
    - hyperalimentation, intravenous fat emulsion (TPN) associated with HPS / thrombocytopenia
    - lipidemia seen in HPS of familial erythrophagocytic lymphohistiocytosis
- Direct suppression of hematopoiesis by some T cell clones (NK and NK-like T cells)

34.11

Subcutaneous Panniculitis-like T Cell Lymphomas

Authors	N	HPS	EBV
Gonzalez *et al.* [1]	8	6/8 *	ns
Medeiros *et al.* [4]	11	8/11 *	0/11
Burg *et al.* [3]	1	prob	ns
Perniciaro *et al.* [5]	2	1/2	ns
Aronson *et al.* [6]	1	1/1	ns
Smith *et al.* [7]	1	1/1	+
Kaplan *et al.* [8]	1	1/1	neg
Summary	**23**	**17/22**	**1/12**

* There was some overlap in these two reports.

ACKNOWLEDGEMENT

This chapter is based on U.S. government work. There are no restrictions on its use.

REFERENCES

1. Gonzalez CL, Medeiros LJ, Braziel RM, Jaffe ES. T-cell lymphoma involving subcutaneous tissue: a clinicopathologic entity commonly associated with hemophagocytic syndrome. *Am J Surg Pathol* 1991; **15**: 1727.

2. Simrell CR, Margolick JB, Crabtree GR, Cossman J, Fauci AS, Jaffe ES. Lymphokine-induced phagocytosis in angio-centric immunoproliferative lesions (AIL) and malignant lymphoma arising in AIL. *Blood* 1985; **65**: 1469-76.

3. Burg G, Dummer R, Wilhelm M *et al*. A subcutaneous delta-positive T-cell lymphoma that produces interferon gamma. *N Engl J Med* 1991; **325**: 1078-81.

4. Medeiros LJ, Greener TG, Gonzalez CL *et al*. T-cell lymphoma involving subcutaneous tissue: An update. *Mod Pathol* 1994; **7**: 116A.

5. Perniciaro C, Zalla MJ, White JW, Menke DM. Subcutaneous T-cell lymphoma: Report of two additional cases and further observations. *Arch Dermatol* 1993; **129**: 1171-6.

6. Aronson IK, West DP, Variakojis D, Ronan SG, Iossifides I, Zeitz HJ. Panniculitis associated with cutaneous T-cell lymphoma and cytophagocytic histiocytosis. *Brit J Dermatol* 1985; **112**: 87-96.

7. Smith KJ, Skelton HG 3d, Giblin WL, James WD. Cutaneous lesions of hemophagocytic syndrome in a patient with T-cell lymphoma and active Epstein-Barr infection. *J Am Acad Dermatol* 1991; **25**: 919-24.

8. Kaplan MA, Jacobson JO, Ferry JA, Harris NL. T-cell lymphoma of the vulva in a renal allograft recipient with associated hemophagocytosis. *Am J Surg Pathol* 1993; **17**: 842-9.

9. Crotty CP, Winkelmann RK. Cytophagic histiocytic panniculitis with fever, cytopenia, liver failure, and terminal hemorrhagic diathesis. *J Am Acad Dermatol* 1981; **4**: 181-94.

10. Winkelmann R, Bowie, EJ. Hemorrhagic diathesis associated with benign histiocytic, cytophagic panniculitis and systemic histiocytosis. *Arch Intern Med* 1980; **140**: 1460-3.

FURTHER READING

Goulet O, Girot R, Maier-Redelsperger M, Bougle D, Virelizier JL, Ricour C. Hematologic disorders following prolonged use of intravenous fat emulsions in children. *J Parenter Enter Nutr* 1986; **10**: 284-8.

POST-SCRIPT

More recent studies have shown that subcutaneous panniculitis-like T-cell lymphoma is derived from cytotoxic T-lymphocytes, nearly always positive for CD8.[11] While most cases are of $\alpha\beta$ T-cell derivation, 25% of cases are derived from $\gamma\delta$ T-cells.

REFERENCES

11. Kumar S, Krenacs L, Medeiros LJ *et al*. Subcutaneous panniculitic T-cell lymphoma is a tumor of cytotoxic T lymphocytes. *Hum Pathol* 1998; **29**: 397-403.

Hepatosplenic gamma delta T cell lymphoma

E S Jaffe

This rare disorder was initially listed in the REAL classification as a provisional malignancy, because very few reports had been published at that time, but there is certainly now convincing evidence that it is a distinctive sub-type of lymphoma. It was initially described by Farcet and colleagues in 1990 as a "hepatosplenic T-cell lymphoma".[1] They identified several patients presenting with striking hepatosplenomegaly and a unique type of T cell lymphoma.

Review of the literature reveals about twenty published cases, all of which conform to a very distinctive clinical presentation [35.1].[2] Nearly all of the patients are males between the ages of 15 and 35. They present with hepatosplenomegaly, and frequently the bone marrow is involved. Tumor cells may be present in low numbers in the peripheral blood, but most patients are not frankly leukemic. Lymphadenopathy is usually absent.

35.1	**Hepatosplenic γδ T Cell Lymphoma**
Clinical features
Young males (Ages 15-35)
Hepatosplenomegaly, positive BM, +/- PB
No lymphadenopathy
Thrombocytopenia, anemia, leukocytosis
Thrombocytopenia persists or recurs following splenectomy
No skin lesions
Aggressive clinical course, median survival < 2 years

A striking clinical feature is thrombocytopenia and, although this may be due in part to the splenomegaly causing hypersplenism, it frequently persists or recurs following splenectomy. In addition, these patients are frequently anemic, but there is often a neutrophil leukocytosis and occasionally an eosinophilia. Skin lesions are usually absent, and the clinical course is very aggressive, with a median survival of less than two years. The only patient the author knows of in continuous complete remission underwent allogeneic bone marrow transplantation from an HLA-matched sibling.

The pathology of this disorder is also very striking and very constant. In the spleen section in [35.2], residual white pulp is present but the red pulp is massively infiltrated by neoplastic cells which distend the sinusoids [35.3]. The infiltrate is very monomorphic, and this is in distinction to peripheral T cell lymphomas, in which pleomorphism is generally the rule. The cells are rather uniform in appearance, being medium sized with a moderate amount of pale cytoplasm. In the liver the sinusoids are distended by a very monomorphic infiltrate [35.4].

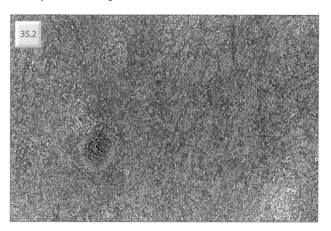

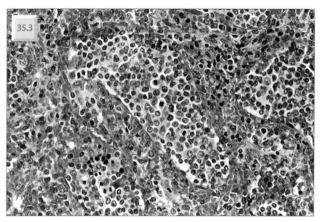

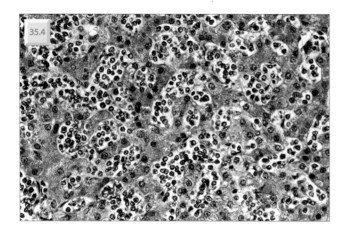

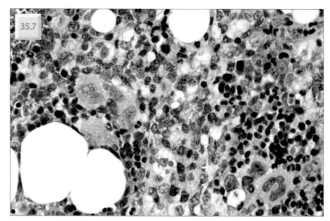

The bone marrow is frequently involved, although at first glance it is frequently hypercellular, and tumor cells may not be obvious [35.5]. However, if one stains for CD3, a striking localization of neoplastic cells within the sinusoids is seen in [35.6] and [35.7].

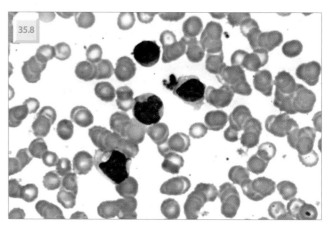

[35.9] shows a frozen section of liver stained for βF1, a marker expressed on αβ T cells, but not on γδ T cells. The normal T cells in the portal triads are positive, but the infiltrating malignant cells on the right are negative. In contrast, the tumor cells are strikingly positive for γδ TCR [35.10]. This γδ T cell phenotype differs from that of most T cell lymphomas, which are of αβ T cell origin.

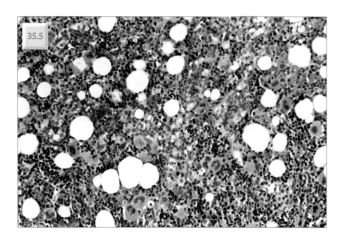

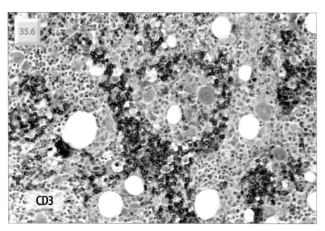

The disease is quite characteristic in its pathology and in its immunophenotype [35.11].[2] The neoplastic γδ T cells express CD2, CD3, CD7 and frequently CD56. Normal γδ T cells are negative for both CD4 and CD8, but in this disease the neoplastic cells may

In aspirates, the cells are medium sized, and many show slight irregularity [35.8]. They usually have a fair amount of abundant cytoplasm, without striking cytologic atypia, and do not contain any cytoplasmic granules (in contrast to large granular lymphocyte leukemia – see Chapter 8).

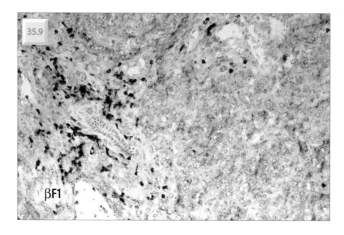

sometimes be CD8-positive. In addition, the cells seem to have features of cytotoxic T cells and stain positively for the cytotoxic granule associated protein (TIA-1), as shown in the section of spleen illustrated in [35.12].

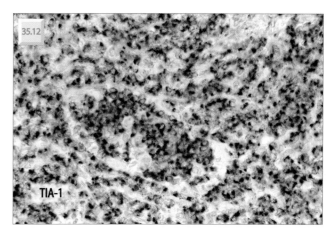

TIA-1

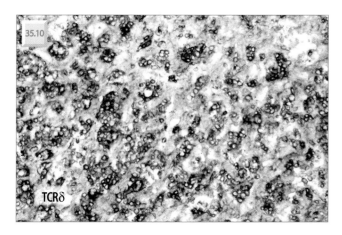

TCRδ

In conclusion [35.13], γδ T cell lymphomas for the most part conform to the entity of hepatic T cell lymphoma as just described. However, there are other rare forms of γδ T cell lymphoma, usually presenting with cutaneous or subcutaneous disease. It is not clear whether the cutaneous cases should be considered in the future as distinct entities, or simply included in the broad group of peripheral T cell lymphomas. The subcutaneous γδ T cell lymphomas conform to subcutaneous panniculitis-like T cell lymphoma (see Chapter 34).

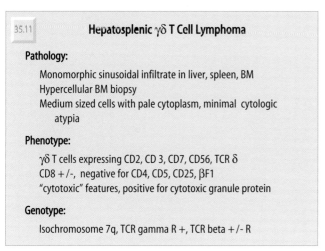

35.11 **Hepatosplenic γδ T Cell Lymphoma**

Pathology:

Monomorphic sinusoidal infiltrate in liver, spleen, BM
Hypercellular BM biopsy
Medium sized cells with pale cytoplasm, minimal cytologic atypia

Phenotype:

γδ T cells expressing CD2, CD 3, CD7, CD56, TCR δ
CD8 +/-, negative for CD4, CD5, CD25, βF1
"cytotoxic" features, positive for cytotoxic granule protein

Genotype:

Isochromosome 7q, TCR gamma R +, TCR beta +/- R

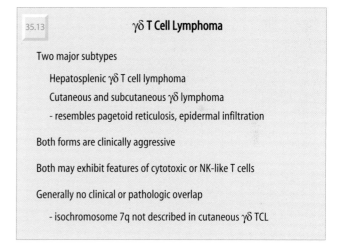

35.13 **γδ T Cell Lymphoma**

Two major subtypes

Hepatosplenic γδ T cell lymphoma

Cutaneous and subcutaneous γδ lymphoma

- resembles pagetoid reticulosis, epidermal infiltration

Both forms are clinically aggressive

Both may exhibit features of cytotoxic or NK-like T cells

Generally no clinical or pathologic overlap

- isochromosome 7q not described in cutaneous γδ TCL

Perhaps the strongest evidence that this is a distinctive clinicopathologic entity comes from recent cytogenetic studies which have identified isochromosome 7q as a characteristic cytogenetic abnormality in all cases thus far studied.[3,4]

ACKNOWLEDGEMENT

This chapter is based on U.S. government work. There are no restrictions on its use.

REFERENCES

1. Farcet JP, Gaulard P, Marolleau J et al. Hepatosplenic T-cell lymphoma: sinusal / sinusoidal localization of malignant cells expressing the T-cell receptor γδ. *Blood* 1990; **75**: 2213-9.

2. Cooke CB, Krenacs L, Stetler-Stevenson M et al. Hepatosplenic T-cell lymphoma: a distinct clinico-pathologic entity of cytotoxic γδ T-cell origin. *Blood* 1996; **88**: 4265-74.

3. Wang CC, Tien HF, Lin MT et al. Consistent presence of isochromosome 7q in hepatosplenic T gamma / delta lymphoma: a new cytogenetic-clinicopathologic entity. *Genes Chromosom Cancer* 1995; **12**: 161-4.

4. Alonsozana EL, Stamberg J, Kumar D et al. Isochromosome 7q: the primary cytogenetic abnormality in hepatosplenic γδ T-cell lymphoma. *Leukemia* 1997; **11**: 1367-72.

FURTHER READING

Burg G, Dummer R, Wilhelm M et al. A subcutaneous delta-positive T-cell lymphoma that produces interferon gamma. *N Engl J Med* 1991; **325**: 1078-81.

Ross CW, Schnitzer B, Sheldon S, Braun DK, Hanson CA. Gamma/delta T-cell post transplantation lymphoproliferative disorder primarily in the spleen. *Am J Clin Pathol* 1994; **102**: 310-5.

Intestinal (enteropathy-associated) T cell lymphoma

P G Isaacson

Although this disease is frequently referred to as a rare T cell lymphoma, it is, in fact, one of the commoner types of T cell neoplasm in Europe, or at least in Northern Europe. In the REAL classification it is listed as "intestinal T cell lymphoma with or without enteropathy" [36.1]. It manifests itself as masses or ulcers in the small intestine, and these are frequently multi-focal. The neoplastic cells usually have a large anaplastic appearance similar to that of anaplastic large cell lymphoma, but medium sized or even small cells may also be present.

36.1	Intestinal T Cell Lymphoma with or without Enteropathy
-	Small intestinal masses or ulcers, frequently multifocal
-	Usually large anaplastic cells but may be medium or small cells
-	Intra-epithelial tumor cells often present – florid intra-epithelial lymphocytosis in some
-	Adjacent mucosa usually shows enteropathy (villous atrophy) but may not
-	Associated "benign" inflammatory ulcers

Intra-epithelial tumor cells are a feature of this condition, and in some cases there is a very florid intra-epithelial lymphocytosis. The adjacent mucosa usually shows enteropathy, taking the form of villous atrophy with cryptic hyperplasia, but in some cases there is no associated histologic evidence of enteropathy. There is a high incidence of associated so-called benign inflammatory ulcers.

Shown in [36.2] is the macroscopic appearance, with multiple ulcerating lesions, of the small intestine. These often have features of malignant ulcers, notably overgrowing of the edges, but they may also be small and fissure-like, and are sometimes very difficult to recognize.

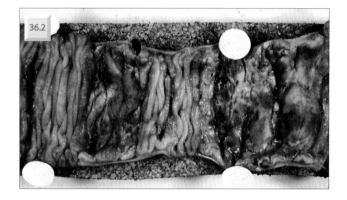

The cytology of the neoplastic cells varies. The appearance in [36.3] on the left is seen in a minority of cases, the neoplastic cells being essentially atypical small lymphocytes. However, the common appearance is on the right, with very large cells, resembling the cells of anaplastic large cell lymphoma.

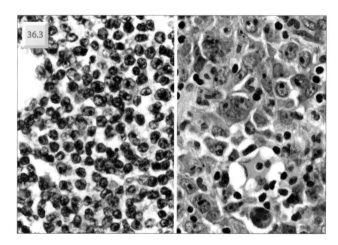

The tumor illustrated in [36.4], which is composed of large cells, shows the presence of neoplastic cells within the epithelium of the intestinal glands, both as single cells and in clusters.

Shown in [36.5] is the mucosa adjacent to a tumor mass. There is an intense intra-epithelial lymphocytosis, with small lymphocytes spilling out into the lamina propria. This type of infiltrate has been shown to be part of the neoplastic process.

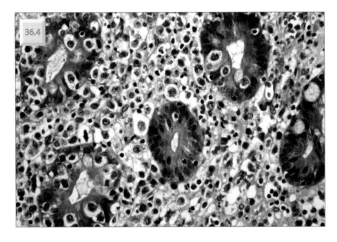

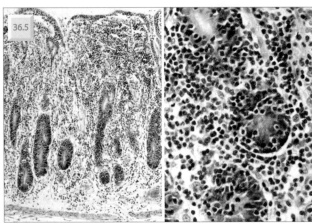

There has been much controversy about enteropathy in this condition, but we have now established that it precedes the lymphoma, and is not a complication of the neoplasm [36.6]. The enteropathy is histologically identical to the enteropathy of gluten sensitivity or celiac disease, and as such it is maximal in the proximal small intestine and fades away distally. In a large study of this lymphoma from Britain, gluten sensitivity could be shown by repeated biopsy studies, before and after a gluten-free diet, in 70% of cases.[1]

36.6	**Enteropathy in Intestinal T Cell Lymphoma**

- Precedes onset of lymphoma
- Histologically identical to celiac disease
- Maximal in proximal small intestine
- Gluten sensitive in 70%
- Associated with celiac-type HLA profile
- Associated with hyposplenism
- May be absent
  - in distal jejunal or ileal lymphomas
  - due to subclinical celiac disease
  - following a gluten free diet

A further important point is that the lymphoma and the enteropathy share with celiac disease both the characteristic HLA profile and also a tendency to hyposplenism. However, enteropathy may be absent in some cases, and this is for at least three reasons. First of all, the neoplasm may occur in the distal jejunum or ileum, where the enteropathy of celiac disease tends to fade out. Furthermore, there has been emphasis recently on so-called latent or sub-clinical celiac disease, in which the enteropathy is extremely subtle or even absent unless provoked with gluten. This could account for some lymphoma cases in which enteropathy appears to be absent. Finally, a small number of cases occur in celiac disease patients in whom the enteropathy has been suppressed or eliminated as a result of a gluten-free diet.

Shown in [36.7] is a case in which a large segment of small bowel had been resected. On the left, the proximal small intestine, the site of the tumor, shows typical crypt hyperplasia, villous atrophy, and an increase in intra-epithelial lymphocytes and inflammatory cells in the lamina propria. These features are typical of a gluten-sensitive enteropathy. On the right, the appearance further down towards the distal jejunum or proximal ileum is seen, and the villi appear normal.

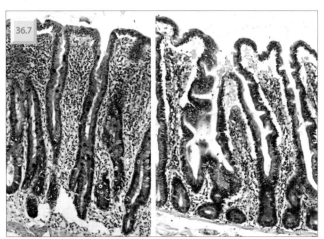

Shown from another case [36.8], one sees on the left, what appear to be normal villi overlying a T cell lymphoma. However, immunostaining for CD3, on the right, shows that these normal villi contain a remarkable excess of intra-epithelial lymphocytes, which is one of the features of gluten-sensitive enteropathy. This case illustrates that the type of enteropathic change present in some cases may be subtle.

Another feature already mentioned, the fact that these lymphomas are frequently accompanied by ulcers in the small intestine, is illustrated in [36.9]. The higher power view of the ulcer (on the right) shows numerous plasma cells, lymphocytes, eosinophils and histiocytes, but no obvious neoplasm. In such cases, ulcers are the only manifestation of the disease, and it is impossible to identify an overt tumor. However, if one analyzes these ulcers for gene rearrangement, using the PCR technique to detect T cell receptor γ chain rearrangement, one can find clear evidence of a clonal T cell population [36.10].

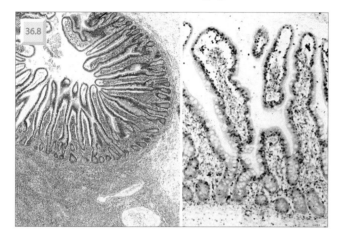

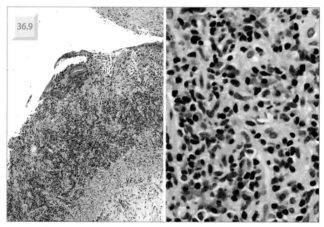

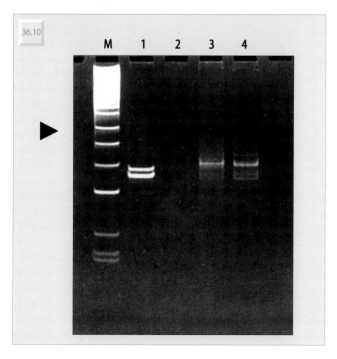

The neoplastic cells of this type of T cell lymphoma usually express CD3, which can be detected in paraffin sections [36.11]. All cases we have studied have been CD7-positive. CD4 is almost always absent, but CD8 is occasionally present. The intestinal lymphocyte antigen, CD103 or HML1, is expressed in most cases. Large anaplastic cells, when present, usually express CD30.

Intestinal T Cell Lymphoma: Immunophenotype	
CD3	+(−)
CD7	+
CD4	−
CD8	−(+)
CD103	+(−)
CD30	+ (large anaplastic)
p53	+

Recently, the Southampton group reported expression of p53 protein as a feature of this disease, and [36.12] shows a recent case from the author's Department. In this section, taken from the large tumor mass, most, if not all, tumor cell nuclei contain p53 protein, and one can also see p53 protein in the intra-epithelial lymphocyte component of the disease, and in occasional cells in the lamina propria.

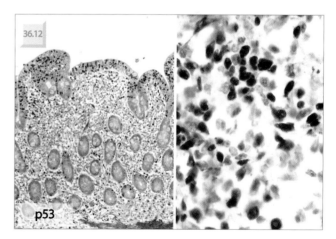

p53

When the genotype of this disease is analyzed [36.13], the T cell receptor β chain gene is rearranged. One can detect TCR γ chain gene rearrangement in the tumor mass, in the intra-epithelial lymphocyte component, and in the so-called benign inflammatory ulcers. Cytogenetic findings are variable and no consistent abnormality has been identified. As yet no data on the sequence of the *p53* gene have been reported to shed light on the mechanism of the over-expression referred to above.

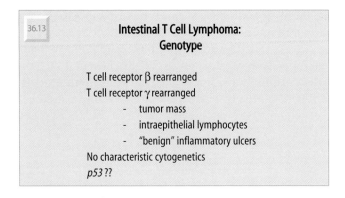

The normal cell counterpart is thought to be the intestinal intra-epithelial T cell [36.14]. The tumor cells are frequently intra-epithelial, and a florid neoplastic intra-epithelial lymphocytosis occurs in some cases. Furthermore, many cases express CD103, which is a feature of intra-epithelial lymphocytes. A recent study has shown the expression of granzyme or perforin by these cells, suggesting that they may be cytotoxic T cells.

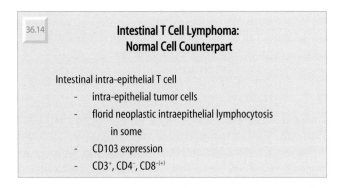

In conclusion [36.15], the disease presents most commonly with acute intestinal perforation, obstruction or hemorrhage. This may or may not be superimposed on a short history of adult celiac disease. In some cases there is a history of conditions associated with celiac disease, such as dermatitis herpetiformis. In the minority of cases there is a classical history of childhood celiac disease. The reason that this is not common is that a gluten-free diet protects against the development of this type of T cell lymphoma. Some cases present as a gradually deteriorating gluten-sensitive enteropathy, in which response to a gluten-free diet is lost. In a minority of cases the disease presents in a disseminated form as an extra-intestinal T cell lymphoma, affecting the lungs, skin or other sites.

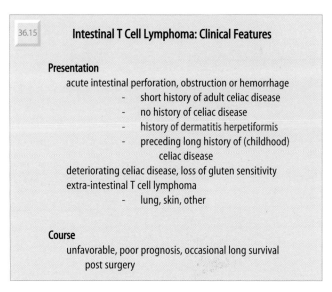

The clinical prognosis is very poor. Therapy is rarely successful - patients may respond at first, but they rapidly relapse, with recurrence of perforation and hemorrhage. The only successes have been in a few cases in which it appears that the disease was localized and surgery resulted in a long term remission.

REFERENCES

1. Swinson CM, Slavin G, Coles EC, Booth CC. Coeliac disease and malignancy. *Lancet* 1983; **i**: 111-5.

FURTHER READING

Isaacson PG. Editorial. Intestinal lymphoma and enteropathy. *J Pathol* 1995; **177**: 111-3.

Murray A, Cuevas EC, Jones DB, Wright DH. A study of the immunohistochemistry and T-cell clonality of enteropathy associated T-cell lymphoma. *Am J Pathol* 1995; **146**: 909-13.

O'Mahony S, Vestey JP, Ferguson A. Similarities in intestinal humoral immunity in dermatitis Herpetiformis without enteropathy and in celiac disease. *Lancet* 1990; **335**: 1487-90.

Spencer J, Cerf-Bensussan N, Jarry A *et al*. Enteropathy associated T cell lymphoma (malignant histiocytosis of the intestine) is recognized by a monoclonal antibody (HML-1) that defines a membrane molecule on human mucosal lymphocytes. *Am J Pathol* 1988; **132**: 1-5

Primary systemic anaplastic large cell lymphoma (ALCL)

H Stein

Anaplastic large cell lymphoma was first identified with the help of antibodies directed against the Ki-1 or CD30 molecule. This molecule was identified in the early 1980s by the author and his collaborators in the course of a search for viral antigens in Hodgkin and Reed-Sternberg cells [37.1].[1,2]

37.1	Hodgkin and Reed-Sternberg Cell-associated Antigens
1982	CD15 (x-Hapten) detected with mAb Tü9 and 3C4;
	1984 detected with Leu-M1
1982	Ki-1 (CD30)
1983	Ki-24 (CDw70)
1983	Ki-27

The Ki-1/CD30 antigen proved to be selectively expressed by these cells, but when normal tissues were studied in more detail it became evident that the Ki-1 antibody also stained a small population of large blastoid cells in the perifollicular region in a normal lymphoid tissue [37.2]. This made it very unlikely that Ki-1/CD30 antigen could represent a Hodgkin's associated virus.

Further studies revealed that expression of Ki-1/CD30 can be induced on lymphoid cells following activation with mitogens. For this reason the molecule is often referred to as a lymphoid activation antigen.

The author's laboratory [3] cloned the CD30 gene, and found its product to be a transmembrane protein which contains six cysteine-rich motives [37.3]. On the basis of these features, it was identified as a cytokine receptor belonging to the TNF receptor family [37.4]. Subsequently, the ligand for CD30 was identified and shown to be a member of the TNF/CD40 ligand family [37.5].[4]

The availability of the CD30 ligand permitted functional studies showing that it can induce proliferation in some cell lines. However, in others apoptosis is induced and in our laboratory we have been able to confirm only the apoptotic effect [37.6].

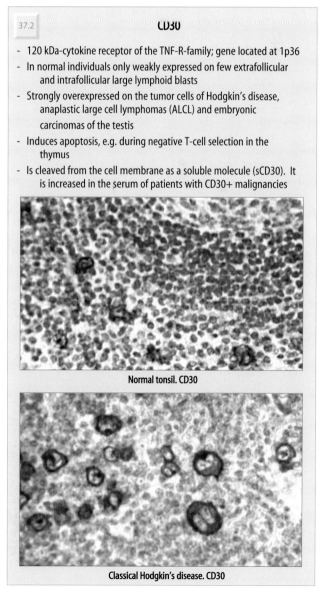

37.2	CD30

- 120 kDa-cytokine receptor of the TNF-R-family; gene located at 1p36
- In normal individuals only weakly expressed on few extrafollicular and intrafollicular large lymphoid blasts
- Strongly overexpressed on the tumor cells of Hodgkin's disease, anaplastic large cell lymphomas (ALCL) and embryonic carcinomas of the testis
- Induces apoptosis, e.g. during negative T-cell selection in the thymus
- Is cleaved from the cell membrane as a soluble molecule (sCD30). It is increased in the serum of patients with CD30+ malignancies

Normal tonsil. CD30

Classical Hodgkin's disease. CD30

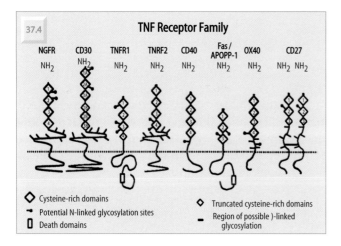

37.3   Features of the CD30 (Ki-1) Molecule*

- Apparent molecular weight 120,000;
- Transmembrane glycoprotein;
- Has 6 cysteine-rich motifs
- Is a member of the TNF-Receptor family;
- The gene is located at 1p36.

* Cloned by Dürkop *et al.* 1992[3]

37.4   TNF Receptor Family

NGFR	CD30	TNFR1	TNRF2	CD40	Fas / APOPP-1	OX40	CD27
NH₂	NH₂	NH₂	NH₂	NH₂	NH₂	NH₂	NH₂ NH₂

◇ Cysteine-rich domains
⊶ Potential N-linked glycosylation sites
◻ Death domains

◇ Truncated cysteine-rich domains
— Region of possible)-linked glycosylation

37.5   Features of the CD30 Ligand*

- Apparent molecular weight 40,000;
- Type II membrane glycoprotein;
- Is a member of the TNF /CD40L family;
- The gene is located at 9q33.

* Cloned by Smith *et al.* 1993[4]

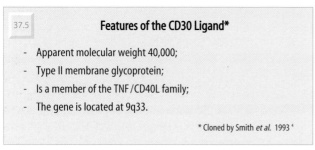

37.6   Biological Activities of the CD30 /CD30 System

CD30L

CD30L+ cell activated peripheral blood T cell activated monocyte or tonsilar T cell

proliferation   proliferation   apoptosis

CD30+ cell
Hodgkin's disease
derived cell line
e.g. HDLM-2

activated T cell

CD30+ cell
ALC lymphoma
derived cell line
e.g. Karpas 299

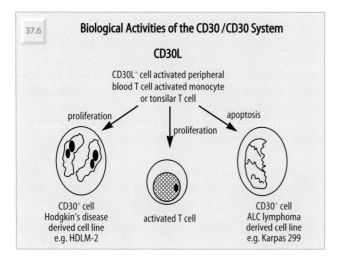

tumors tend to disseminate within lymph node sinuses, and for this reason many of these cases had been diagnosed before the availability of CD30 staining as metastatic carcinoma. Furthermore, in some cases large cells that have engulfed erythrocytes are seen, and in consequence many hematopathologists regarded this tumor as macrophage derived, and called it malignant histiocytosis [37.9].

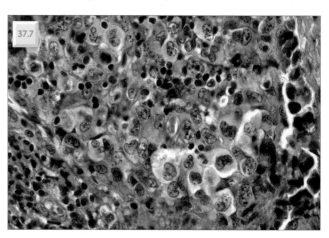

37.7

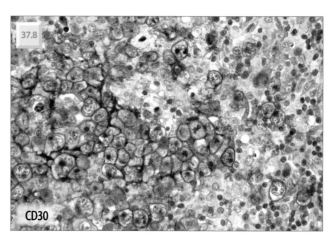

37.8

CD30

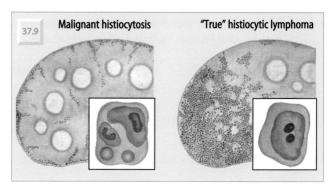

37.9   **Malignant histiocytosis**   **"True" histiocytic lymphoma**

Prior to these molecular and functional studies, our laboratory investigated the diagnostic value of the CD30 antigen by staining a wide variety of malignancies, and had found strong positivity in tumors made up of anaplastic large cells with bizarre looking nuclei and abundant cytoplasm [37.7].[5] The staining for CD30 is shown in [37.8]. Ki-1/CD30-positive

A case with an extreme degree of erythrophagocytosis is shown in [37.10]. The sinuses are filled with large cells, many of which contain erythrocytes in their cytoplasm. Immunostaining with an anti-macrophage antibody, e.g. directed at the CD68 antigen, reveals that the cells which contain the phagocytosed erythrocytes are indeed macrophages.

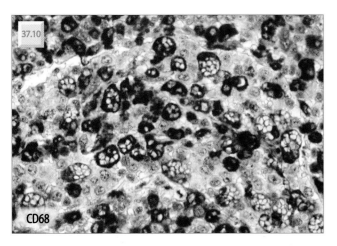

CD68

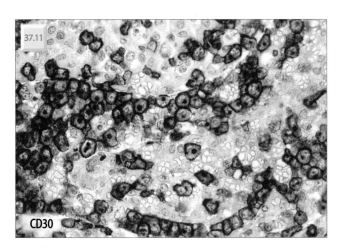

CD30

However, the cells in mitosis and with atypical nuclei are negative for the macrophage marker, but positive for CD30 [37.11], indicating that the CD30-positive cells, and not the macrophages, represent the neoplastic population. The latter cells are reactive bystander cells, possibly attracted by the tumor cells.

The idea that CD30-positive anaplastic large cell tumors represent a previously unrecognized tumor entity derived from lymphoid cells was confirmed by subsequent immunohistochemical studies which showed that these tumors constantly lack histiocytic markers and frequently express T cell markers and more rarely B cell markers. This new lymphoid tumor category was therefore named "anaplastic large cell lymphoma", or ALCL for short.

Further clinicopathologic studies have shown that anaplastic large cell morphology and CD30-positivity is not specific for a single disease entity, since this morphology, sometimes accompanied by CD30 expression, can be observed in some cases of diffuse large cell B cell lymphoma, of adult T cell leukemia/lymphoma, and of intestinal T cell lymphoma [37.12]. In such cases anaplastic morphology is interpreted as representing morphologic variation, rather than a link with true ALCL.

37.12 **ALCL Morphology**

CD30 anaplastic large cell (ALC) morphology can represent a(n)

- anaplastic variant of
  diffuse large B cell lymphoma
  ATL/L
  intestinal T cell lymphoma
- primary cutaneous ALC lymphoma
- primary systemic ALC lymphoma
- secondary ALC Lymphoma

It has also been observed that other types of non-Hodgkin's lymphoma can transform into lymphomas which resemble ALCLs morphologically – sometimes referred to as "secondary" ALCLs. However, the majority of ALCLs arise *de novo* as primary neoplasms. Among these, two main types can be distinguished – one arises in the skin, and the other in lymph nodes or soft tissue. The latter are referred to as primary systemic ALCL and this is the subject of this chapter.

Sinusoidal spread is highly characteristic of ALCL and is regularly seen if a lymph node is only partially invaded [37.13]. An additional characteristic is the homing of the tumor cells around the follicles. These features are seen when a section is immunostained for CD30. In some cases, it is very difficult to diagnose ALCL in a H & E section of a lymph node biopsy when the infiltration is discrete, but the ALCL cells are easy to identify when the biopsy is labeled for CD30 antigen [37.14].

In 1986 Morgan and colleagues described a new chromosome abnormality, the (2;5) translocation, in cases of malignant histiocytosis [37.15].[6] Some years later Mason and colleagues, and other research groups, reinvestigated cases with the (2;5) translocation and found that all cases had the morphology of ALCL, expressed CD30, and lacked histiocytic markers.[7] Approximately half of these cases expressed T cell antigens – the rest were devoid of B and T cell antigens. This correlation between phenotypic and cytogenetic data strengthened the idea that ALCL is a distinct entity, but left the question open as to whether there are cases of ALCL which do not carry the (2;5) translocation.

The latter question could be addressed when the breakpoints of the (2;5) translocation were cloned. This led to the identification of a known gene on the breakpoint at chromosome 5, the nucleophosmin or *NPM* gene. A new gene was discovered at the chromosome 2 breakpoint which received the designation anaplastic lymphoma kinase or *ALK* gene [37.16]. The *NPM* gene is active in nearly all human tissues, including lymphoid tissues. In contrast, the *ALK* gene is not transcribed in most tissues including the lymphoid system, but it is activated when juxtaposed to the *NPM* gene. This means that expression of the *ALK* gene indicates the presence of the (2;5) translocation. In consequence, we can now detect (2;5) translocation by labeling sections for the mRNA or the protein encoded by the *ALK* gene sequence present in the t(2;5) fusion gene.

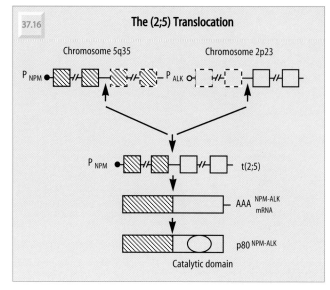

The (2;5) Translocation

The author's laboratory has performed such studies by *in situ* hybridization and by immunohistology.[8] Other laboratories have analyzed the presence of the t(2;5) using the RT-PCR technique. An ALCL hybridized with a probe specific for *ALK* mRNA is seen in [37.17]. The tumor cells are strongly labelled. In [37.18] immunostaining of the same ALCL is shown with a polyclonal antiserum against the ALK protein (from Dr Mori, Japan). The immunostaining proved to be restricted to the ALCL cells as expected.

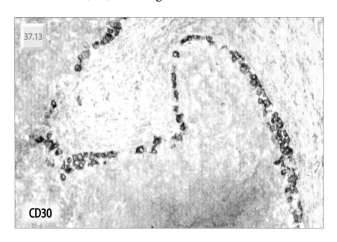

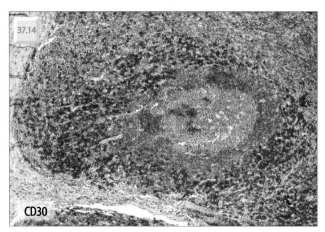

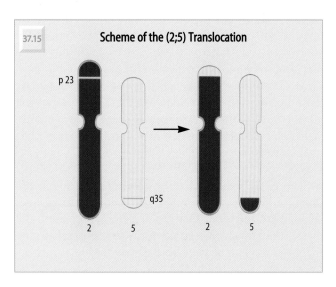

Scheme of the (2;5) Translocation

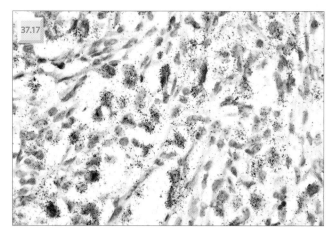

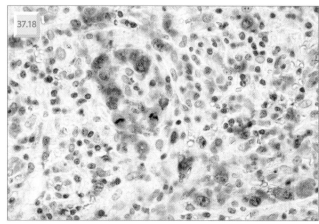

If our *in situ* hybridization and immunohistologic labeling findings are compared with the results of other studies, it is clear that the (2;5) translocation can be detected in a significant proportion of primary systemic ALCL. However, there is no consensus about the exact frequency, for which estimates range between 10 and 70%.

We have not been able to detect the (2;5) translocation in the primary cutaneous category of ALCL, supporting the idea that this is a different disease. Moreover, we could not detect the (2;5) translocation in any lymphoma type other than primary systemic ALCL. However, it has been reported that some T cell lymphomas and one B cell lymphoma were positive for the (2;5) translocation, so there is still some controversy in this field.

Primary systemic ALCLs show a very characteristic bimodal age distribution, with the major peak in the second decade, providing further support for the idea that it represents a distinct entity [37.19].

In conclusion, primary systemic ALCL is a neoplasm in which there is a proliferation of large bizarre strongly CD30-positive blasts. They grow around lymphoid follicles, often in a cohesive manner [37.20], and tend to disseminate within sinuses. The age distribution is bimodal. The tumor cells exhibit T or null-cell immunophenotype but are never of B cell type. Primary systemic ALCL may be associated with the t(2;5) translocation. Bone marrow is rarely involved, but extranodal tissues are frequently affected.

On these grounds the neoplasm appears to represent a distinct clinicopathologic entity, about which we may hope to learn much more in the next few years.

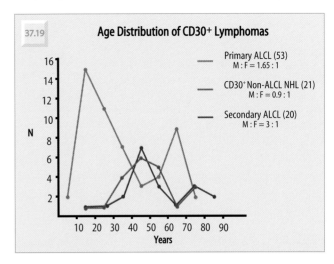

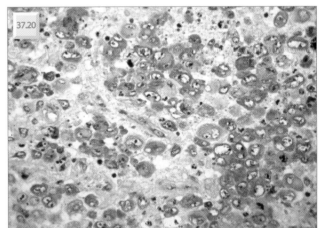

REFERENCES

1. Stein H, Gerdes J, Schwab U *et al.* Identification of Hodgkin and Sternberg-reed cells as a unique cell type derived from a newly-detected small-cell population. *Int J Cancer* 1982; **30**: 445-59.

2. Schwab U, Stein H, Gerdes J *et al.* Production of a monoclonal antibody specific for Hodgkin and Sternberg-Reed cells of Hodgkin's disease and a subset of normal lymphoid cells. *Nature* 1982; **299**: 65-7.

3. Dürkop H, Latza U, Hummel M, Eitelbach F, Seed B, Stein H. Molecular cloning and expression of a new member of the nerve growth factor receptor family that is characteristic for Hodgkin's disease. *Cell* 1992; **68**: 421-27.

4. Smith CA, Gruss HJ, Davis T *et al.* CD30 antigen, a marker for Hodgkin's lymphoma, is a receptor whose ligand defines an emerging family of cytokines with homology to TNF. *Cell* 1993; **73**: 1349-60.

5. Stein H, Mason DY, Gerdes J *et al.* The expression of the Hodgkin's disease associated antigen Ki-1 in reactive and neoplastic lymphoid tissue: evidence that Reed-Sternberg cells and histiocytic malignancies are derived from activated lymphoid cells. *Blood* 1985; **66**: 848-58.

6. Morgan R, Hecht BK, Sandberg AA, Hecht F, Smith SD. Chromosome 5q35 breakpoint in malignant histiocytosis. *N Engl J Med* 1986; **314**: 1322.

7. Mason DY, Bastard C, Rimokh R *et al.* CD30-positive large cell lymphomas ('Ki-1 lymphoma') are associated with a chromosomal translocation involving 5q35. *Br J Haematol* 1990; **74**:161-8.

8. Herbst H, Anagnostopoulos J, Heinze B, Dürkop H, Hummel M, Stein H. ALK gene products in anaplastic large cell lymphomas and Hodgkin's disease. *Blood* 1995; **86**: 1694-1700.

Primary CD30+ cutaneous lymphomas (including lymphomatoid papulosis)

M E Kadin

This chapter is concerned with tumors that arise in the skin without extracutaneous localization at presentation, and that are characterized by papules, nodules or tumors derived from activated T lymphocytes [38.1].

38.1   **Defining Criteria**

Papules, nodules and tumors of the skin derived from activated T lymphocytes without extracutaneous localization at presentation.

Peak incidence in 5th decade.

Both adults and children affected.

Similar frequency in males and females.

The peak incidence is in the fifth decade and both adults and children are affected, with similar frequency in males and females. As in the case of other T cell disorders, these disorders constitute a spectrum, ranging from the benign to the highly malignant [38.2]. The benign end of the spectrum is known as lymphomatoid papulosis, of which there are two major histologic types. The large cell lymphomas can be either anaplastic neoplasms or non-anaplastic lymphomas, which are usually pleomorphic in morphology. There are also of course borderline cases which do not easily fit into either type.

The pie chart shown in [38.3] is based on data from Dr. Vonderheid in Philadelphia, to give a perspective on the frequency of these disorders. It shows that lymphomatoid papulosis and CD30-positive lymphomas comprise as many as 20% of the cases that we normally refer to as cutaneous T cell lymphomas.

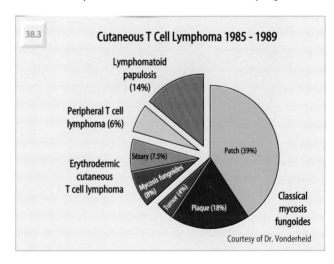

38.3   Cutaneous T Cell Lymphoma 1985 - 1989

Lymphomatoid papulosis (14%)

Peripheral T cell lymphoma (6%)

Erythrodermic cutaneous T cell lymphoma

Sézary (7.5%)

Mycosis fungoides (8%)

Tumor (4%)

Patch (39%)

Plaque (18%)

Classical mycosis fungoides

Courtesy of Dr. Vonderheid

The example of lymphomatoid papulosis in a child illustrated in [38.4][1] shows the characteristic feature of spontaneous regression, which is seen in virtually all cases. Lymphomatoid papulosis can be localized or, as shown in [38.5], generalized.

38.2   Primary Cutaneous CD30+ Lymphoproliferative Disease Spectrum

Borderline cases

Lymphomatoid papulosis

Ki-1 Lymphoma

A   B   ALCL   Other

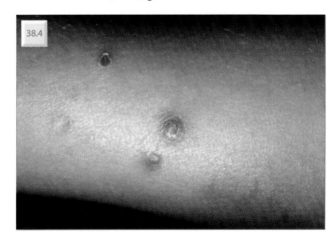

38.4

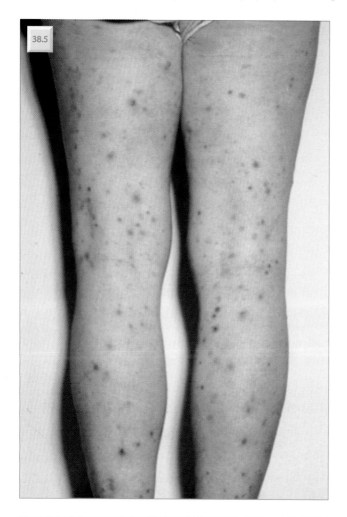

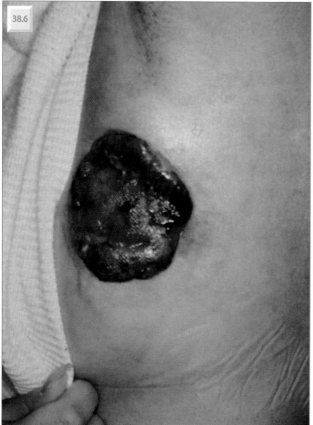

At the other end of the spectrum are CD30-positive large cell lymphomas [38.6], which usually occur as solitary masses. Some individuals have both lymphomatoid papulosis and large cell lymphoma [38.7],[1] illustrating the continuous spectrum linking these disorders.

If we turn to the histopathology of lymphomatoid papulosis [38.8], it occurs as a perivascular or wedge-shaped dermal infiltrate, and generally does not extend into the subcutis. It contains atypical cells with the cytology of immunoblasts, anaplastic cells and/or cerebriform cells. Variable numbers of inflammatory cells are present, and atypical cells are dispersed and in the minority.

The commonest type of lymphomatoid papulosis has been termed "type A" by Dr. Willemze [38.9].[2,3] It resembles Hodgkin's disease, is generally non-epidermotropic and contains large blasts which often resemble Reed-Sternberg cells. There is an admixture of neutrophils, eosinophils and small lymphocytes. Mitoses are frequent.

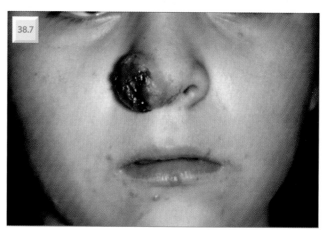

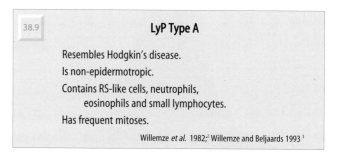

Morphology of LyP

Perivascular or wedge-shaped dermal infiltrate which does not extend to subcutis.

Contains atypical cells (immunoblasts, anaplastic cells and/or cerebriform cells).

Contains variable numbers of inflammatory cells.

Atypical cells are always in the minority.

LyP Type A

Resembles Hodgkin's disease.

Is non-epidermotropic.

Contains RS-like cells, neutrophils, eosinophils and small lymphocytes.

Has frequent mitoses.

Willemze et al. 1982;[2] Willemze and Beljaards 1993 [3]

Shown in [38.10] is a typical example of type A morphology. There is a wedge-shaped infiltrate sparing the epidermis. At higher magnification [38.11] one sees Reed-Sternberg-like cells, with abnormal mitoses, and a generous admixture of neutrophils and eosinophils. It appears as though these inflammatory cells are being actively recruited into the lesion, because one typically sees many of them in the blood vessels [38.12]. This may be due to recruitment by cytokines secreted by the CD30-positive cells. One example is TNF, as revealed in [38.13] by immunohistochemistry.

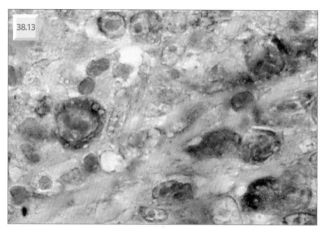

Type B lesions are much less common [38.14]. They resemble mycosis fungoides and are often epidermotropic. They contain cerebriform mononuclear cells and inflammatory cells, and mitoses are less prominent than in type A lesions. [38.15] is an example of a perivascular epidermotropic infiltrate in type B lymphomatoid papulosis. [38.16] is another case showing a band-like subepidermal infiltrate with exocytosis which would be difficult, without clinical correlation, to distinguish from mycosis fungoides.

In [38.17], the presence of cerebriform cells in the upper dermis is clearly seen.

The regressing papules shown in [38.18] from a patient with type B lymphomatoid papulosis, make the point that we need clinical information to reach the correct diagnosis.

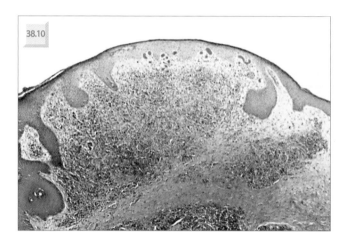

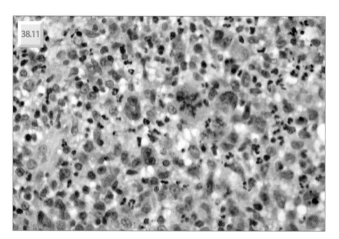

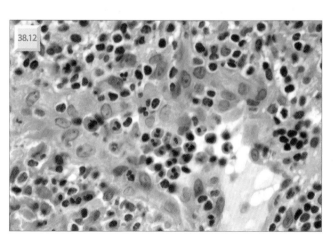

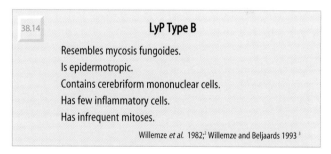

LyP Type B

Resembles mycosis fungoides.

Is epidermotropic.

Contains cerebriform mononuclear cells.

Has few inflammatory cells.

Has infrequent mitoses.

Willemze *et al.* 1982;[2] Willemze and Beljaards 1993 [3]

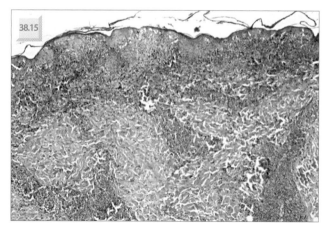

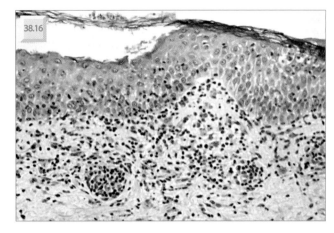

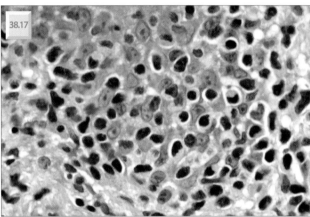

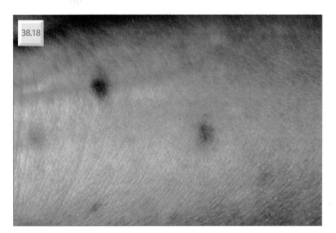

recurrent anomaly has been identified, perhaps because of the small numbers studied. We have been unable to detect the (2;5) translocation, characteristic of primary nodal CD30-positive lymphomas.

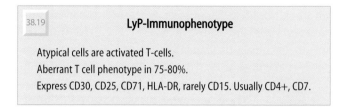

LyP-Immunophenotype

Atypical cells are activated T-cells.
Aberrant T cell phenotype in 75-80%.
Express CD30, CD25, CD71, HLA-DR, rarely CD15. Usually CD4+, CD7.

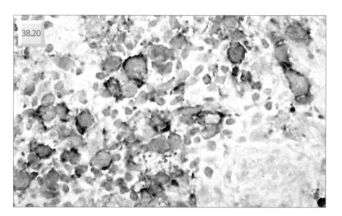

LyP-Genetics

TCRβ and γ chain genes are clonally rearranged in most cases.

The same T cell clone is present in separate skin lesions of most cases.

Multiple chromosome abnormalities but no consistent abnormality found.

The t(2;5)(p23;q35) is absent or rare.

The immunophenotype in lymphomatoid papulosis [38.19] is that of activated helper T cells, generally expressing CD4, and lacking CD7. In the great majority of cases there is an aberrant T cell phenotype, and in about 20% no T cell antigens can be detected. The most consistent marker is CD30 on the large atypical cells, which are numerous in the type A lesions [38.20].

One can detect clonal rearrangements of T cell receptor β and γ chain genes even in the T cell antigen-silent cases [38.21]. We have found that in most cases the same T cell clone is present in the separate skin lesions. We also find, even in regressing lesions, multiple chromosome abnormalities, but so far no

Illustrated in [38.22] is a study, performed by Andreas Chott in our group, of multiple skin lesions from two patients with lymphomatoid papulosis.[4] One patient, shown on the left, had only polyclonal T cells, and these were detected in two separate lesions (tracks 1 and 2). On the right one sees three separate skin lesions from the second patient (tracks 3-5). Interestingly, they were of different histologic types - type A, type B and one mixed type A/type B. A dominant clonal band is present in all three lesions, showing that they are clonally related. This pattern was found in nine out of eleven patients.

As already mentioned, multiple chromosome abnormalities are found, even in regressing lesions. This is illustrated in [38.23] in which trisomy 7, an interstitial deletion on chromosome 10, additional chromosomal material on chromosome 12 and a deletion of chromosome 19 are all present. The presence of abnormal karyotypes in these cases has been a consistent observation.

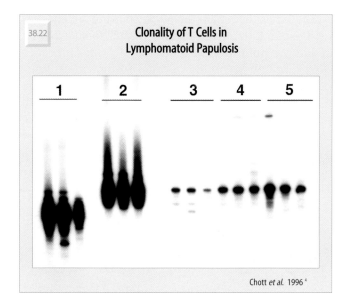

38.22

Clonality of T Cells in Lymphomatoid Papulosis

1　2　3　4　5

Chott *et al.* 1996 [4]

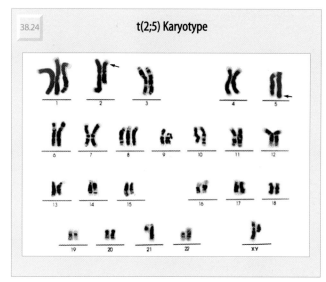

38.24

t(2;5) Karyotype

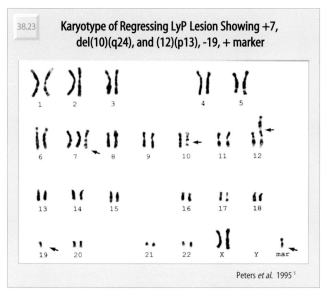

38.23

Karyotype of Regressing LyP Lesion Showing +7, del(10)(q24), and (12)(p13), -19, + marker

Peters *et al.* 1995 [5]

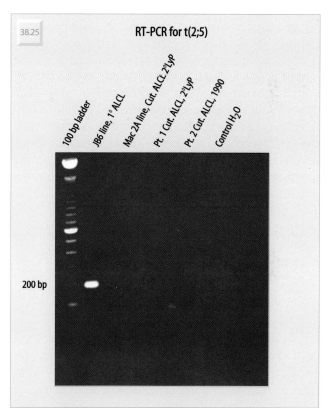

38.25

RT-PCR for t(2;5)

100 bp ladder
J86 line, 1° ALCL
Mac 2A line, Cut. ALCL 2°LyP
Pt. 1 Cut. ALCL 2°LyP
Pt. 2 Cut. ALCL, 1990
Control H₂O

200 bp

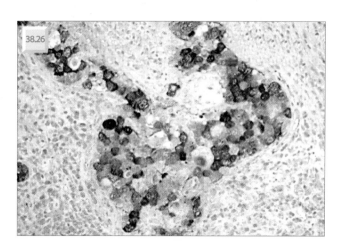

38.26

The (2;5) translocation, as shown in [38.24] in a cell line that we derived from an anaplastic large cell lymphoma of nodal origin, has not been found in any of our cases of lymphomatoid papulosis. This has been confirmed by RT-PCR. In [38.25], the second track shows the predicted product from the (2;5)-positive cell line, but no bands are seen in material from cell lines or primary explants from lymphomatoid papulosis or primary cutaneous CD30-positive lymphomas.

We have also looked in lymphomatoid papulosis or primary cutaneous CD30-positive lymphoma for expression of the p80 protein. This protein is encoded by the *NPM:ALK* fusion gene, and [38.26] shows the typical staining pattern of a t(2;5)-positive ALCL. However, we have not found evidence of its production in lymphomatoid papulosis or primary CD30-positive cutaneous lymphoma by either immunohistochemistry or RT-PCR [38.27].

38.27	p80 and t(2;5) Results		
Disease		**p80+**	**t(2;5)+**
Lymphomatoid papulosis		0/10	0/10
Primary cutaneous CD30⁺ LCL		0/3	0/3
Nodal CD30⁺ ALCL		17/25	3/3
Nodal CD30⁻ LCL		3/15	ND
Hodgkin's disease, syncytial variant		0/4	ND
Secondary CD30⁺ LCL		0/1	0/1

It is interesting that there is a high frequency, estimated at 10 - 20% from the literature, of associated lymphomas in patients with lymphomatoid papulosis [38.28]. When these are subtyped, the commonest lymphomas are mycosis fungoides, Hodgkin's disease and CD30-positive large cell lymphomas. Rare B cell lymphomas are also seen. Represented in [38.29] is a patient with co-existent lymphomatoid papulosis and mycosis fungoides in whom we found, as in other cases, the same rearrangement in both the mycosis plaque lesion and the lymphomatoid papulosis, suggesting that they are related via a common T cell precursor.

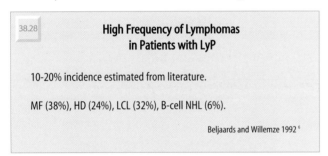

38.28

High Frequency of Lymphomas in Patients with LyP

10-20% incidence estimated from literature.

MF (38%), HD (24%), LCL (32%), B-cell NHL (6%).

Beljaards and Willemze 1992 [6]

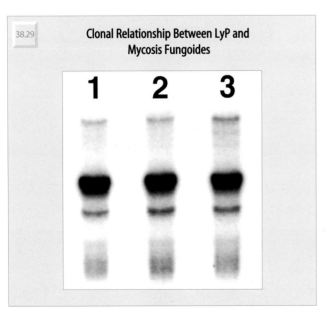

38.29

Clonal Relationship Between LyP and Mycosis Fungoides

Shown in [38.30] are the negative results of analysis for Epstein Barr virus.[7] Case 8 in this Table, from an article we published in the *New England Journal of Medicine*,[8] is particularly interesting, since lymphomatoid papulosis, mycosis fungoides, Hodgkin's disease and anaplastic large cell lymphoma were all present. Epstein Barr virus was not found, even in the Hodgkin's tissues, and we have evidence from other patients with mycosis fungoides that when Hodgkin's disease develops it is unassociated with Epstein Barr virus and may be of a special type.

38.30	Staining for EBER and LMP-1 in Lymphomatoid Papulosis and Associated Lymphomas				
Patient no.	**Age /sex**	**Specimen**	**Diagnosis**	**EBER**	**LMP-1**
1	75 M	Papule, thigh	LyP, type A	Neg	U
2	39 M	Papule, arm	LyP, type A	Neg	Neg
		Papule, arm	LyP, type A	Neg	Neg
3	27 F	Papule, hip	LyP, type B	Neg	Neg
4	48 M	Papule, arm	LyP, type B	Neg	U
5	54 F	Papule, thigh	LyP, type A	Neg	Neg
		Papule, wrist	LyP, type B	Neg	U
6	57 F	Papule, back	LyP, type A	Neg	U
		Patch, back	LyP, type B	Neg	Neg
		Papule, thumb	LyP, type A	Neg	U
		Papule, wrist	LyP, type B	Neg	U
7	28 M	Nodule, face	LyP, type A	Neg	Neg
		Nodule , thigh	LyP, type A	Neg	Neg
8	32 M	Retroperitoneal LN	ALCL	Neg	U
		Inguinal LN	HD	Neg	Neg
		Papule, trunk	LyP, type A	Neg	Neg
9	41 F	Papule, thigh	LyP, type A	Neg	Neg
		Patch, thigh	LyP, type B	Neg	Neg
		Papule, abdomen	LyP, type A	Neg	U

ALCL = Anaplastic large cell lymphoma; HD = Hodgkin's disease, mixed cellularity type; U = uninterpretable due to background staining.

Kadin et al. 1993 [7]

Turning now to the primary cutaneous CD30-positive lymphomas [38.31], in these tumors the infiltrate extends throughout the dermis into the subcutis, and the epidermis is usually spared. Sheets of immunoblastic, pleomorphic or anaplastic cells are seen. Inflammatory cells are largely confined to the periphery of the lesion, although there may be numerous neutrophils in some lesions, and pseudo-epitheliomatous hyperplasia is often present.

38.31

Primary CD30+ Cutaneous Lymphomas

Infiltrate extends throughout dermis into subcutis; epidermis often spared.

Contains sheets of immunoblastic, pleomorphic, or anaplastic cells.

Inflammatory cells at periphery.

May contain many neutrophils.

Pseudoepitheliomatous hyperplasia often present.

Shown in [38.32] is an example of a primary cutaneous CD30-positive lymphoma. One sees sheets of tumor cells, and only secondary involvement of the epidermis, which is ulcerated. The infiltrate extends down into the subcutaneous fat [38.33] and the inflammatory cells are confined to the periphery [38.34]. The neoplastic cells in these primary CD30-positive lymphomas can be anaplastic [38.35], or pleomorphic [38.36].

In some instances, they may resemble large immunoblasts, with oval or round nuclei [38.37]. In all cases, the percentage of CD30-positive cells exceeds 75% [38.38].

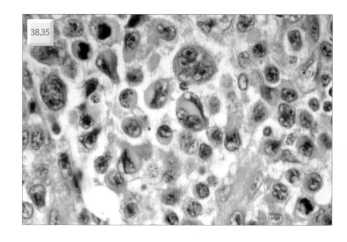

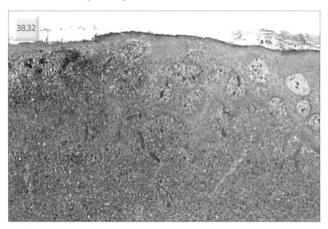

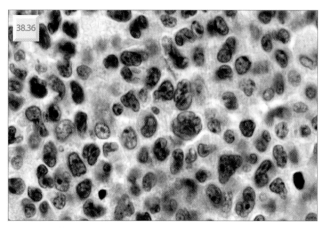

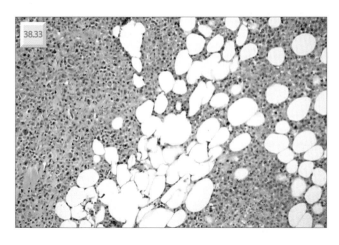

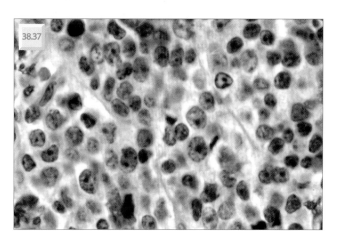

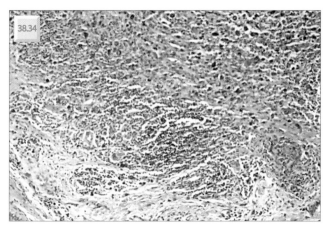

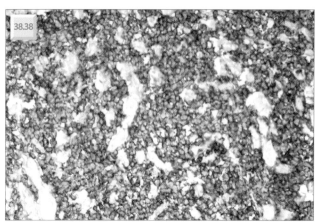

Regardless of the cytologic appearance, survival for patients with CD30-positive lymphomas is significantly better than for CD30-negative ones [38.39]. The other poor prognostic indicator is the development of extracutaneous disease [38.40].

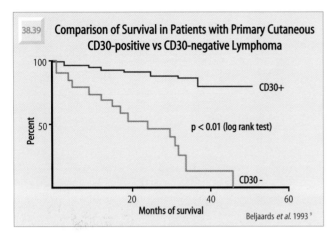

38.39 **Comparison of Survival in Patients with Primary Cutaneous CD30-positive vs CD30-negative Lymphoma**

CD30+

p < 0.01 (log rank test)

CD30 -

Percent

Months of survival

Beljaards *et al.* 1993 [9]

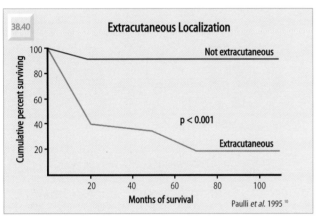

38.40 **Extracutaneous Localization**

Not extracutaneous

p < 0.001

Extracutaneous

Cumulative percent surviving

Months of survival

Paulli *et al.* 1995 [10]

Finally, borderline lesions, which have an ambiguous clinical appearance and/or histology, and which are not readily classifiable as either lymphomatoid papulosis or lymphoma should be mentioned. The patient illustrated in [38.41] might well have been diagnosed as having lymphoma, but the lesion regressed spontaneously.

Shown in [38.42] is a biopsy from a patient who had clusters of CD30-positive cells in a lesion clinically resembling lymphomatoid papulosis. It has emerged from a co-operative study that patients with borderline lesions have a prognosis which is favorable and similar to that of lymphomatoid papulosis.[10]

In [38.43] a comparison is seen between lymphomatoid papulosis and CD30-positive lymphoma. In lymphomatoid papulosis the CD30-positive cells are dispersed and admixed with inflammatory cells, whereas in CD30-positive lymphoma one sees sheets of CD30-positive cells. Clinically, lymphomatoid papulosis generally presents as papules, whereas one sees nodules or tumors in lymphoma. The distribution

in lymphomatoid papulosis is generalized or regional, and solitary or localized in lymphoma. Self-healing is an essential feature of lymphomatoid papulosis, but is seen only occasionally in large cell lymphoma. Extracutaneous spread is rare in lymphomatoid papulosis, whereas it occurs in about 95% of patients with large cell lymphoma.

Finally, the author would like to acknowledge his colleagues who provided valuable clinical specimens and follow-up data, and also the people who have worked on this project in the laboratory with me [38.44].

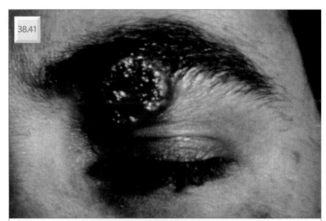

38.41

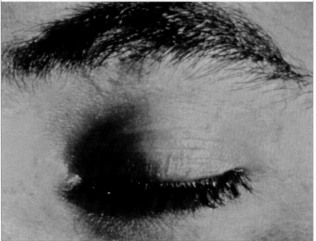

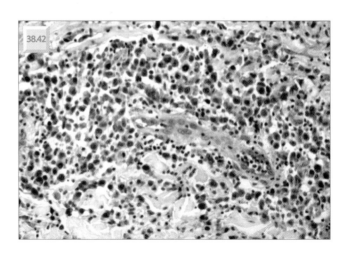

38.42

38.43	Comparison of LyP and CD30+ LCL	
	LyP	CD30+ LCL
Histology	Few CD30+ cells, many inflammatory cells	Clusters of CD30+ cells
Morphology	Papules	Nodules
Distribution	Generalized or regional	Localized
Self-healing	Always	Variable
Extracutaneous spread	< 5%	Frequent

38.44 Acknowledgements

Eric Vonderheid, M.D.   Andreas Chott, M.D.

Suzanne Olbricht, M.D.   John De Coteau, M.D.

Howard Koh, M.D.   Joan Knoll, Ph.D.

Stephen Balk, M.D., Ph.D.

ACKNOWLEDGEMENTS

Figures [38.3], [38.5] and [38.41] were kindly provided by Dr. E C Vonderheid.

Figures [38.4] and [38.7] are reproduced from Kadin ME. Lymphomatoid papulosis, Chapter 157. In: Arndt KA, LeBoit PE, Robinson JK and Wintroub BU (eds.). *Cutaneous Medicine and Surgery. An Intergrated Program in Dermatology*. 1996, vol. 2: 1631-38, with copyright permission from W.B. Saunders Company.

Figure [38.22] is reprinted from *The Journal of Investigative Dermatology*, 1996; 106: 696-700. Chott A, Vonderheid EC, Olbricht S, Miao NN, Balk SP, Kadin ME. The same dominant T cell clone is present in multiple regressing skin lesions and associated T cell lymphomas of patients with lymphomatoid papulosis. Reproduced with permission.

Figure [38.23] is reprinted from *Cancer Genetics Cytogenetics*, vol. 80, Peters K, Knoll JH, Kadin ME, Cytogenetic findings in regressing skin lesions of lymphomatoid papulosis., 13-16, 1995, with permission from Elsevier Science.

Figure [38.30] is reprinted from *The Journal of Pathology*, Kadin ME; Vonderheid EC; Weiss LM. Absence of Epstein-Barr viral RNA in lymphomatoid papulosis. 1993; 170: 145-8. Copyright © John Wiley & Sons Limited. Reproduced with permission.

Figure [38.39] is reproduced from *Cancer* vol. 71, No. 6, 1993, 2097-104. Copyright © 1993 American Cancer Society. Reprinted by permission of Wiley-Liss, Inc., a subsidiary of John Wiley & Sons, Inc.

Figure [38.40] is reproduced from *The Journal of Clinical Oncology* 1995; 13: 1343-1354, with copyright permission from W.B. Saunders Company.

REFERENCES

1. Kadin ME. Lymphomatoid papulosis. In: Arndt KA, Robinson JK LeBoit PE, and Wintroub BU, eds. *Cutaneous Medicine and Surgery. An Intergrated Program in Dermatology*. W.B. Saunders 1996; 1631-8.

2. Willemze R, Meyer CJ, Van Vloten WA, Scheffer E. The clinical and histological spectrum of lymphomatoid papulosis. *Br J Dermatol* 1982; **107**: 131-144.

3. Willemze R, Beljaards RC. Spectrum of primary cutaneous CD30 (Ki-1)-positive lymphoproliferative disorders. A proposal for classification and guidelines for management and treatment. *J Am Acad Dermatol* 1993; **28**: 973-80.

4. Chott A, Vonderheid EC, Olbricht S, Miao NN, Balk SP, Kadin ME. The same dominant T cell clone is present in multiple regressing skin lesions and associated T cell lymphomas of patients with lymphomatoid papulosis. *J Invest Dermatol* 1996; **106**: 696-700.

5. Peters K, Knoll JH, Kadin ME. Cytogenetic findings in regressing skin lesions of lymphomatoid papulosis. *Cancer Genet Cytogenet* 1995; **80**: 13-16.

6. Beljaards RC and Willemze R. The prognosis of patients with lymphomatoid papulosis associated with malignant lymphomas. *Br J Dermatol* 1992; **126**: 596-602.

7. Kadin ME, Vonderheid EC, Weiss LM. Absence of Epstein-Barr viral RNA in lymphomatoid papulosis. *J Pathol* 1993; **170**: 145-8.

8. Davis TH, Morton CC, Miller-Cassman R, Balk SP, Kadin ME. Hodgkin's disease, lymphomatoid papulosis, and cutaneous T-cell lymphoma derived from a common T-cell clone. *N Engl J Med* 1992; **326**: 1115-22.

9. Beljaards RC, Kaudewitz P, Berti E *et al*. Primary cutaneous CD30-positive large cell lymphoma: definition of a new type of cutaneous lymphoma with a favorable prognosis. A European Multicenter Study of 47 patients. *Cancer* 1993; **71**: 2097-104.

10. Paulli M, Berti E, Rosso R *et al*. CD30/Ki-1-positive lymphoproliferative disorders of the skin - Clinicopathological correlation and statistical analysis of 86 cases: A multicentric study from the European Organization for Research and Treatment of Cancer Cutaneous Lymphoma Project Group. *J Clin Oncol* 1995; **13**: 1343-54.

FURTHER READING

De Coteau JF, Butmarc JR, Kinney MC, Kadin ME. The t(2;5) chromosomal translocation is not a common feature of primary cutaneous CD30+ lymphoproliferative disorders: Comparison with anaplastic large cell lymphoma of nodal origin. *Blood* 1996; **87**: 3437-41.

Is anaplastic large cell lymphoma (ALCL) clinically distinct from diffuse large B cell lymphoma?

L N Shulman

Two editorials published three years apart [39.1] demonstrate the way in which anaplastic large cell lymphoma has become increasingly accepted. However, there are still many unanswered questions. It is noteworthy that in 1991 it was an entity followed by a question mark. The question mark was dropped in 1994, but the writer still refers to "maturation of a clinical entity".

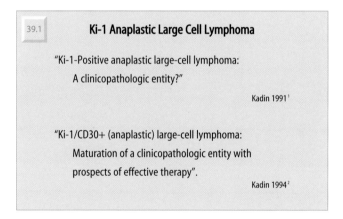

39.1 Ki-1 Anaplastic Large Cell Lymphoma

"Ki-1-Positive anaplastic large-cell lymphoma: A clinicopathologic entity?"

Kadin 1991 [1]

"Ki-1/CD30+ (anaplastic) large-cell lymphoma: Maturation of a clinicopathologic entity with prospects of effective therapy".

Kadin 1994 [2]

These disorders present a confusing clinical picture [39.2]. They appear to comprise a group of large cell lymphomas, of which some are CD30-positive, some are of B cell type, some are derived from T cells, and some have the t(2;5) translocation. There appears to be some overlap between CD30-positivity and the translocation, as well as with the T cell lymphomas. The question of whether this entity in children differs from the disease seen in adults also remains unanswered.

This tumor strongly expresses CD30, and is usually of T cell origin, but it can be of B cell origin [39.3]. It is believed to be relatively rare, its frequency in different series varying between 5 and 10% of non-Hodgkin's lymphomas. It has some very distinct clinical features, including a high incidence of extranodal involvement, particularly in the skin, even in the systemic form [39.4].

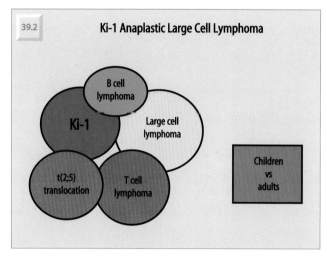

39.2 Ki-1 Anaplastic Large Cell Lymphoma

B cell lymphoma

Ki-1

Large cell lymphoma

t(2;5) translocation

T cell lymphoma

Children vs adults

39.3 Ki-1 Anaplastic Large Cell Lymphoma

"This tumor was originally recognized by application of the Ki-1 (CD30) antibody ... Although other lymphomas of either T-cell or B-cell type may strongly express CD30, we believe there is sufficient evidence that the anaplastic type is a distinct clinicopathologic entity to warrant its inclusion in any lymphoma categorization attempt."

Harris et al. 1994 [3]

39.4 Ki-1 Anaplastic Large Cell Lymphoma

"ALCL is a relatively rare tumor, but may be diagnosed with increasing frequency as its features are more widely recognized ... Most cases arise 'de novo'; however, some patients have a history of other lymphomas including MF or HD. There is growing evidence for two distinct forms of primary ALCL: a systemic form, which may involve lymph nodes or extranodal sites, including the skin, ... and a primary cutaneous form, without extracutaneous spread at the time of the diagnosis."

Harris et al. 1994 [3]

The series summarized in [39.5] is from Vanderbilt, and it included both children and adults, with a median age of 35 years. There was a very slight male predominance, half the patients had B symptoms, and peripheral adenopathy was very common, as was retroperitoneal adenopathy. The skin was involved in 23% cases. Some patients had bone and liver involvement and bone marrow involvement was present in a single patient. Three quarters of the cases were of T cell phenotype, a small percentage had B cell markers, and some of the tumors expressed neither B cell nor T cell antigens.

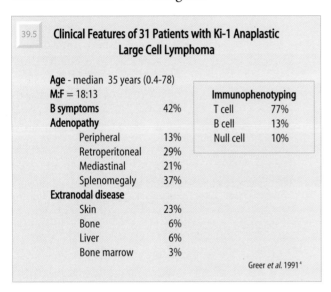

39.5   Clinical Features of 31 Patients with Ki-1 Anaplastic Large Cell Lymphoma

Age - median 35 years (0.4-78)
M:F = 18:13

		Immunophenotyping	
B symptoms	42%		
Adenopathy		T cell	77%
Peripheral	13%	B cell	13%
Retroperitoneal	29%	Null cell	10%
Mediastinal	21%		
Splenomegaly	37%		
Extranodal disease			
Skin	23%		
Bone	6%		
Liver	6%		
Bone marrow	3%		

Greer *et al.* 1991[4]

Illustrated in [39.6] is the age distribution of the Vanderbilt patients, showing a peak in childhood and early adulthood, and a second peak in later adulthood. Most of the other series referred to below are confined either to children or to adults.

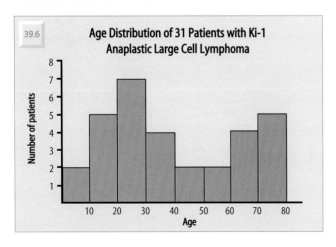

39.6   Age Distribution of 31 Patients with Ki-1 Anaplastic Large Cell Lymphoma

Shown in [39.7] is the overall survival and the disease-free survival from the Vanderbilt series. These patients received a variety of different treatments, and it is difficult to draw specific conclusions, other than that its survival is not very different from that of large cell lymphoma. Although the numbers

are small, the curve appears to reach a plateau. Not unexpectedly, there was a difference in overall survival between patients with Stage I and II disease, and those with Stage III and IV disease [39.8].

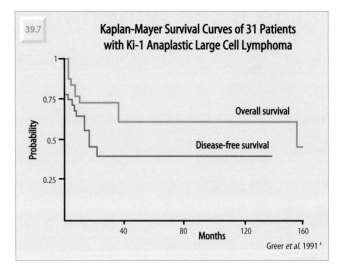

39.7   Kaplan-Mayer Survival Curves of 31 Patients with Ki-1 Anaplastic Large Cell Lymphoma

Greer *et al.* 1991[4]

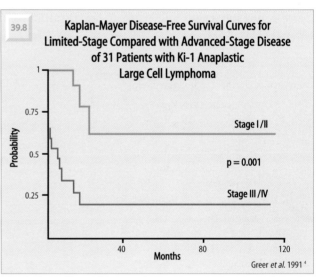

39.8   Kaplan-Mayer Disease-Free Survival Curves for Limited-Stage Compared with Advanced-Stage Disease of 31 Patients with Ki-1 Anaplastic Large Cell Lymphoma

Greer *et al.* 1991[4]

Summarized in [39.9] is a prospective analysis of children treated in three German trials over a period of several years. A total of 62 patients with CD30-positive anaplastic large cell lymphoma were reported, with a median age of ten years. Again, there was a male predominance of about two to one. About 60% of the patients had advanced disease, soft tissue and bone involvement being common. Skin involvement was a little less frequent, and spread to the bone marrow was not seen. Most tumors were of T cell phenotype, a small number were of B cell type, and again there was a substantial number of cases which expressed neither B nor T cell markers.

Patients were treated with three different chemotherapy schedules, all of which were intensive regimens that included multi-drug chemotherapy [39.10]. They received no radiation therapy. The great majority of patients achieved remission, and 50 of the 62 patients had a continuing remission. A total of 56 of the 62 patients were alive, indicating that, with appropriate therapy, this is a lymphoma type which carries a good prognosis.

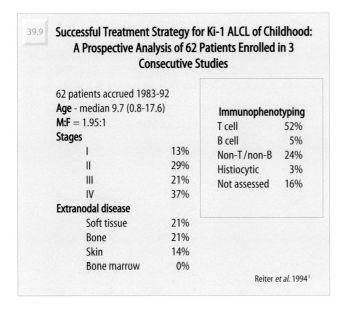

39.9 Successful Treatment Strategy for Ki-1 ALCL of Childhood: A Prospective Analysis of 62 Patients Enrolled in 3 Consecutive Studies

62 patients accrued 1983-92
Age - median 9.7 (0.8-17.6)
M:F = 1.95:1
Stages

I	13%
II	29%
III	21%
IV	37%

Extranodal disease

Soft tissue	21%
Bone	21%
Skin	14%
Bone marrow	0%

Immunophenotyping

T cell	52%
B cell	5%
Non-T/non-B	24%
Histiocytic	3%
Not assessed	16%

Reiter et al. 1994 [5]

39.10 Successful Treatment Strategy for Ki-1 ALCL of Childhood: A Prospective Analysis of 62 Patients Enrolled in 3 Consecutive Studies

All patients treated with intensive chemotherapy including CTX, MTX, VP-16, Ara-C, Doxorubicin, VCR, Prednisone and others.
No XRT
CR - 58/62 (4 remission failures)
CCR - 50/62
Relapses 7/58 (1 death in remission)
56/62 alive

Reiter et al. 1994 [5]

The curves for both progression-free survival and overall survival are shown in [39.11].

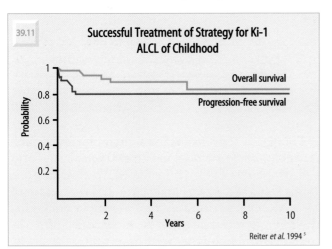

39.11 Successful Treatment of Strategy for Ki-1 ALCL of Childhood

A series of pediatric large cell lymphomas [39.12], both CD30-positive and CD30-negative, was published in 1994 from St Jude Hospital.[6] A total of 300 children with non-Hodgkin's lymphoma were studied, of whom 91 had large cell neoplasms. Forty five of these had adequate tissue for analysis, and 18 were CD30-positive, but the age profile was identical in the two groups. As in the study from Germany, there was a male predominance in the CD30-positive patients. There was a slightly lower incidence of early stage disease in the CD30-positive group. Skin involvement was present in a quarter of the CD30-positive large cell lymphoma patients, but in none of the patients with CD30-negative lymphomas. Adenopathy was common in both groups, and mediastinal involvement was present in about a third of the CD30-positive cases. Marrow involvement was very uncommon. The t(2;5) translocation was found in three of 18 patients in the CD30-positive group, but was also found in two of 27 CD30-negative cases.

39.12 Clinical Features and Treatment Outcome for Children with CD30+ Large Cell NHL

300 children with NHL, 91 with large cell, 45 analyzed

	CD30+	CD30-
Patients	18	27
Age	13 (2-20)	13 (1-29)
Male	72%	52%
Stage I/II	22%	48%
Skin involvement	28%	0%
Nodes	89%	63%
Mediastinum	33%	15%
Bone marrow	6%	4%
t(2;5) (p23;q35)	3/18	2/27

Sandlund et al. 1994 [6]

Analysis of event-free [39.13] and overall survival [39.14] suggested that, at least for Stage III or IV disease, patients with CD30-positive tumors have a survival advantage as compared to patients with CD30-negative tumors.

39.13 Clinical Features and Treatment Outcome for Children with CD30+ Large Cell NHL

5-year EFS according to CD30 status

Stage	CD30+	CD30-
I/II	75% (N = 4)	92% (N = 13)
III/IV	57% (N = 14)	29% (N = 14)

Sandlund et al. 1994 [6]

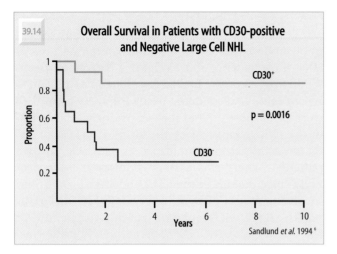

Overall Survival in Patients with CD30-positive and Negative Large Cell NHL

CD30+

p = 0.0016

CD30−

Sandlund et al. 1994 [6]

In another study [39.15], looking specifically at the t(2;5) translocation, 115 patients with large cell lymphoma were reviewed over 18 years.[7] In 18 patients with abnormal karyotypes, nine had the t(2;5) translocation. All were children, and the majority had Stage III or IV disease. Using Working Formulation criteria, seven had immunoblastic, and two had diffuse large cell neoplasms. Six tumors had anaplastic large cell lymphoma according to the Kiel criteria. Six of the eight patients tested were CD30-positive. The majority were of T cell phenotype, but there was one B cell neoplasm and three non-B, non-T cell tumors [39.16]. The treatment outcome was quite good for the patients, in keeping with the other studies.

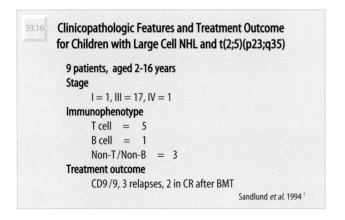

Clinicopathologic Features and Treatment Outcome for Children with Large Cell NHL and t(2;5)(p23;q35)

115 patients with large cell lymphoma 1975-1993
9/18 with abnormal karyotype t(2;5)
Working Formulation
7 large cell immunoblastic
2 diffuse large cell
Kiel classification
6 anaplastic
2 immunoblastic
1 centroblastic
CD30+ in 6/8 tested

Sandlund et al. 1994 [7]

Clinicopathologic Features and Treatment Outcome for Children with Large Cell NHL and t(2;5)(p23;q35)

9 patients, aged 2-16 years
Stage
I = 1, III = 17, IV = 1
Immunophenotype
T cell = 5
B cell = 1
Non-T/Non-B = 3
Treatment outcome
CD9/9, 3 relapses, 2 in CR after BMT

Sandlund et al. 1994 [7]

Our own series [39.17], from the Harvard Medical Area, reviewed 31 cases of adult CD30-positive anaplastic large cell lymphomas.[8] The median age was 44, with a span of 16 to 86 years, and again we saw a male predominance. About 70% of our patients had advanced stage disease, 32% had skin involvement, and only a couple of patients had bone marrow involvement. Overall, extranodal involvement was very common. As in other studies, a T cell phenotype was the commonest finding, but B cell and null phenotypes were also seen.

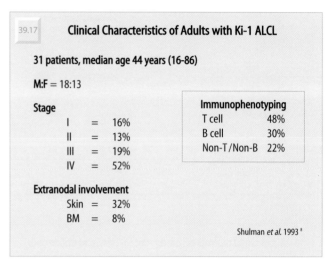

Clinical Characteristics of Adults with Ki-1 ALCL

31 patients, median age 44 years (16-86)

M:F = 18:13

Stage		Immunophenotyping	
I	= 16%	T cell	48%
II	= 13%	B cell	30%
III	= 19%	Non-T/Non-B	22%
IV	= 52%		

Extranodal involvement
Skin = 32%
BM = 8%

Shulman et al. 1993 [8]

Shown in [39.18] are our disease-free and overall survival curves, which revealed a relatively good prognosis. Not surprisingly the early Stage patients do very well, and the later Stage patients have a poorer prognosis [39.19]. It is hard to say, however, with these small numbers, if they differ from large cell lymphoma patients.

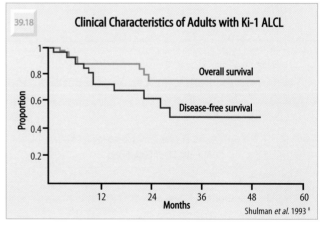

Clinical Characteristics of Adults with Ki-1 ALCL

Overall survival

Disease-free survival

Shulman et al. 1993 [8]

Finally, a few comments may be made on Hodgkin's-like or Hodgkin's-related anaplastic large cell lymphoma [39.20]. In the REAL classification, this is listed as a provisional entity. It is characterized by a number of features that resemble Hodgkin's disease. It was said that the disease is primarily found in young adults, who have aggressive nodal disease and often bulky mediastinal masses. Cases are said to respond poorly to conventional therapy for Hodgkin's disease, but to do much better with therapy for high grade, non-Hodgkin's lymphoma [39.21].

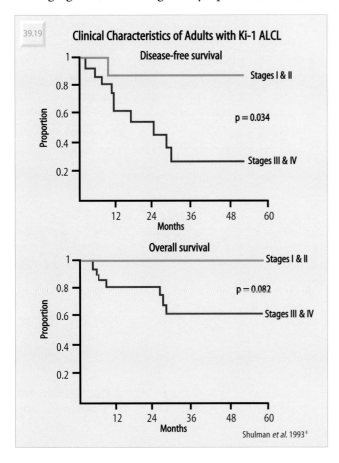

Shulman et al. 1993[8]

39.20

Ki-1 + ALCL - Hodgkin's-like
(Hodgkin's-related - Provisional Entity)

Morphologic features:

" … confluent sheets of tumor cells, and a cohesive, often sinusoidal growth pattern, similar to classic ALCL; but with architectural features that resemble HD of the NS type, such as capsular thickening, nodular growth of tumor cells, and sclerotic bands."

Harris et al. 1994[3]

39.21

Ki-1 + ALCL - Hodgkin's-like
(Hodgkin's-related - Provisional Entity)

Clinical features:

" … young adults with aggressive nodal disease, often with bulky mediastinal masses; according to European studies they do not do well with conventional therapy for HD, but may have a good response to very aggressive therapy, such as third generation chemotherapy regimens for high-grade NHLs. We believe that further study is required to define this possible entity and its relationship to HD on the one hand and classic ALCL on the other."

Harris et al. 1994[3]

Summarized in [39.22] is the study from Italy and Germany, which compared 41 conventional anaplastic large cell lymphoma patients with 28 cases of the putative Hodgkin's-related form of the disease.[9] Their ages and stage distribution were relatively similar. There were slightly more early stage patients in the Hodgkin's-related category, but B symptoms were similar in frequency. Bulky disease was commoner in the Hodgkin's-related group, and mediastinal involvement was present in all 28 patients. Bone marrow involvement was rare in both groups.

39.22

Ki-1 + ALCL - Hodgkin's-like (Hodgkin's-related - Provisional Entity)		
	ALCL-CT	ALCL-HR
N patients		41 28
Age	34 (16-59)	27 (15-55)
Stage		
I	0	0
II	46%	68%
III	34%	11%
IV	20%	21%
B symptoms	54%	50%
Bulky disease	24%	57%
Bone marrow +	7%	4%
Mediastinal mass	58%	100%

Pileri et al. 1994[9]

If one looks at how these patients fared on therapy, the complete remission rates were the same [39.23]. The continued complete remission rates were very similar, although slightly more patients in the conventional anaplastic large cell lymphoma group were alive at last follow-up.

39.23

Ki-1 + ALCL - Hodgkin's-like (Hodgkin's-related - Provisional Entity) Response to MACOP-B or F-MACHOP		
	ALCL-CT	ALCL-HR
N patients	41	28
CR	68%	68%
PR	24%	14%
CCR	46%	54%
DOD	34%	32%
AWD	20%	14%

Pileri et al. 1994[9]

Shown in [23.24] are the event-free survival curves. They suggest that the Hodgkin's-related cases did slightly better. However, the numbers are very small and these differences are not statistically significant.

Finally, if one looks at overall survivals [23.25], and compares them with large cell high grade lymphomas, there are no obvious differences.

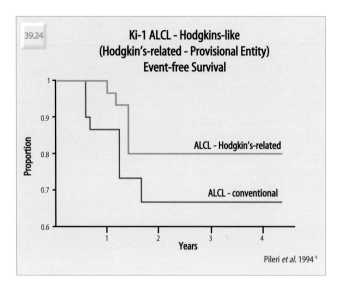

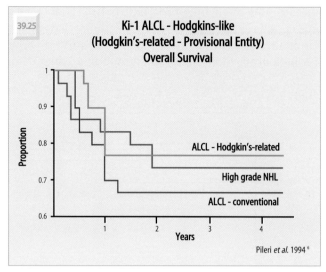

REFERENCES

1. Kadin ME. Ki-1-positive anaplastic large-cell lymphoma: a clinicopathological entity? *J Clin Oncol* 1991; **9**: 533-6.

2. Kadin ME. Ki-1 / CD30+ (anaplastic) large-cell lymphoma: maturation of a clinicopathological entity with prospects of effective therapy. *J Clin Oncol* 1994; **12**: 884-7.

3. Harris NL, Jaffe ES, Stein H *et al.* A revised European-American classification of lymphoid neoplasms: a proposal from the International Lymphoma Study Group. *Blood* 1994; **84**: 1361-92.

4. Greer JP, Kinney MC, Collins RD *et al.* Clinical features of 31 patients with Ki-1 anaplastic large-cell lymphoma. *J Clin Oncol* 1991; **9**: 539-47.

5. Reiter A, Schrappe M, Tiemann M *et al.* Successful treatment strategy for Ki-1 anaplastic large-cell lymphoma of childhood: a prospective analysis of 62 patients enrolled in three consecutive Berlin-Frankfurt-Munster Group studies. *J Clin Oncol* 1994; **12**: 899-908.

6. Sandlund JT, Pui C-H, Santana VM *et al.* Clinical features and treatment outcome for children with CD30+ large-cell non-Hodgkin's lymphoma. *J Clin Oncol* 1994; **12**: 895-8.

7. Sandlund JT, Pui C-H, Roberts WM *et al.* Clinicopathologic features and treatment outcome of children with large-cell lymphoma and the t(2;5)(p23;q35). *Blood* 1994; **84**: 2467-2471.

8. Shulman LN, Frisard B, Antin JH *et al.* Primary Ki-1 anaplastic large-cell lymphoma in adults: clinical characteristics and therapeutic outcome. *J Clin Oncol* 1993; **11**: 937-42.

9. Pileri S, Bocchia M, Baroni CD *et al.* Anaplastic large cell lymphoma (CD30+/Ki-1+): results of a prospective clinico-pathological study of 69 patients. *Brit J Haematol* 1994; **86**: 513-23.

FURTHER READING

1. Kadin ME, Sako D, Berliner N *et al.* Childhood Ki-1 lymphoma presenting with skin lesions and peripheral lymphadenopathy. *Blood* 1986; **68**: 1042-9.

POST-SCRIPT

Since the writing of this chapter, additional clinical studies have been published confirming the clinical characteristics of pediatric and adult patients with anaplastic large cell lymphoma (ALCL) and the outcome of treatment for these patients. [1-3]

Additional work has been done in an attempt to distinguish subcategories of ALCL, particularly in relation to the presence of the t(2;5) chromosomal abnormality in the malignant cells. [4-7] These data remain of unclear significance at this time, though it appears that this translocation occurs most commonly in the lymphoma cells of pediatric patients with the T cell or null cell subtype of ALCL, and in those patients with primary nodal, rather than primary cutaneous disease. Implications for treatment based on the presence or absence of t(2;5) are unclear at this time. In addition, the occurrence of this chromosomal translocation in other malignant lymphomas has been a subject of study without consistent results at this time.

REFERENCES

1. Zinzani PL, Bendandi M, Martelli M *et al.* Anaplastic large-cell lymphoma: clinical and prognostic evaluation of 90 adult-patients. *J Clin Oncol* 1996;**14**: 955-62.

2. Tilly H, Gaulard P, Lepage E *et al.* Primary anaplastic large-cell lymphoma in adults: clinical presentation, immunophenotype, and outcome. *Blood* 1997; **90**: 3727-34.

3. Filippa DA, Ladanyi M, Wollner N *et al.* CD30 (Ki-1)-positive malignant lymphomas: clinical, immunophenotypic, histologic, and genetic characteristics and differences with Hodgkin's disease. *Blood* 1996; **87**: 2905-17.

4. DeCoteau JF, Butmarc JR, Kinney MC, Kadin ME. The t(2;5) chromosomal translocation is not a common feature of primary cutaneous CD30+ lymphoproliferative disorders: comparison with anaplastic large-cell lymphoma of nodal origin. *Blood* 1996; **87**: 3437-41.

5. Weisenburger DD, Gordon BG, Vose JM *et al.* Occurrence of the t(2;5)(p23;q35) in non-Hodgkin's lymphoma. *Blood* 1996; **87**: 3860-8.

6. Sarris AH, Luthra R, Papadimitracopoulou V *et al.* Amplification of genomic DNA demonstrates the presence of the t(2;5)(p23;q35) in anaplastic large cell lymphoma, but not in other non-Hodgkin's lymphomas, Hodgkin's disease, or lymphomatoid papulosis. *Blood* 1996; **88** :1771-9.

7. Benharroch D, Meguerian-Bedoyan Z, Lamant L *et al.* ALK-positive lymphoma: a single disease with a broad spectrum of morphology. *Blood* 1998; **91**: 2076-84.

Morphologic, immunologic and genetic features of HTLV-1-positive adult T cell lymphoma/leukemia

E S Jaffe

Adult T cell leukemia/lymphoma is found throughout the world [40.1], but is concentrated in areas in which HTLV-1 is endemic. It was first described in South Western Japan, and on the island of Kyushu more than 10% of normal individuals have antibodies to the virus. HTLV-1 is also frequently found in the Caribbean basin, where there are clusters of this disease. However, the risk of developing ATL/L for sero-positive people is only about one in a thousand, so that many individuals exposed to the virus do not develop lymphoma or leukemia.

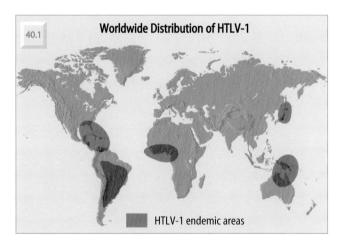

Worldwide Distribution of HTLV-1

HTLV-1 endemic areas

In the United States the disease tends to be clustered in the South Eastern region and also in urban areas, such as New York city [40.2], where there is significant immigration from the Caribbean. In North America the disease is found almost exclusively in black patients, in contrast to the patients in Japan.

[40.3], kindly provided by Dr. Hanaoka of Kyoto University, illustrates the characteristic pleomorphic polylobated cells seen in the peripheral blood in this disease. They vary considerably in size and the larger cells have sometimes been called "flower" cells. In lymph nodes [40.4], the tumor often shows a leukemic pattern of infiltration. If one looks closely, the sinuses are open and infiltrated by neoplastic cells.

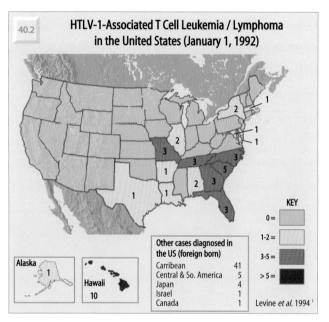

HTLV-1-Associated T Cell Leukemia / Lymphoma in the United States (January 1, 1992)

Alaska 1

Hawaii 10

Other cases diagnosed in the US (foreign born)

Carribean	41
Central & So. America	5
Japan	4
Israel	1
Canada	1

KEY

0 =
1-2 =
3-5 =
> 5 =

Levine *et al.* 1994 [1]

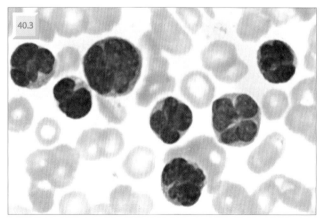

The cytologic spectrum is very variable within lymph nodes. Shown in [40.5] are small polymorphic cells, resembling those seen in the peripheral blood, within a sinus. The cells can be small and polymorphic in appearance, as in this case. In other cases [40.6], there is a mixture of small and larger transformed cells. In some cases [40.7], the cells are predominantly large and relatively monomorphic. A case such as this might be difficult to distinguish from a large B cell lymphoma. Finally, in some cases [40.8] the cells are markedly pleomorphic, and large giant cell forms are seen among the other cellular appearances.

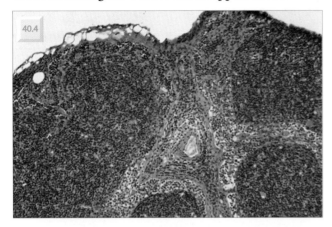

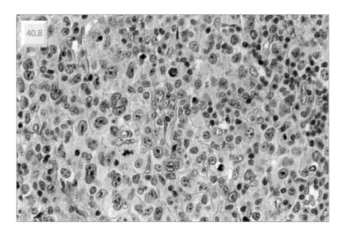

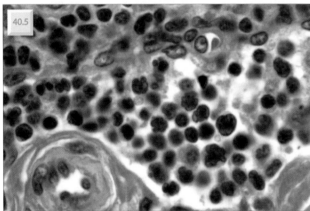

Because of this cytologic heterogeneity, adult T cell leukemia was not identified as a single subgroup in the Kiel scheme [40.9]. It was described as either "pleomorphic small cell", "pleomorphic medium and large cell" or "immunoblastic", with or without HTLV-1 positivity. However, in the REAL classification it was felt that this disease should be designated as a discrete pathologic entity, regardless of cell morphology.

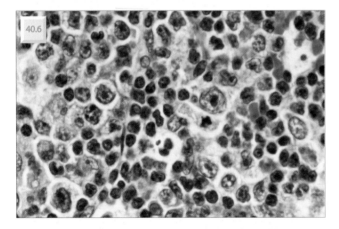

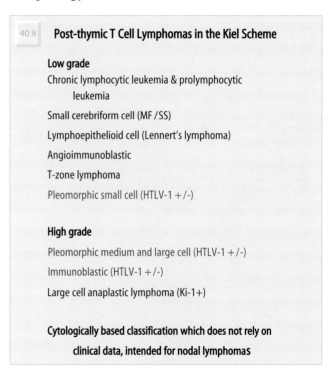

40.9   **Post-thymic T Cell Lymphomas in the Kiel Scheme**

Low grade

Chronic lymphocytic leukemia & prolymphocytic
       leukemia

Small cerebriform cell (MF/SS)

Lymphoepithelioid cell (Lennert's lymphoma)

Angioimmunoblastic

T-zone lymphoma

Pleomorphic small cell (HTLV-1 +/-)

High grade

Pleomorphic medium and large cell (HTLV-1 +/-)

Immunoblastic (HTLV-1 +/-)

Large cell anaplastic lymphoma (Ki-1+)

**Cytologically based classification which does not rely on
clinical data, intended for nodal lymphomas**

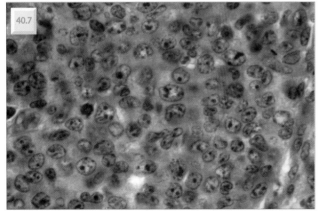

This disorder [40.10] always has a T cell phenotype. The cells are usually CD3 and CD4-positive, and, as with many T cell lymphomas, there is often loss of CD7.

A highly characteristic feature [40.11] is strong expression of CD25 (IL-2 receptor). This has been used as a target for immunotherapy by Dr. Waldmann at the NCI. In addition, levels of soluble CD25 in the peripheral blood correlate closely with disease activity.

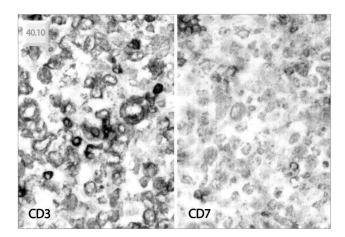

CD3   CD7

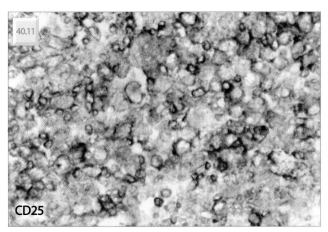

CD25

nuclear irregularity is much more subtle than that seen in ATL/L. In addition, in ATL/L the neoplastic cell cytoplasm is typically quite basophilic, in contrast to Sézary cells, in which the cytoplasm is less intensely stained.

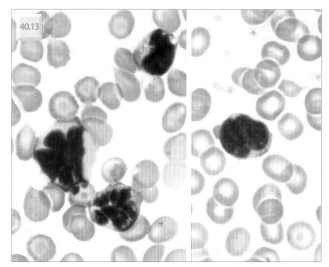

If one looks at hematologic parameters in ATL/L [40.14], the white cell count may be markedly elevated, due to large numbers of circulating malignant cells, but other findings are frequently normal. These patients are usually not anemic or thrombocytopenic. This suggests that the bone marrow is not a primary target organ for this disease and is only secondarily involved. Patients with ATL/L often show eosinophilia and polymorphonuclear leukocytosis.

Clinically, ATL/L is a systemic disorder and virtually all patients are at Stage IV at presentation. Leukemia is seen initially in the majority of patients [40.12], and, at least in the NCI series, developed in all patients at some point during their clinical course. Other frequent clinical findings are hypercalcemia, with or without lytic bone lesions, lymphadenopathy, hepatosplenomegaly and skin lesions, which are seen in about two thirds of patients.

Hematologic Parameters in ATL/L

WBC ranges from normal to 100,000 per μL
  Lymphocytosis of 15 to 93% (med 46 %), 80% of patients
    have abnormal lymphs in PB
  Frequent eosinophilia and PMN leukocytosis
BM-positive in only a fraction of those with blood involvement
Hgb /Hct and platelet count usually normal

Bunn et al. 1983 [2]

Skin involvement is seen in about two thirds of patients, and can have a number of clinical manifestations. Ulcerating tumors can be seen [40.15]. In other patients small nodules and papules are seen [40.16], and sometimes there is a diffuse exfoliative rash [40.17], which can be very difficult to distinguish from mycosis fungoides. Histologically, the lesions can also simulate mycosis fungoides, with infiltration of the epidermis to form Pautrier's microabscesses [40.18]. Indeed, the case in which Dr. Gallo's laboratory first identified the HTLV-1 virus had been diagnosed as an aggressive form of mycosis fungoides. It is still controversial whether HTLV-1 or a related retrovirus is associated with mycosis fungoides. A number of

Adult T Cell Leukemia /Lymphoma Clinical Manifestations - NCI Series

Clinical feature	At presentation (%)	During course (%)
Leukemia	62	100
Hypercalcemia	73	83
Lytic bone lesions	36	—
Lymphadenopathy	61	85
Hepatosplenomegaly	61	—
Skin lesions	61	—
Bone marrow +	58	—
Stage IV	100	—

In [40.13], the appearance of ATL/L cells in the peripheral blood, on the left, is contrasted with a case of Sézary syndrome, on the right. Although Sézary cells are cerebriform and irregular in appearance, the

studies using PCR-based techniques have shown sequences homologous to portions of HTLV-1 in typical mycosis fungoides.

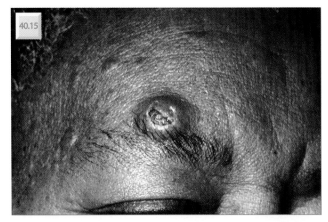

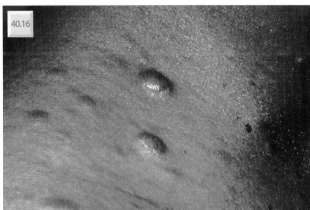

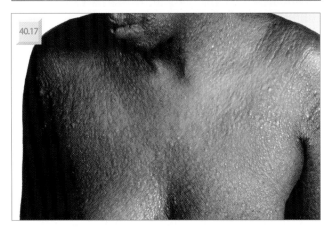

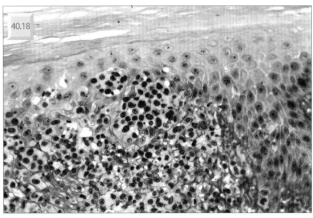

Hypercalcemia is another common clinical manifestation. This can be very dramatic in its presentation. This radiograph [40.19] is from a South American patient who was referred to the NCI with a presumptive diagnosis of hyperparathyroidism. He had undergone a parathyroid exploration prior to the diagnosis of ATL/L.

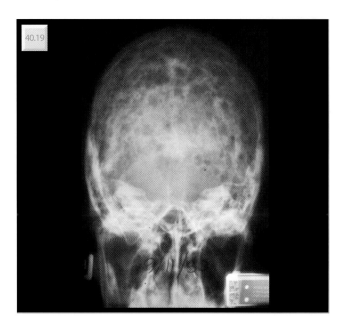

The histologic section [40.20] is from another patient who presented with lytic bone disease, and a bone biopsy was performed in an attempt to make a diagnosis. The biopsy did not show any tumor but marked osteoclastic activity was evident. [40.21] gives data from a study by Kiyokawa et al [3] and shows that the osteoclastic proliferation correlates closely with the levels of hypercalcemia. When the serum calcium is markedly elevated, one sees osteoclastic proliferation not only in lytic bone lesions, but also in bone marrow biopsies without evidence of lytic bone disease.

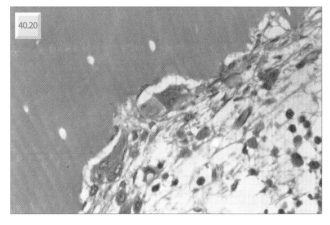

More indolent forms of the disease have been described in Japan. These are termed smoldering ATL/L or chronic ATL/L [40.22]. In these disorders the survival is longer and there are less striking clinical manifestations - minimal lymphadenopathy, minimal hepatosplenomegaly and only rare circulating neoplastic cells. In these more indolent forms, there are frequently cutaneous manifestations [40.23], with an exfoliative scaly rash.

Histologically the infiltrates in smoldering ATL/L are surprisingly benign in appearance, as shown in the skin biopsy illustrated [40.24] from a Jamaican patient. Infiltrating lymphoid cells are seen in the dermis, and focal exocytosis in the epidermis, but one would not suspect that this was a malignant process. However, these cells contained clonal HTLV-1 virus. Interestingly, immunophenotyping on that biopsy [40.25] showed that these infiltrating cells were CD3-positive T cells, expressing IL-2 receptor (CD25), supporting the concept that the infiltrate is a manifestation of ATL/L.

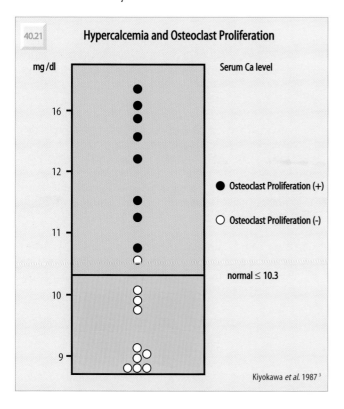

40.21 Hypercalcemia and Osteoclast Proliferation

mg/dl — Serum Ca level

- Osteoclast Proliferation (+)
- ○ Osteoclast Proliferation (−)

normal ≤ 10.3

Kiyokawa *et al*. 1987 [3]

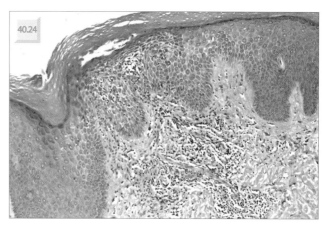

40.24

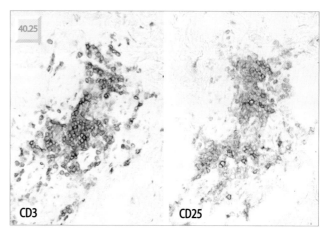

40.25

CD3   CD25

40.22 Indolent Forms of ATL/L

Smoldering ATL/L	Chronic ATL/L
Normal WBC	Increased WBC
ATL cells < 3%	ATL cells > 10%
No lymphadenopathy	Mild lymphadenopathy
No hepatosplenomegaly	Slight hepatosplenomegaly
Skin rash: erythema papules	Skin rash variable
Normal LDH, Ca^{++}	Slight inc. LDH, Normal Ca^{++}
Survival: > 2 years	Survival: usually > 2 years

Despite its benign clinical and histologic features, the smoldering forms of the disease can undergo blastic transformation, and develop an acute crisis, with all the aggressive clinical and histologic features of typical ATL/L syndrome [40.26].[4]

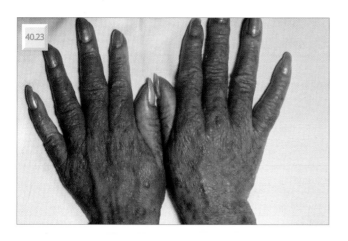

40.23

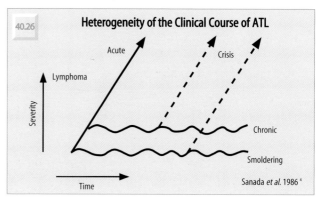

40.26 Heterogeneity of the Clinical Course of ATL

Acute — Crisis

Lymphoma

Severity

Chronic

Smoldering

Time

Sanada *et al*. 1986 [4]

ACKNOWLEDGEMENT

This chapter is based on U.S. government work. There are no restrictions on its use.

REFERENCES

1. Levine PH, Manns A, Jaffe ES *et al*. The effect of ethnic differences on the pattern of HTLV-1-associated T-cell leukemia/lymphoma (HATL) in the United States. *Int J Cancer* 1994; **56**: 177-81.

2. Bunn PA Jr, Schechter GP, Jaffe E *et al*. Clinical course of retrovirus-associated adult T-cell lymphoma in the United States. *N Engl J Med* 1983; **309**: 257-64.

3. Kiyokawa T, Yamaguchi K, Takeya M *et al*. Hypercalcemia and osteoclast proliferation in adult T-cell leukemia. *Cancer* 1987; **59**: 1187-91.

4. Sanada I, Nakada K, Furugen S *et al*. Chromosomal abnormalities in a patient with smoldering adult T-cell leukemia: evidence for a multistep pathogenesis. *Leuk Res* 1986; **10**: 1377-82.

FURTHER READING

Abrams M, Sidawy M, Novich M. Smoldering HTLV-associated T cell leukemia. *Arch Intern Med* 1985; **145**: 2257-8.

Chadburn A, Athan E, Wieczorek R, Knowles D. Detection and characterization of HTLV-1 associated T neoplasms in an HTLV-1 nonendemic region by polymerase chain reaction. *Blood* 1991; **70**: 1500-8.

Duggan D, Ehrlich G, Davey F *et al*. HTLV-1 induced lymphoma mimicking Hodgkin's disease. Diagnosis by polymerase chain reaction amplification of specific HTLV-1 sequences in tumor DNA. *Blood* 1988; **71**: 1027-32.

Jaffe ES, Blattner WA, Blayney DW *et al*. The pathologic spectrum of adult T-cell leukemia/lymphoma in the United States. *Am J Surg Pathol* 1984; **8**: 263-75.

Kikuchi M, Mitsui T, Takeshita M, Okamura H, Naitoh H, Eimoto T. Virus associated adult T-cell leukemia (ATL) in Japan: clinical, histological and immunological studies. *Hematol Oncol* 1987; **4**: 67.

Levine PH, Cleghorn F, Manns A *et al*. Adult T-cell leukemia/lymphoma: a working point-score classification for epidemiological studies. *Int J Cancer* 1994; **59**: 491-3.

Manns A, Cleghorn FR, Falk RT *et al*. Role of HTLV-1 in development of non-Hodgkin lymphoma in Jamaica and Trinidad and Tobago. The HTLV Lymphoma Study Group. *Lancet* 1993; **342**: 1447-50.

Poiesz B, Ruscetti F, Gazdar A. Detection and isolation of type C retrovirus particles from fresh and cultured lymphocytes of a patient with cutaneous T-cell lymphoma. *Proc Natl Acad Sci USA* 1980; **77**: 7415-9.

Swerdlow S, Habeshaw J, Rohatiner A, Lister T, Stansfeld A. Caribbean T-cell lymphoma/leukemia. *Cancer* 1984; **54**: 687-96.

Uchiyama T, Yodoi J, Sagawa K, Takatsuki K, Uchino H. Adult T-cell leukemia: clinical and hematologic features of 16 cases. *Blood* 1977; **50**: 481-92.

Morphologic, immunologic and genetic features of Burkitt's and Burkitt-like lymphomas

T M Grogan

This chapter is concerned with two entities – Burkitt's and Burkitt-like lymphoma. One curious aspect of this topic is that we all feel very familiar with the definition of Burkitt's lymphoma, and yet in the everyday practice of medicine in the United States we almost never encounter it. In contrast, we feel uncomfortable with this provisional category of Burkitt-like lymphoma, and yet we see it all the time.

The features of the endemic entity known as Burkitt's lymphoma are very familiar [41.1]. There is a "starry sky" pattern at low power [41.2], and typically the neoplasm is a diffuse extranodal process. Follicular involvement is rare. The tumor is monomorphic in appearance, the cells are medium-sized and round, with blastic features. They contain two to five basophilic nucleoli and their cytoplasm is basophilic and vacuolated [41.3]. The cytoplasm is abundant and "squared off", giving a jig-saw puzzle pattern.

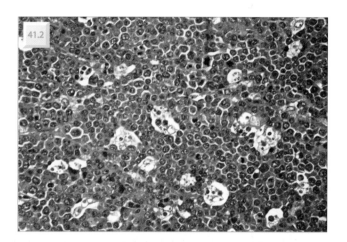

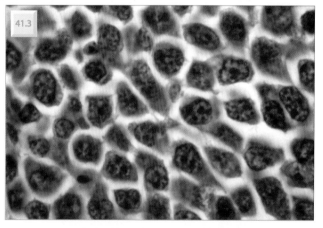

41.1	**Burkitt's Lymphoma**
	Morphology

- Monomorphic, medium-sized cells
- Round nuclei, blastic chromatin
- Multiple (2-5) basophilic nucleoli
- Touch prep: cytoplasm basophilic, vacuolated
- Abundant amphophilic cytoplasm
- "Squared-off" cytoplasm; jig-saw puzzle pattern
- "Starry sky" pattern; high mitotic rate
- Diffuse, extranodal, with rare follicle involvement

In the touch preparations in [41.4] and [41.5], the effete apoptotic lymphoid cells, a phagocytic histiocyte, and the basophilic vacuolated cytoplasm of the tumor cells are all seen.

If a large number of Burkitt's lymphomas are reviewed, one occasionally finds involvement of germinal centers, but this is rare [41.6].

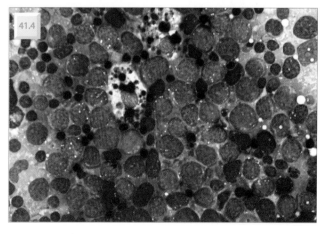

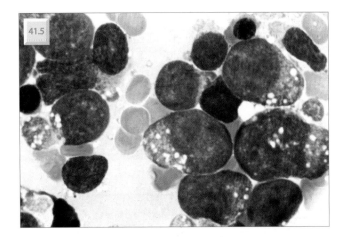

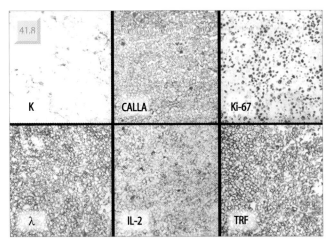

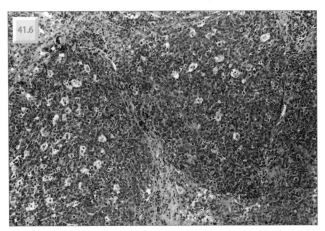

In terms of the phenotype [41.7], Burkitt's lymphoma fits squarely in the middle of the B cell differentiation scheme. It expresses monotypic Ig and a range of pan B markers. Typically there is strong reactivity for CD10 and expression of CD21, a receptor for Epstein-Barr virus, at least in the endemic African cases. The proliferative rate, as measured by Ki-67, is typically greater than 80%, making it the most rapidly proliferating of all lymphomas.

41.7	**Burkitt's Lymphoma**
	Phenotype

- Monoclonal Ig (IgM > D > G > A)
- Pan B antigens: CD19, 20, 22, 79a
- Strong CD10 expression; absent CD5, 23, 44
- Early B cell in maturation scheme
- CD21+: EBVr (endemic African cases)
- Proliferative rate > 80% (Ki67)

Shown in [41.8] is a typical phenotype. Interestingly there is a tendency for lambda light chains to be expressed more often than kappa chains. CD10 (CALLA) is also commonly expressed and the high proliferative rate, as measured by Ki-67, is evident. Activation-associated antigens can also be found.

The genotype is very much part of the definition of this entity [41.9]. Translocation of the *c-MYC* gene is due typically to the (8;14) translocation involving the Ig heavy chain gene, but occasionally the (2;8) or (8;22) translocations are seen, involving, respectively, the lambda and kappa Ig genes [41.10] and [41.11]. There is a difference between endemic and non-endemic forms of the disease in terms of whether the Ig joining region or switch region is involved. The association with Epstein-Barr virus varies: virtually all endemic cases are associated with Epstein-Barr virus; whereas in the USA the figure differs, depending on the patient population. The Epstein-Barr viral termini typically show a clonal homogeneous pattern on Southern blotting, suggesting early infection of a single B cell.

41.9	**Burkitt's Lymphoma**
	Genotype

- Ig gene rearrangement
- *c-MYC* translocated and overexpressed
- Translocations: t(8;14), t(2;8), t(8;22)
- Africa: Ig joining region (early B cell)
- Non-African: Ig switch region (later B cell)
- EBV genomes: 95% African, 20% nonendemic, 40% HIV; clonally homogeneous

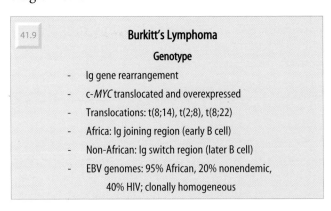

C-*MYC* Translocation in Burkitt's Lymphoma with t(8;14)

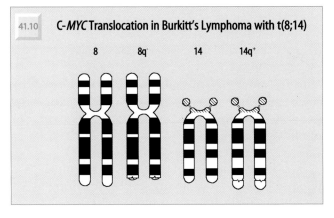

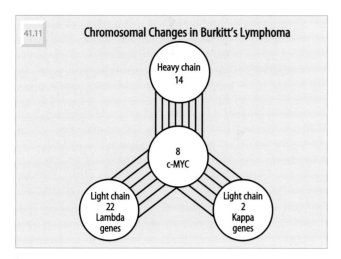

Chromosomal Changes in Burkitt's Lymphoma

The clinical picture varies depending on the patients' origin [41.12]. Children are affected in the endemic regions, but in the USA patients may be adults. The disease tends to be extranodal, and has the interesting property of involving bilateral sites. In the non-endemic areas, gut-associated lesions are common. There is a high cure rate in the endemic areas and it appears that prognosis relates to the bulk and stage of disease.

Burkitt's Lymphoma

Clinical

- Endemic: common in children
- Non-endemic: adults (HIV associated)
- Sex: M > F (2.5 / 1) Stage: majority IV
- Sites (bilaterality)
    Africa: jaw, ovaries, breasts, kidneys
    Non-Africa: gut, mesentery, jaw
- Rare PB L3-ALL; complication FL
- Endemic BL, high cure rate
- Prognosis ~ bulk of disease, stage

Illustrated in [41.13] is a Burkitt's lymphoma involving the mesentery, and it shows a frequently seen feature of interest. On the right, a lymph node with a few germinal centers and widely open sinuses is seen. This tissue, however, shows no involvement by the Burkitt's lymphoma, which is seen at the center, spreading into adjacent fat. This figure emphasizes the tumor's tendency to remain as an extranodal lesion.

Show in [41.14] is a virtually complete replacement of the bone marrow by Burkitt's lymphoma, a feature usually seen as a terminal complication.

To turn now to the "poor cousin", "Burkitt-like" lymphoma [41.15], its features are intermediate between the description just given of Burkitt's

lymphoma and large cell B cell lymphoma. It is more pleomorphic, and it is not as monomorphous. There are fewer nucleoli, which tend to be eosinophilic. However, one does see vacuolated basophilic cytoplasm, and it is common to see a "starry sky" pattern and a high proliferative rate.

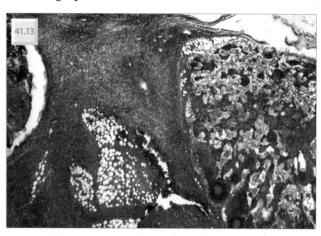

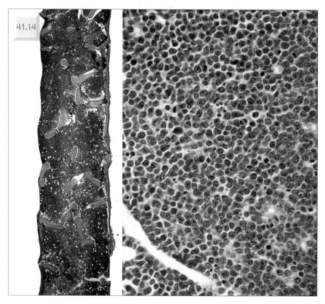

Provisional Entity: High-Grade B Cell Lymphoma, Burkitt-like

Morphology

- Size between BL and LCL
- Pleomorphic, not monomorphic
- Few eosinophilic nucleoli (1-2)
- Basophilic, vacuolated cytoplasm
- "Starry-sky" and high proliferative rate

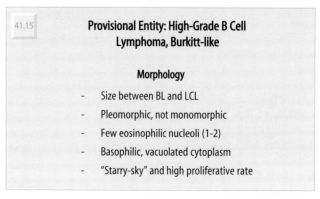

A "starry sky" pattern at low power, such as that seen in [41.16], immediately evokes a diagnosis of Burkitt's lymphoma. There is a moderate nuclear:cytoplasmic ratio, and "squared off" cytoplasm giving the jig-saw like pattern [41.17].

There tend to be one or two eosinophilic nucleoli. Cells vary in size and there may even be some multi-nucleation.   If one looks at a touch preparation [41.18], it has many Burkitt-like features, including basophilic cytoplasm, vacuolation, and histiocytes containing apoptotic lymphocytes.

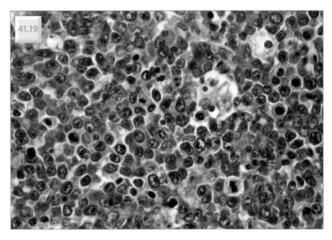

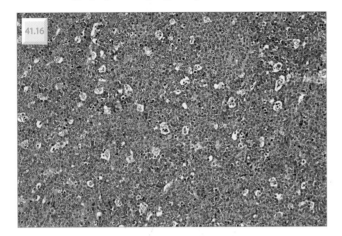

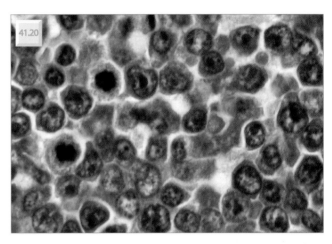

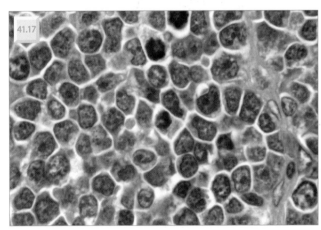

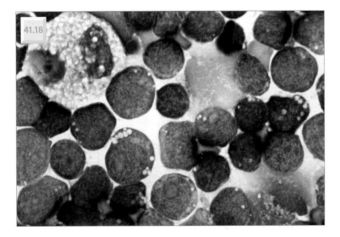

Illustrated in [41.21] is the appearance of Burkitt's lymphoma and Burkitt-like lymphoma side by side, making the point that features such as cell size, nuclear cytoplasmic ratio, cytoplasmic basophilia and vacuolation are very similar.   The electron microscopic appearances are shown in [41.22], with Burkitt's in the left half of the electron micrograph and Burkitt-like on the right.   If one compares the degree of pleomorphism and the nucleolar frequency in the two diseases by image analysis one can confirm that Burkitt's cases have more nucleoli and are very monomorphic [41.23].

In the case shown in [41.19], there is more variation in terms of the size of the lymphoid cells, but their average size is similar to that of Burkitt's cells, and again they have a moderate nuclear cytoplasmic ratio.   A "starry sky" appearance is also present. Shown in [41.20] is the same case at higher magnification.

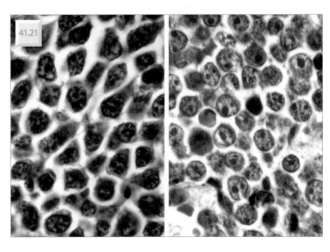

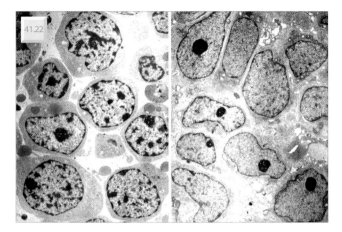

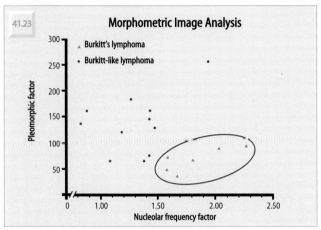

Morphometric Image Analysis

infiltrating T lymphocytes. There is light and heavy chain restriction, as is always seen. Expression of BCL-2 and p53 is also illustrated.

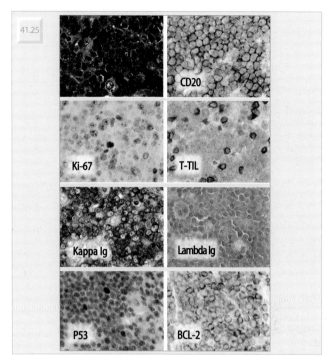

In terms of the phenotype [41.24], there are similarities. There are rare cases of T cell Burkitt-like lymphoma, and occasional CD21-positive cases. They also have a high proliferative rate. Although cases with *c-MYC* and t(8;14) are described, they are rare. A more constant finding, as described by Yano *et al.*, is *BCL-2* rearrangement,[1] and *BCL-2* over-expression related to translocation is described in one third of these cases. Over-expression of p53 has also been described in more than 40% of cases. The association with Epstein-Barr virus is less constant in this entity.

An illustration from a case classified as Burkitt-like lymphoma is shown in [41.26], and [41.27] shows the basophilic vacuolated cytoplasm. However, this case had a T cell phenotype and was CD7-positive and CD20-negative [41.28]. It also contained infiltrating myeloid elements, as commonly happens with peripheral T cell lymphomas, so that there was quite a complex phenotype.

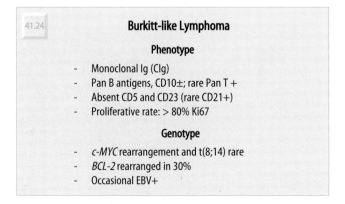

Burkitt-like Lymphoma

Phenotype

- Monoclonal Ig (CIg)
- Pan B antigens, CD10±; rare Pan T +
- Absent CD5 and CD23 (rare CD21+)
- Proliferative rate: > 80% Ki67

Genotype

- *c-MYC* rearrangement and t(8;14) rare
- *BCL-2* rearranged in 30%
- Occasional EBV+

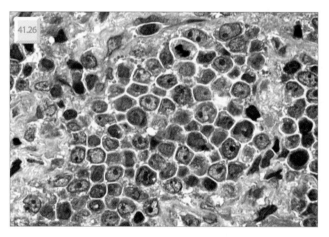

Shown in [41.25] is an example of the phenotype of a case. There is pan-B antigen expression, a high proliferative rate, and only a small number of

In the case of suspected Burkitt-like lymphoma shown in [41.29], one sees, on the left, the typical features in a touch preparation – basophilic cytoplasm, vacuoles, and a "starry sky" pattern. However, on the right, in the tissue section, there were coherent islands of cells which proved, following immunohistochemical labeling, to be a neuroendocrine carcinoma.

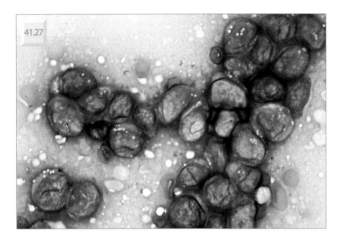

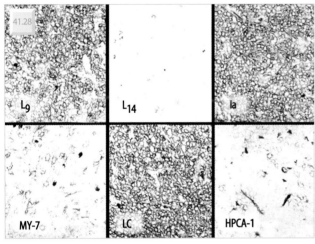

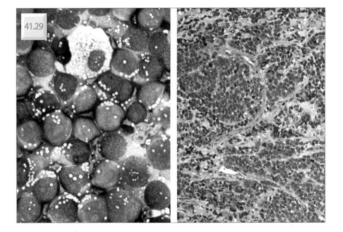

In summary, Burkitt-like lymphomas, as seen in this country, tend to recur in adults, and may be associated with HIV infiltration [41.30]. There was even an epidemic, described in the *Lancet*, in San Francisco in the early 1980s, in which there is a high incidence of jaw tumors.[2-4] Furthermore, some of the CNS tumors seen in immunodeficient patients are Burkitt-like. We see more nodal involvement in this entity than in Burkitt's lymphoma. Gut involvement occurs and it can complicate a follicular lymphoma. In children, it can be highly responsive as Burkitt's lymphoma would be, whereas in adults its response is more like that of a large cell lymphoma.

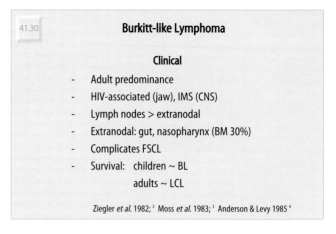

Burkitt-like Lymphoma

Clinical

- Adult predominance
- HIV-associated (jaw), IMS (CNS)
- Lymph nodes > extranodal
- Extranodal: gut, nasopharynx (BM 30%)
- Complicates FSCL
- Survival: children ~ BL
  adults ~ LCL

Ziegler *et al.* 1982;[2] Moss *et al.* 1983;[3] Anderson & Levy 1985[4]

Shown in [41.31] is an example of an HIV-associated Burkitt-like lymphoma, the most common lymphoma type complicating HIV infection.

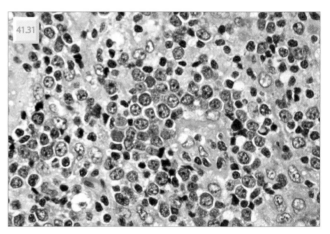

Presented in [41.32] are data from our SWOG studies showing survival in group category J, in which 98% of cases are Burkitt-like lymphomas. The response to therapy is essentially that of a large cell lymphoma.

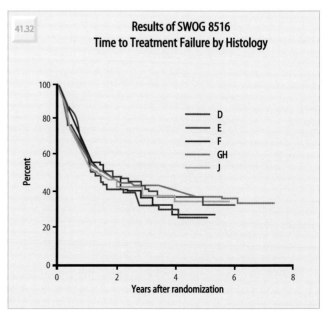

Results of SWOG 8516
Time to Treatment Failure by Histology

Compared in [41.33] are the features of the two disorders.

Finally, is Burkitt-like lymphoma an entity? In the author's view there is something very distinctive about this disorder, but we have yet to identify its defining characteristics. For the time being we will have to continue to use the name "Burkitt-like" - but maybe in a year or so we will know what accounts for its distinctive nature.

41.33	Burkitt's versus Burkitt-like Lymphoma		
	BURKITT'S		BURKITT-LIKE
	Endemic	Non-endemic	
Median age	7 years	30 years	55 years
M/F	2.5/1	2.5/1	2/1
EBV	95%	< 30%	Rare
Sites	Jaw, facial bones, ovary, testis, kidney, breast, CNS	Abdominal, jaw facial bones, testis, LN	LN, nasopharynx, GI, jaw
BM involvement	8%	10-30%	40%

REFERENCES

1. Yano T, van Krieken JH, Magrath IT, Longo DL, Jaffe ES, Raffeld M. Histogenetic correlations between subcategories of small non-cleaved cell lymphomas. *Blood* 1992; **79**: 1282-90.

2. Ziegler JL, Drew WL, Miner RC *et al*. Outbreak of Burkitt's lymphoma in homosexual men. *Lancet* 1982; **2**: 631-3.

3. Moss AR, Bacchetti P, Gorman M *et al*. AIDS in the "gay" areas of San Francisco [letter]. *Lancet* 1983; **1**: 923-4.

4. Anderson RE & Levy JA. Prevalence of antibodies to AIDS-associated retrovirus in single men in San Francisco. *Lancet* 1985; **1**: 217.

FURTHER READING

Garcia CF, Weiss LM, Warnke RA. Small noncleaved cell lymphoma: An immunophenotypic study of 18 cases and comparison with large cell lymphoma. *Hum Pathol* 1986; **17**: 454-61.

Grogan TM, Warnke RA, Kaplan HS. A comparative study of Burkitt's and non-Burkitt's "undifferentiated" malignant lymphoma: immunologic, cytochemical, ultrastructural, cytologic, histopathologic, clinical and cell culture features. *Cancer* 1982; **49**: 1817-28.

Hutchison RE, Murphy SB, Fairclough DL *et al*. Diffuse small non-cleaved cell lymphoma in children, Burkitt versus non-Burkitt types - results from the Pediatric Oncology Group and St. Jude Childrens Research Hospital. Cancer 1989; **64**: 23-7.

Magrath IT, Shiramizu B. Biology and treatment of small non-cleaved cell lymphoma. *Oncology* 1989; **3**: 41-53.

Neri A, Barriga F, Knowles DM, Magrath IT, Dalla-Favera R. Different regions of the immunoglobulin heavy-chain locus are involved in chromosomal translocations in distinct pathogenetic forms of Burkitt lymphoma. *Proc Natl Acad Sci USA* 1988; **85**: 2748-52.

Pelicci PG, Knowles DM, Magrath I, Dalla-Favera R. Chromosomal breakpoints and structural alterations of the c-myc locus differ in endemic and sporadic forms of Burkitt lymphoma. *Proc Natl Acad Sci USA* 1986; **83**: 2984-8.

Clinical aspects and treatment of Burkitt's and Burkitt-like lymphomas in children

42

H J Weinstein

This chapter is concerned with the current status of therapy for children suffering from Burkitt's, or small non-cleaved cell, lymphomas. An initial point to make is that, for protocol purposes, no differentiation is made between Burkitt-like lymphoma and Burkitt's lymphoma [42.1]. In children with small non-cleaved cell lymphomas, there does not appear to be a significant difference in immunophenotype or clinical presentation between the Burkitt's and Burkitt-like subgroups.

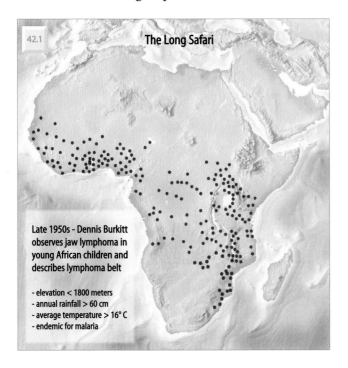

The Long Safari

Late 1950s - Dennis Burkitt observes jaw lymphoma in young African children and describes lymphoma belt

- elevation < 1800 meters
- annual rainfall > 60 cm
- average temperature > 16° C
- endemic for malaria

The unique staging system of non-Hodgkin's lymphoma that is uniformly accepted for the pediatric population is shown in [42.2]. Modifications from the Ann Arbor system are underlined. Patients with resected ileocecal tumors are classified as Stage II, and those with mediastinal disease or an unresectable abdominal mass as Stage III. If the bone marrow is involved but there are less than 25% blasts, the lymphoma is considered Stage IV. However, if there are more than 25% blasts in the bone marrow, a diagnosis is made of acute lymphoblastic leukemia, which is subcategorized into precursor B, precursor T or mature B (L3) subtypes. CNS lymphoma without bone marrow involvement is classified as Stage IV.

Pediatric NHL Staging System (St. Jude)

Stage	Features
I.	Single nodal or extranodal tumor
II.	Two nodal areas or extranodal tumors (same side of diaphragm)
	Resected ileocecal tumor
III.	Nodal or extranodal on both sides of diaphragm.
	Mediastinum
	Unresectable abdominal
IV.	Any of the above with:
	< 25% bone marrow blasts
	CNS positive

Burkitt's lymphoma accounts for 40% of childhood non-Hodgkin's lymphoma. Only 30% of these children have early stage disease (Stage I and II) [42.3]. The early stage patients have the same immunophenotype as the advanced stage cases [42.4]. The most common immunophenotype is CD10- and CD19-positive, associated with either kappa or lambda light chain expression.

Pediatric NHL Histology and Stage

	Stages I / II	Stages III / IV
Lymphoblastic (30%)	15%	85%
Burkitt's (40%)	30%	70%
Large cell (20%)	35%	65%

42.4	**Burkitt's or Small Non-cleaved Cell Lymphoma**	
	Stages I / II	Stages III / IV
Frequency	30%	70%
Immunophenotype	sIgM, CD19, 20, +/-10	same
Primary Sites	Waldeyer's ring cervical nodes, jaw, ileocecal	abdomen, ascites, kidney, ovary, bone, BM-20%, CNS-5 to 8%

The primary sites of disease in early stage patients include Waldeyer's ring, cervical nodes, jaws (similar to the presentation in endemic areas), and the ileocecal region. Patients with ileocecal Burkitt's lymphoma invariably present with intestinal obstruction or abdominal pain and usually have completely resectable disease. In contrast, patients with advanced stage abdominal disease most often present with a rapidly enlarging abdominal girth secondary to ascites. In addition to gastrointestinal tract tumors with extensive nodal disease, there is often diffuse renal enlargement, or multifocal nodules in the kidneys and ovarian involvement. The appendicular skeleton may be infiltrated by tumor, and about 20% of patients have bone marrow involvement. CNS disease is defined by either Burkitt cells in the CSF or a cranial nerve palsy, and occurs in about 5% to 8% of children.

To appreciate the treatment of Burkitt's lymphoma, it is necessary to go back to the early 1970s when a number of important principles were established by Drs Ziegler, McGrath and Burkitt [42.5].[1] These were, firstly, that cyclophosphamide, vincristine, and methotrexate are very active single agents. Secondly, controlled clinical trials showed that combination regimes were superior to single agent therapy.

42.5	**Protocols 74-0 and 75-6 for the treatment of American Burkitt's Lymphoma**		
Drug	Dose mg / m^2	Route	Schedule
Protocol 74-0			
Cyclophosphamide	1,000	IV	Day 1
Vincristine	1.4	IV	Day 1
Methotrexate	15	IT	Day 1, 4
Methotrexate	15	IV	Day 2, 3
Protocol 75-6			
Cyclophosphamide	1,000	IV	Day 1
Vincristine	1.4	IV	Day 1
Methotrexate	12.5	IV	Day 1, 3, 4
Methotrexate	12.5	IT	Day 2, 5
Prednisolone	1,000	IV	Day 1-5

In the early 1970s, Dr Ziegler studied two different cyclophosphamide/vincristine/methotrexate regimens in U.S. children with Burkitt's lymphoma.[2] In the upper left panel of [42.6], one sees the outcome after three cycles of chemotherapy by disease stage. Patients with Stage A (I) and B (II) disease or resected ileocecal disease (AR) had an 80% survival. These patients also received whole abdominal radiotherapy and CNS prophylaxis with intrathecal methotrexate. Patients with unresectable abdominal disease (C) had about a 40% long term survival. Almost no patients with either CNS or bone marrow involvement survived.

This short term chemotherapy regimen has become the cornerstone of therapy for early stage Burkitt's lymphoma.

About 10 years ago, the Pediatric Oncology Group began studying CHOP chemotherapy (cytoxan/vincristine/prednisolone/doxorubicin) for children with early stage non-Hodgkin's lymphoma of all histologies.[3] The subgroup of patients with Burkitt's or small non-cleaved cell lymphoma and large cell lymphoma had about a 90% survival after treatment with three cycles of CHOP chemotherapy [42.7].

The Pediatric Oncology Group completed several NHL studies over that decade [42.8]. In a prospectively controlled trial, there was no benefit when involved field radiotherapy was added to CHOP for any histologic type of non-Hodgkin's lymphoma. Nine weeks of chemotherapy was then compared with eight months of chemotherapy, and no difference in outcome was found for children with Burkitt's or large cell lymphoma.[4]

For patients with advanced stage Burkitt's lymphoma, a CHOP regimen or a Ziegler COMP regimen failed for patients with Stage IV disease and resulted in about 40% survival for patients with Stage III (C) disease. Chemotherapy protocols that were successful in treating acute lymphoblastic leukemia, such as LSA$_2$L$_2$ Sloan-Kettering regimen and the APO regimen used at the Dana-Farber Cancer Institute, included little or no cyclophosphamide and were not effective in advanced stage Burkitt's lymphoma [42.9].

However, regimens that included fractionated or single high dose cyclophosphamide, high dose methotrexate with cytosine arabinoside and aggressive intrathecal chemotherapy, increased event-free survival for children with Stage III and Stage IV Burkitt's lymphoma to 70-85%. These results were achieved with two to four months of

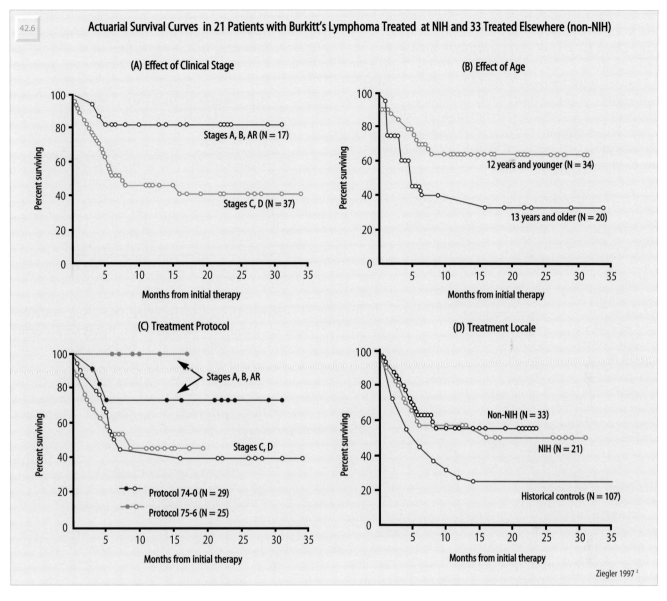

42.6 Actuarial Survival Curves in 21 Patients with Burkitt's Lymphoma Treated at NIH and 33 Treated Elsewhere (non-NIH)

(A) Effect of Clinical Stage

Stages A, B, AR (N = 17)

Stages C, D (N = 37)

(B) Effect of Age

12 years and younger (N = 34)

13 years and older (N = 20)

(C) Treatment Protocol

Stages A, B, AR

Stages C, D

Protocol 74-0 (N = 29)
Protocol 75-6 (N = 25)

(D) Treatment Locale

Non-NIH (N = 33)

NIH (N = 21)

Historical controls (N = 107)

Ziegler 1997 [2]

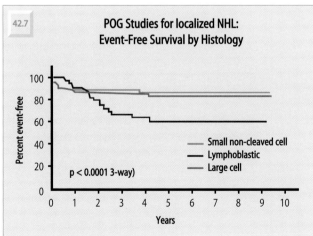

42.7 POG Studies for localized NHL: Event-Free Survival by Histology

Small non-cleaved cell
Lymphoblastic
Large cell

p < 0.0001 3-way)

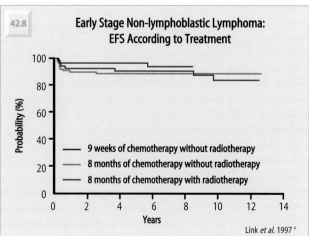

42.8 Early Stage Non-lymphoblastic Lymphoma: EFS According to Treatment

9 weeks of chemotherapy without radiotherapy
8 months of chemotherapy without radiotherapy
8 months of chemotherapy with radiotherapy

Link et al. 1997 [4]

therapy, and this approach is now uniformly accepted. I should point out that these protocols are based on three of the original drugs that were shown by Drs Ziegler, McGrath and Burkitt to be most active in the treatment of this disease.

Tumor lysis syndrome has always been a major issue in the treatment of Burkitt's lymphoma especially for children with advanced stage disease. The data in [42.10] were provided by Dr Schwenn of the Pediatric Oncology Group, who reviewed patient outcomes in terms of the frequency of tumor lysis syndrome and the need for dialysis. A number of patients, especially with Stage III and IV disease, underwent dialysis, but the majority of patients received induction chemotherapy without requiring dialysis. Patients with Stage III/IV Burkitt's are at particular risk for the tumor lysis syndrome because, in addition to their large tumour burden, they often have renal involvement or retroperitoneal, lymphadenopathy resulting in hydronephrosis.

Stages III / IV Burkitt's Lymphoma Treatment

42.9	Protocol	Signature	EFS
	LSA$_2$L$_2$	10 drug Cytoxan-day 1 only	29%
	APO	Doxorubicin / L-asp No cytoxan	< 10%
	St Jude Total B POG 8617 (4 months)	Fractionated cytoxan HDmtx and Ara-C IT ara-C / mtx	70-85%
	LMB-86	Fractionated cytoxan HDmtx, ara-C, VP16	80-90%

Tumor Lysis Syndrome - Incidence

42.10		Total number	Dialysis	Non-dialysis	Total TLS
	Stage III / IV NHL	81	13	10	23 (28%)
	B-ALL	17	1	1	2 (12%)
	Totals	98	14	11	25 (26%)

The most consistent prognostic factor in Burkitt's lymphoma [42.11] is Stage of disease, but, as already noted, patients with advanced stage disease are now enjoying survivals which approach those seen in patients with early stage disease. Serum LDH is also, with some therapy regimes, an independent prognostic variable. In some studies, CNS disease at diagnosis is an unfavorable prognostic indicator. In recent studies, time to complete remission has tended to correlate with overall survival - the faster remission is achieved, the longer it is likely to last.

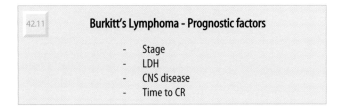

Burkitt's Lymphoma - Prognostic factors

- Stage
- LDH
- CNS disease
- Time to CR

Shown in [42.12] is a life table analysis of a Pediatric Oncology Group trial for Stage III small non-cleaved cell lymphomas. The regimen, that included fractionated cytoxan, high-dose methotrexate

with cytosine arabinoside, was superior to cytoxan and high-dose methotrexate. Very few relapses were observed after the first nine months of treatment.[5]

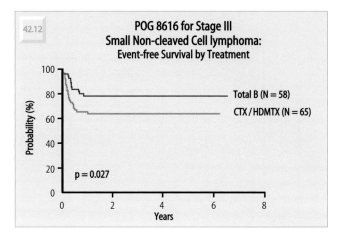

Presented in [42.13] is data from the Pediatric Oncology Group for patients with B cell, or L3, acute lymphoblastic leukemia. The two graphs show the clear improvement from the period 1981 to 1986, when long-term survival was less than 20%, to the subsequent period (1986-1991). This change directly reflects the introduction of Burkitt lymphoma treatment regimens.[6]

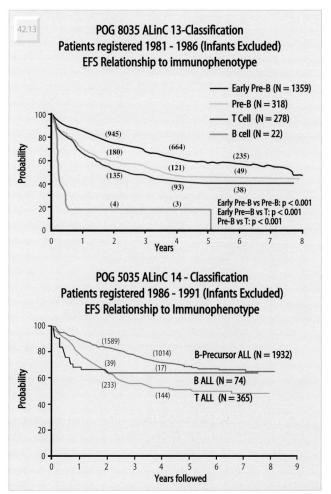

REFERENCES

1. Burkitt D. Long-term remissions following one and two-dose chemotherapy for African lymphoma. *Cancer* 1967; **20**: 756-9.

2. Ziegler JL. Treatment results of 54 American patients with Burkitt's lymphoma are similar to the African experience. *N Engl J Med* 1977; **297**: 75-80.

3. Link MP, Donaldson SS, Berard CW, Shuster JJ, Murphy SB. Results of treatment of childhood localized non-Hodgkin's lymphoma with combination chemotherapy with or without radiotherapy. *N Engl J Med* 1990; **322**: 1169-74.

4. Link MP, Shuster JJ, Donaldson SS, Berard CW, Murphy SB. Treatment of children and young adults with early-stage non-Hodgkin's lymphoma. *N Engl J Med* 1997; **337**: 1259-66.

5. Brecher ML, Schwenn MR, Coppes MJ *et al.* Fractionated cyclophosphamide and back to back high dose methotrexate and cytosine arabinoside improves outcome in patients with stage III high grade small non-cleaved cell lymphomas (SNCCL): a randomized trial of the Pediatric Oncology Group. *Med Pediatr Oncol* 1997; **29**: 526-33.

6. Bowman WP, Shuster JJ, Cook B *et al.* Improved survival for children with B-cell acute lymphoblastic leukemia and stage IV small noncleaved-cell lymphoma: a pediatric oncology group study. *J Clin Oncol* 1996; **14**: 1252-61.

Morphologic, immunologic and genetic features of precursor T and B cell neoplasms

D M Knowles

In the Rappaport classification lymphoblastic lymphoma was subdivided morphologically into convoluted and non-convoluted cell types [43.1]. In the Lukes-Collins classification, which was a combined morphologic and immunologic classification, it was subdivided into "convoluted", which was supposed to indicate a T cell origin, and "unclassified", which was supposed to correlate with a null cell phenotype.

43.1	Terminology of Lymphoblastic Lymphoma	
Classification system	**Terminology**
Rappaport	Lymphoblastic lymphoma Convoluted cell Non-convoluted cell
Lukes-Collins	Malignant lymphoma Convoluted Unclassified
Working Formulation	Lymphoblastic lymphoma Convoluted cell Non-convoluted cell
REAL	Precursor T lymphoblastic leukemia/lymphoma Precursor B lymphoblastic leukemia/lymphoma

These terms "convoluted" and "non-convoluted" were carried forward into the Working Formulation, but they do not appear in the REAL classification. There are several reasons for this. One is that we now know that "convoluted" and "non-convoluted" morphology does not correlate with phenotype. Furthermore, to the best of the author's knowledge, there is no correlation between convoluted or non-convoluted morphology and clinical features or prognosis.

Lymphoblastic neoplasms are of either precursor T or precursor B cell lineage, and can hence be objectively assigned to one or the other of these categories. There is evidence that precursor T cell neoplasms have different features from precursor B cell neoplasms, and this provides the justification for separating them. Lymphoblastic lymphoma and acute lymphoblastic leukemia have overlapping morphologic, clinical, cytogenetic and phenotypic features, which accounts for the use of the "leukemia/lymphoma" nomenclature.

What is the justification for distinguishing precursor lymphoblastic lymphoma/leukemia from other non-Hodgkin's lymphomas? The simple answer is that lymphoblastic lymphoma has a rather distinctive clinical presentation and course [43.2]. Lymphoblastic lymphoma is usually a disease of childhood and young adults. It comprises about one third or slightly more of childhood non-Hodgkin's lymphomas, but only about 5% or less of non-Hodgkin's lymphoma in adults. It tends to occur in the second and third decades of life, and in many series there is a marked male predominance. It usually presents with Stage III or IV (advanced) disease, and it has very distinctive patterns of presentation. About 75% of patients have bulky lymphadenopathy, which is above the diaphragm. It is often associated with a mediastinal mass, which can be very large, and patients sometimes present with acute respiratory distress.

43.2	Clinical Characteristics of Lymphoblastic Lymphoma	
Age:	Second and third decades (children > 10; adults < 30)
Sex:	Males predominate (2:1 to 10:1)
Stage:	Majority present with stage III or IV disease
Sites:	75% Supradiaphragmatic lymphadenopathy 67% Mediastinal mass 33% Peripheral blood and/or bone marrow 20% Central nervous system 5% Primarily osseous 5% Primarily cutaneous
B SX:	50%

About one third of patients at examination will have peripheral blood or bone marrow involvement, and this is one of the parameters for distinguishing lymphoblastic lymphoma from acute lymphoblastic leukemia. If one uses the St. Jude's criteria, the patients are classified as having acute lymphoblastic leukemia if more than 25% of the marrow cells are lymphoblasts. If the number is less than 25%, the disease is classified as a lymphoma.

This disease also has a tendency to involve the central nervous system, and there is a small subset of patients who have a primarily osseous or cutaneous presentation. A very high proportion of patients have B symptoms.

The natural history of lymphoblastic lymphoma is to develop a leukemic phase, and to spread widely throughout the body [43.3]. Patients tend to develop bone marrow replacement and involvement of the central nervous system and gonads. Therapy is also different in that these patients' lesions tend to respond better to protocols developed for acute lymphoblastic leukemia than to non-Hodgkin's lymphoma regimens.

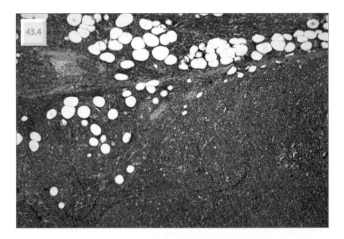

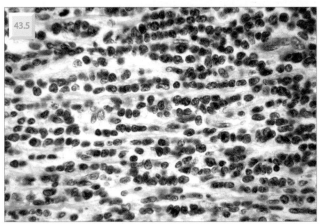

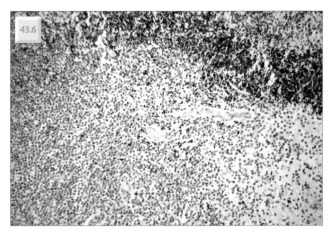

43.3	**Clinical Characteristics of Lymphoblastic Lymphoma**	
Natural HX:	Leukemic conversion	
	Bone marrow replacement	
	Spread to CNS	
	Spread to gonads	
Therapy:	Responds best to multi-drug	
	anti-ALL protocols	

Morphologically these are rather distinctive disorders. Shown in [43.4][1] is a precursor lymphoblastic lymphoma involving a lymph node, and what remains of the subcapsular sinus and capsule is still discernible. The neoplastic cells grow diffusely, not just within the lymph node, but also into the perinodal tissue, giving a broadly infiltrative appearance. The neoplasm tends to infiltrate rather than to destroy - and the cells often follow the path of least resistance, giving an "Indian file" pattern of progression between the collagen fibres [43.5].[1]

Often the cells show striking crush artefact, and this can pose a problem when only a very small tissue sample is available for diagnosis [43.6]. A similar artefact is also seen in tumors such as oat cell carcinomas and neuroendocrine carcinomas, so this feature of lymphoblastic lymphoma can cause practical problems.

At low power [43.7][1] one sees a starry sky pattern in about 25% of cases of lymphoblastic lymphoma, although it is usually not as prominent as in Burkitt's lymphoma.

The cell morphology in lymphoblastic lymphoma is quite different from that of other non-Hodgkin's lymphomas, but is indistinguishable from that of acute lymphoblastic leukemia [43.8]. About 85% of the acute lymphoblastic lymphomas will have a cytologic appearance that corresponds to the cells of L1 acute lymphoblastic leukemia in the FAB scheme, and the remainder correspond to the L2 acute lymphoblastic leukemia category. The neoplastic cells are generally small and rather monotonous. They do not have very much cytoplasm, and have a thin nuclear membrane. One sees cases in which the cells have a perfectly round appearance, and others in which the nuclear configuration is much more convoluted. However, an important feature is that the chromatin is very finely stippled and evenly dispersed. Nucleoli are inconspicuous.

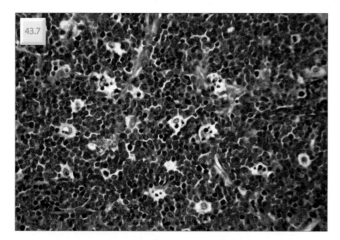

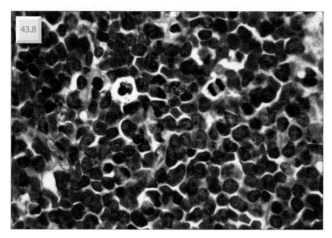

Phenotypically, these neoplasms are of either precursor T or precursor B type [43.9]. The important marker is terminal deoxynucleotide transferase (TdT), which is present in virtually every case. Precursor T cell lymphoblastic lymphoma, and also T cell acute lymphoblastic leukemia, express cytoplasmic CD3, and a variety of pan-T cell antigens, such as CD2, CD5 and CD7. They may or may not express CD4 and/or CD8.

In general, the various T cell phenotypes, which may be associated with different maturation stages, do not have clinical significance. This is not the case, however, for precursor B cell neoplasms [43.10]. Once again, all cases are TdT-positive. They may have an early pre-B cell phenotype, in which there is expression of class II HLA-DR, CDl9, CD22 and CD34. A subset of cases, known as common type ALL, expresses the common ALL antigen (CD10).

There is also a subtype that expresses cytoplasmic μ chain, so-called pre-B cell lymphoblastic neoplasms. Each of these subtypes tend to have distinct clinical courses.

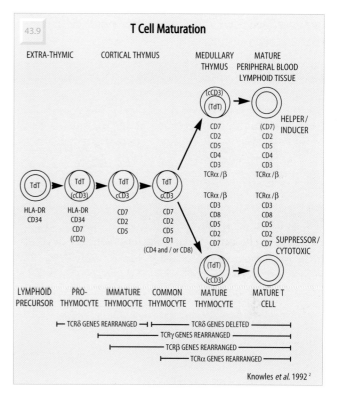

Knowles *et al.* 1992 [2]

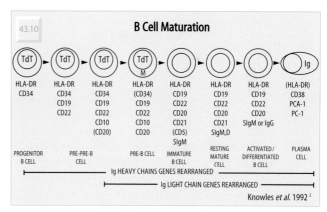

Knowles *et al.* 1992 [2]

TdT is an important diagnostic marker, and lymphoblastic lymphoma is the only non-Hodgkin's lymphoma that expresses this marker. Some acute leukemias which are not lymphoblastic express TdT, for example, mixed lineage leukemias and occasional acute myeloblastic leukemias, but among lymphoid proliferations TdT is specific for lymphoblastic tumors. TdT can be immunostained in cytospin preparations, or by flow cytometry or, as shown here, in [43.11], in tissue sections.

About 95% or more of precursor T cell lesions show rearrangements of T cell receptor β chain and γ chain genes, but there is a subset of cases which also have rearranged Ig heavy chain genes [43.12]. If one looks at the precursor B cell lesions, most have immunoglobulin heavy chain gene rearrangements, but again there is a subset that have clonal rearrangement of the T cell receptor genes. These cases, from the genetic point of view, are therefore promiscuous, and there are a fair number of cases that are bigenotypic.

suggestions in the literature that E rosette-negative (CD2-negative) precursor T cell lesions may have a worse prognosis. There is a subset, which is rare, of precursor T cell lesions which express antigens associated with NK cells, and these are said to have a worse prognosis.

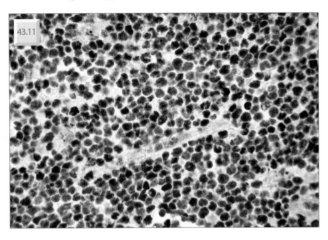

43.13	Clinical Characteristics of Lymphoblastic Lymphoma	
	Precursor T cell	**Precursor B cell**
	Children > 10; adults < 30	< 6; > 60
	M:F 10:1	M:F 1:1 - 2:1
	Stage III, IV	Stage I$_e$, III, IV
	Mediastinal mass	Skin (head & neck)
	Lymph nodes	Bony lytic lesion
	Leukemic conversion, spread to marrow, blood, CNS and gonads. Responds best to anti-all multi-drug therapy	
	Worse prognosis	Better prognosis

43.12	Antigen Receptor Gene Rearrangements in Precursor T- and B- Lymphoblastic Lymphoma	
Gene	**Precursor T cell**	**Precursor B cell**
IgH	20%	95%
Igk	rare	40%
Igl	rare	20%
TCRβ	> 90%	25%
TCRγ	> 90%	40%
TCRδ	> 95%	75%
TCRα	?	40%
		Medeiros *et al.* 1992[3]

43.14	Acute Lymphoblastic Leukemia Phenotypes Associated with Unfavorable Prognosis
	Precursor T cell
	E rosette negative pre-T
	Natural killer (CD16, CD57) positive
	Precursor B cell
	Pre-B cell - t(1;19)
	CD10 negative - t(4;11)
	CD34 negative
	CD24 negative
	CD13, CD33 positive

What is the justification for distinguishing subtypes of precursor lymphoblastic leukemia/lymphoma [43.13]? About 85 - 90% of precursor lymphoblastic lymphomas seen by the pathologist are of T cell type, so that most of the clinical features presented earlier correlate with this form of the disease. The precursor B lymphoblastic lymphomas tend to occur in slightly younger children or older adults, and the male predominance is not seen. A number of precursor B cell cases present with Stage I disease, for example with primarily osseous lesions, or, in children, with isolated skin lesions, usually involving the head and neck. However, in both precursor T and precursor B cell neoplasms there is the tendency to become leukemic, with spread to the marrow, central nervous system and gonads.

In general, the phenotypic features of precursor T cell neoplasms do not correlate, as already noted, with clinical outcome [43.14]. There have been some

Among the precursor B cell neoplasms, a number of antigens are said to relate to outcome. Those that have the pre-B cell phenotype, a CD10-negative phenotype (and these are associated with certain cytogenetic abnormalities), are CD24- or CD34-negative or express myeloid antigens have all been claimed to be associated with an unfavorable prognosis.

Numerous cytogenetic abnormalities have been found in association with precursor T cell lesions [43.15]. Many of these are translocations involving T cell receptor genes, but to the best of the author's knowledge none of these abnormalities is associated with a particularly unfavorable prognosis. However, in the precursor B cell neoplasms a few chromosomal abnormalities are associated with an unfavorable prognosis, for example the (9;22), (1;19) and (4;11) translocations.

In conclusion [43.16], lymphoblastic lymphoma displays very distinctive clinical, morphologic, immunologic and molecular characteristics. This justifies its recognition as a distinct entity, certainly distinct from other forms of non-Hodgkin's lymphoma.

43.15 Cytogenetic Abnormalities Associated with Unfavorable Prognosis in Precursor Lymphoblastic Leukemia /Lymphoma	
Precursor B cell	**Precursor T cell**
t(9;22) (q34;q11)	None
t(1;19) (q23;p13)	
t(4;11) (q21;q23)	

The clinical characteristics, the natural history, and the prognosis of precursor B cell and T cell lymphoblastic lymphoma/leukemia are sufficiently different to justify their recognition as distinct sub-categories. There are a variety of immunophenotypic

markers and karyotypic abnormalities which may yet prove to have prognostic implications and allow these cases to be subdivided in a clinically meaningful way in the future.

43.16 Conclusions
- Lymphoblastic lymphoma displays unique clinical, morphologic, immunologic and molecular characteristics that justify its recognition as a distinct entity.
- The clinical characteristics, natural history, and prognosis of precursor B and T cell lymphoblastic lymphoma are sufficiently distinctive to justify their recognition as distinct subcategories.
- Several immunophenotypic profiles and karyotypic abnormalities may have prognostic implications suggesting that the further subcategorization of precursor B and T cell lymphoblastic lymphoma may be justified.

ACKNOWLEDGEMENT

Figures [43.4], [43.5], [43,7], [43.8], [43,9] and [43.10] were reproduced from DM Knowles (ed) *Neoplastic Hematopathology*, 1992, with copyright permission from Williams and Wilkins.

REFERENCES

1. Knowles DM. Lymphoblastic lymphoma. In Knowles DM (ed). *Neoplastic Hematopathology*. Baltimore: Williams and Wilkins, 1992: 715-747.

2. Knowles DM, Chadburn A, Inghirami G. Immunophenotypic markers useful in the diagnosis and classification of hematopoietic neoplasms. In Knowles DM (ed). *Neoplastic Hematopathology*. Baltimore: Williams and Wilkins, 1992: 73-167.

3. Medeiros LJ, Bagg A, Cossman J. Application of molecular genetics to the diagnosis of hematopoietic neoplasms. In Knowles DM. *Neoplastic Hematopathology*. Baltimore: Williams and Wilkins, 1992: 263-298.

Treatment and prognostic factors in childhood precursor T and B cell neoplasms 44

H J Weinstein

Lymphoblastic lymphomas account for about 30% of childhood non-Hodgkin's lymphoma. Stage I and Stage II lymphoblastic lymphoma is a very rare entity, and most children have advanced stage disease, as evaluated by the St. Jude staging system [44.1].

44.1	Pediatric NHL Histology and Stage	
	Stages I / II	Stages III / IV
Lymphoblastic (30%)	15%	85%
Burkitt's (40%)	30%	70%
Large cell (20%)	35%	65%

Early stage patients differ in clinical presentation and immunophenotype from those with advanced disease [44.2]. Most patients with early stage lymphoblastic lymphoma have precursor B cell neoplasms, and the primary sites of disease include peripheral nodes, Waldeyer's ring, and occasionally, the skin and solitary bone lesions.

44.2	Lymphoblastic Lymphoma	
	Stages I / II	Stages III / IV
Distribution	15%	85%
Immunophenotype	Precursor B	Precursor T
Primary Sites	Peripheral nodal, Waldeyer's ring, cutaneous	Mediastinum nodal, bone, CNS (3%) BM (13%)

The majority of patients with advanced stage disease have precursor T cell neoplasms with mediastinal involvement. Other presentations include multifocal bone disease or peripheral nodal disease. About 13% of patients have 5 - 25% blasts in the marrow and therefore have Stage IV lymphoblastic lymphoma. A very small number of patients have clinically detectable central nervous system involvement at the time of diagnosis.

The Pediatric Oncology Group and the Children's Cancer Study Group have been investigating the use of either cytoxan/vincristine/methotrexate/prednisolone, or CHOP regimens for children with early stage non-Hodgkin's lymphoma. The outcome after three cycles of CHOP for small non-cleaved and large cell lymphoma is excellent, with event-free survival of about 90%.

In contrast, the event-free survival is 60-70% for children with lymphoblastic lymphoma on identical therapy [44.3]. A subsequent study showed that three cycles of CHOP (9 weeks) without continuation therapy (6-mercaptopurine and methotrexate) was inferior to the eight month treatment regime that included continuation therapy. However, the overall survival of these patients is excellent [44.4]. This reflects the high salvage rate after relapse using intensive multi-agent acute lymphoblastic leukemia protocols. The author's bias has been to recommend "standard or average risk" acute lymphoblastic leukemia therapy for these children, rather than CHOP, plus maintenance mercaptopurine and methotrexate.

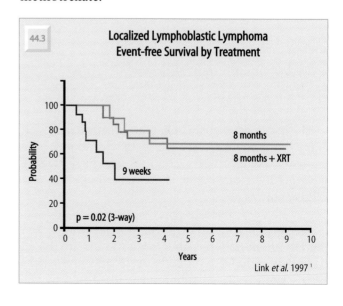

44.3 Localized Lymphoblastic Lymphoma Event-free Survival by Treatment

Link *et al.* 1997 [1]

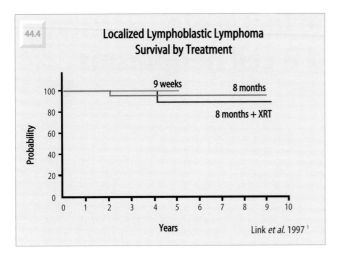

44.4 Localized Lymphoblastic Lymphoma Survival by Treatment

Link *et al.* 1997 [1]

presence of cytoplasmic immunoglobulin. In very young children with ALL, CALLA (CD10) is expressed in only about 50% of infants, whereas it is found in the majority of early pre-B cell leukemia patients aged more than 18 months. One sees a greater frequency of T cell precursor acute lympho-blastic leukemia in adolescents compared to younger children. B cell (FAB L3) acute lymphoblastic leukemia remains very rare, regardless of age.

44.6	Distinguishing ALL from NHL	
	Stage IV NHL	**ALL**
	Biopsy proven lymphoma and	
	1) 5 to 25 % BM blasts	> 25% BM blasts
	2) CSF blasts or cranial	
	nerve palsy	

For advanced stage lymphoblastic lymphoma, the use of multi-agent high risk acute lymphoblastic leukemia protocols has proven very successful. The four different regimens outlined in [44.5] result in event-free survivals ranging from 64% to almost 90%. One of the major lessons learned over the past two decades has been that antimetabolite-based therapy (6-mercaptopurine or methotrexate) is insufficient for these children and that drugs such as doxorubicin and L-asparaginase are very effective. The other important component of therapy is central nervous system prophylaxis. There is controversy as to whether intrathecal methotrexate alone is adequate in this high risk population. The current trend favors regimens that omit cranial irradiation but use intensive intrathecal therapy during induction and for extended periods during continuation therapy.

44.7	Immunophenotypes of ALL Distribution by Age		
Immunophenotype	**< 1.5 years**	**1.5 -10**	**>10**
Early Pre-B	64%	68%	58%
CALLA +	*(49%)*	*(94%)*	*(87%)*
Pre-B (cIg)	26%	18%	18%
T	6%	13%	23%
B	4%	1%	1%

Shown in [44.8] is a scheme from some years ago to show the classic "backbone" of therapy for child-hood acute lymphoblastic leukemia. Three drugs, vincristine, prednisolone, L-asparaginase, are used for induction, accompanied by central nervous system prophylaxis. Maintenance involves 6-mercaptopurine and methotrexate, with pulses of vincristine and prednisolone.

44.5	Stage III / IV Lymphoblastic Lymphoma Treatment	
Protocol	**Signature / CNS**	**5yr EFS**
LSA2L2	10-drug / IT mtx	64%
DFCI 81-87	Doxorubicin,	75%
	L-asparaginase,	
	cranial 18 Gy + IT	
BFM-NHL 86	Pre-induction	79%
	cranial 12 GY + IT	
POG 9296	Ara-C / cytoxan	88%
	ID mtx / IV 6MP TIT	

The remainder of this chapter is concerned with acute lymphoblastic leukemia in childhood. By current staging criteria, children are diagnosed as having ALL if more than 25% of the bone marrow cells are blasts [44.6].

Several immunophenotypes of ALL can be identified [44.7]. About 80% of patients have precursor B cell ALL, that includes both early pre-B and pre-B sub-type. The pre-B cell subgroup is identified by the

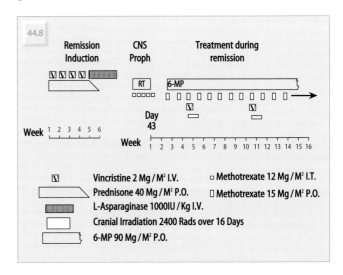

This core regimen is sufficient therapy for only a small subgroup of patients with acute lymphoblastic leukemia. As previously mentioned, an anti-metabolite based maintenance regimen for T precursor is insufficient, and would result in a survival of less than 20%. However, about 10% of children with precursor B acute lymphoblastic leukemia would have a 90% cure rate with such a regimen. This very favorable group includes children who are between 1 and 9 years of age with a WBC of less than 50,000/ml and hyperdiploid blasts. However, the vast majority of patients with precursor B ALL need more intensive chemotherapy.

Shown in [44.9] are two examples of more intensive treatment protocols. One is from the Dana-Farber Cancer Institute/Children's Hospital and the other is from the German BFM group. One common theme in these protocols is the use of multiple drugs during induction. It is clear that the "road to remission" predicts long-term survival - the quicker leukemic cells are killed in the initial stages of therapy, the better the long-term survival. For this reason, multi-agent induction is currently used in all protocols for children with higher risk acute leukemia.

44.9	Acute Lymphoblastic Leukemia - Treatment	
Protocol	Unique features / CNS	5-year EFS
DFCI 81-87	5-drug induction. L-asparaginase doxorubicin (HR) IT mtx (SR) cranial 18 Gy + IT	SR-85% HR-70% T-75%
ALL BFM-86	8-drug induction. Re-induction IT mtx (SR) cranial 12-18 Gy + IT for HR	SR-87% HR-70% T-73%
	Reiter et al. 1994;[2] Schorin et al. 1994[3]	

The Dana-Farber protocols have featured L-asparaginase and doxorubicin, whereas the German BFM studies feature re-induction and intensification therapy shortly after inducing remission. All patients receive intrathecal methotrexate for CNS prophylaxis, but those with higher risk features also receive cranial irradiation. The five year event-free survival (which in the pediatric population is not very different from the 10 and 15 year figures) is 85% for standard risk patients. For high risk patients, including those with T cell ALL, the cure rate is 70%.[4]

Many prognostic variables have been identified for children with ALL [44.10]. The most powerful prognostic factors that have withstood the test of time are age and white blood cell count - age between one and nine is favorable, as is a white count of less than 50,000/ml. The next most important risk factor is the DNA index. Acute lymphoblastic leukemia patients with hyperdiploid cells (greater than 50 chromosomes per cell) have a very favorable prognosis. However, most of the patients in this group also have a good prognosis based on age and white blood cell count. Trisomies for chromosomes 4 and 10 are very favorable findings and are also associated with a DNA index greater than 1.6, and favorable age and white count parameters. T cell phenotype has long been recognized as an adverse variable, but it is correlated with unfavorable age and white count, so it remains unclear if it has independent prognostic significance.

44.10	ALL Prognostic Variables	
Favorable		Unfavorable
Age 1-9 years WBC<50,000 / ml DNA index >1.16 Trisomy for chromosomes 4, 10 TEL / AML1 fusion		t(9;22), t(4;11) Slow response to therapy CNS-3, ?CNS-2 ? T cell Black race L2 morphology
		Smith et al. 1996 [5]

The presence of the Philadelphia chromosome or the (4;11) translocation (causing rearrangement of the MLL gene) are independent adverse prognostic variables. Slow response to therapy, as measured by day 8 response to prednisolone in BFM studies or the day 14 bone marrow response, is also an adverse prognostic indicator.

There has recently been a re-classification of CNS disease. The standard definition of CNS leukemia is based both on CSF WBC (> five white cells) plus blasts. The new classification includes leukemic blasts independent of the cell count in the CSF. The prognostic significance of having fewer than five white cells but with definite CSF blasts remains controversial.

A number of chromosome rearrangements involving the core binding transcription factor (CBF) complex have been identified in both AML and ALL [44.11]. In ALL a small number of patients have a translocation involving chromosomes 12 and 21, in which the breakpoints involve the TEL gene, an ets-like transcription factor on chromosome 12, and the AML1 gene on chromosome 21.[6] The latter gene is also involved in AML. The t(12;21), resulting in the TEL-AML1 fusion, accounts for only 1% of the cytogenetically detected chromosome abnormalities in ALL. However, RT-PCR analysis has shown that it is found in 25-30% of cases of precursor B acute lymphoblastic leukemia. Drs. Golub and Gilliland have shown that the *TEL-AML1* fusion is an independent favorable prognostic factor in ALL [44.12]. These data are of interest because they indicate how molecular probes will redefine prognostic factors in the not too distant future.

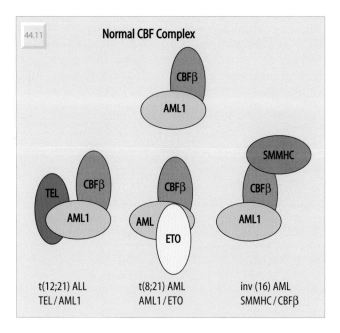

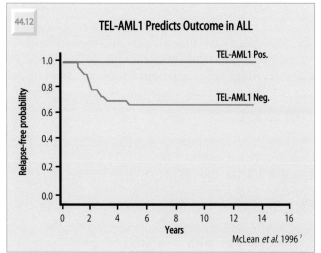

This review will be concluded with comments on the role of bone marrow transplantation in childhood acute lymphoblastic leukemia [44.13]. It is seldom used in first remission, but most pediatric oncologists would agree that allogeneic marrow transplantation is a reasonable experimental option

for a child with either the t(9;22) or t(4;11) translocations. In contrast, transplantation is not justifiable for children simply on the basis of high white count or a slow induction response, because of the relatively favorable results achieved with chemotherapy. There are preliminary data to suggest that allogeneic transplantation for children with the (9;22) translocation offers a better survival than does intensive chemotherapy. The role of marrow transplantation in ALL is mainly limited to second or subsequent remission.

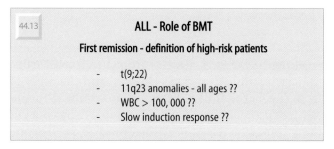

If one compares allogeneic bone marrow transplantation from an HLA-matched sibling in second remission with chemotherapy, the most important prognostic factor for either treatment is the duration of the first remission. When first remissions are less than 24 months, bone marrow transplantation in three studies outlined in [44.14] was superior to chemotherapy. If the first remission was greater than 24 months, bone marrow transplantation was also superior to chemotherapy in two of the three studies. The trend is therefore to recommend an allogeneic marrow transplant for a child with acute lymphoblastic leukemia in second remission. The use of unrelated bone marrow donors is becoming more successful in this setting.[8] The role of autologous transplantation is yet to be defined and requires further evaluation. For children with ALL in second remission who have had a very long first remission (e.g. three to four years), chemotherapy alone is a reasonable option.

44.14	**ALL in 2nd Remission**			
Allogeneic BMT vs Chemotherapy				
Study	"Short" 1st CR BMT	chemo	"Long" 1st CR BMT	chemo
GITMO:AIEOP	33%	16%	55%	40%
BFM;CoALL	56%	22%	47%	52%
IBMTR;POG	35%	10%	53%	32%
				Barrett *et al.* 1994 [9]

REFERENCES

1. Link MP, Shuster JJ, Donaldson SS, Berard CW, Murphy SB. Treatment of children and young adults with early-stage non-Hodgkin's lymphoma. *N Engl J Med* 1997; **337**: 1259-66.

2. Reiter A, Schrappe M, Ludwig WD *et al*. Chemotherapy in 998 unselected childhood acute lymphoblastic leukemia patients. Results and conclusions of the multicenter trial ALL-BFM 86. *Blood* 1994; **84**: 3122-33.

3. Schorin MA, Blattner S, Gelber RD *et al*. Treatment of childhood acute lymphoblastic leukemia: results of Dana-Farber Cancer Institute/Children's Hospital Acute Lymphoblastic Leukemia Consortium Protocol 85-01. *J Clin Oncol* 1994; **12**: 740-7.

4. Niemeyer CM, Gelber RD, Tarbell NJ *et al*. Low-dose versus high-dose methotrexate during remission induction in childhood acute lymphoblastic leukemia (Protocol 81-01 update). *Blood* 1991; **78**: 2514-9.

5. Smith M, Arthur D, Camitta B *et al*. Uniform approach to risk classification and treatment assignment for children with acute lymphoblastic leukemia. *J Clin Oncol* 1996; **14**: 18-24.

6. Golub TR, Barker GF, Bohlander SK *et al*. Fusion of the TEL gene on 12p13 to the AML1 gene on 21q22 in acute lymphoblastic leukemia. *Proc Natl Acad Sci USA* 1995; **92**: 4917-21.

7. McLean TW, Ringold S, Neuberg D *et al*. TEL/AML-1 dimerizes and is associated with a favorable outcome in childhood acute lymphoblastic leukemia. *Blood* 1996; **88**: 4252-8.

8. Hongeng S, Krance RA, Bowman LC *et al*. Outcomes of transplantation with matched-sibling and unrelated-donor bone marrow in children with leukaemia. *Lancet* 1997; **350**: 767-71.

9. Barrett AJ, Horowitz MM, Pollock BH *et al*. Bone marrow transplants from HLA-identical siblings as compared with chemotherapy for children with acute lymphoblastic leukemia in a second remission. *N Engl J Med* 1994; **331**: 1253-8.

Treatment and prognostic factors in adult precursor T and B cell neoplasms

C N Coleman

This chapter reviews precursor B and T cell neoplasms in the adult [45.1]. One problem when considering these diseases in adults is that there are not as much data available as for pediatric disorders, and most therapeutic results are from single arm studies. The approach has generally been similar to that used for pediatric patients, but there are fewer results from randomized trials. Essentially the regimens are similar to those used for acute lymphoblastic leukemia in children, but the major questions for adult cases are, firstly, whether treatment should take prognostic factors into account, and, secondly, whether bone marrow transplantation has a role to play in primary treatment.

> **45.1 Precursor B and T Cell Neoplasms in Adults: Lymphoblastic Lymphoma**
>
> Most results from single arm studies
>
> Approach similar to pediatric patients
>
> - more randomized studies available
>
> Regimens similar to ALL
>
> - ? treat by prognostic factors

If the topic is considered from a historic viewpoint, it is evident this is one of the entities that benefited dramatically from pathologic classification [45.2]. Before 1975 there was an entity with a very poor prognosis called "Sternberg sarcoma" or "mediastinal diffuse lymphocytic lymphoma". Patients were treated with pulsed chemotherapy, had transient responses and tended to relapse at many sites.

Barcos and Lukes categorized this as a malignant lymphoma of convoluted lymphocytes.[1] In 1976 Nathwani et al. then described what they called "lymphoblastic lymphoma",[2] and in 1981 published the first paper describing this clinicopathologic entity in 95 adult patients.[3] A paper by Rosen et al. in 1978 also described "convoluted lymphocytic lymphoma" in adults.[4] This disease was therefore only recognized as a separate entity about 20 years ago.

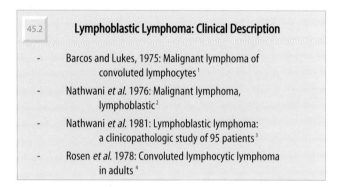

> **45.2 Lymphoblastic Lymphoma: Clinical Description**
>
> - Barcos and Lukes, 1975: Malignant lymphoma of convoluted lymphocytes[1]
> - Nathwani et al. 1976: Malignant lymphoma, lymphoblastic[2]
> - Nathwani et al. 1981: Lymphoblastic lymphoma: a clinicopathologic study of 95 patients[3]
> - Rosen et al. 1978: Convoluted lymphocytic lymphoma in adults[4]

The treatment used for this disorder evolved from pulsed CHOP towards lymphoma/leukemia-like protocols.[5] The first protocols for adults were developed in collaboration with Drs. Cohen and Bertino at Stanford, and they followed to some extent Dr. Weinstein's APO protocol. They used CHOP-like drugs, although in much more intensive regimens, consolidated with intrathecal high dose methotrexate [45.3]. There was then some brief reinforcement, and the total period of therapy lasted about one year.

This protocol was started at a time when median survivals were about three to six months, and showed for the first time that lymphoblastic lymphoma in adults was a curable entity. Total treatment "Therapy" lasted one year. The freedom from relapse and survival rates from this protocol were close to what they are today, at about 50% [45.4]. Not entirely surprisingly, what emerged from these studies, and from pediatric data as well, is that CNS relapse was frequent and rapid, and that prophylaxis against this complication was ineffective if it was delayed by even a few months.

What evolved as a result was a more intensive protocol [45.5]. The chemotherapy is basically modified CHOP therapy, but in this regimen CNS

45.3 Stanford University Hospital Original Lymphoblastic Lymphoma Protocol

	Induction	CNS prophylaxis x 5 weeks	Consolidation	Maintenance
Week	1 2 3 4 5 6 7	8 9 10 11 12 13	14 15 16 17 18 19 20	21 22 23 to 52
Cyclophosphamide 400 mg/m² orally x 4 d	x x x		x x x	
Doxorubicin 50 mg/m² IV	x x x		x x x	
Vincristine 2 mg IV	x x x x x x		x x x	
Prednisone 40 mg/m² d orally	Daily Taper		5d 5d 5d	
		Each week 1 2 3 4 5 6 7		
L-asparaginase 6,000 U/m² IM		x		
Methotrexate 12 mg IT		x		
Methotrexate 1 g/m² IV		x		
Leucovorin 25 mg/ m² every 6 hrs orally		x x x		
6-Mercaptopurine 75 mg/m² orally				daily
Methotrexate 30 mg/m² orally				weekly

Coleman et al. 1986 [6]

prophylaxis was used earlier. Again total therapy lasted about a year, with about six or seven months of intensive treatment.

With this regime survival rates were about 60-70%. Response rates were very high, at about 95% complete responses, and what emerged as a major prognostic factor was bulk of disease [45.6]. Patients with advanced stage disease, associated with LDH levels more than one and a half times normal, did worse in terms of survival and freedom from relapse.

About two thirds of the patients fell into the high risk group when analyzed in terms of bulk of disease [45.7]. The one third in the low risk category did surprisingly well with a regimen which was a very modest one by leukemia standards, requiring only a year of therapy. However, the high risk group did poorly. Unfortunately, the Northern California Oncology Group, which performed this study, is no longer funded, so no long-term follow-up of this patient population is available. However, the median follow-up was about three or four years, so that these curves are probably representative for low and high risk groups.

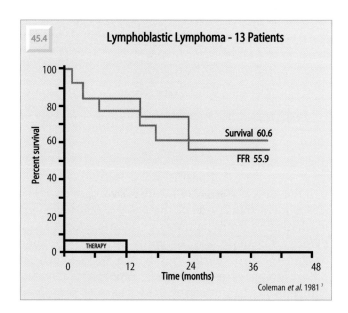

45.4 Lymphoblastic Lymphoma - 13 Patients

Coleman et al. 1981 [7]

The third protocol [45.8] is a very complicated regime which was developed in collaboration with a hematologist, Dr. Picozzi.[5] We used a very intensive induction protocol, with CHOP, VM26/cytosine arabinoside for the high risk groups, and the less intense regimen of Protocol 2 for the low risk group.

45.5

LBL - Stanford /NCOG Protocol

Week	Induction				CNS prophylaxis					Consolidation														Maintenance
	1	2	3	4	5	6	7	8	9	10	11	12	13	14	15	16	17	18	19	20	21	22	23 to 52
Cyclophosphamide 400 mg/m² x 3 d orally	x		x						x			x			x			x					
Doxorubicin 50 mg/m² IV	x		x						x			x			x			x					
Vincristine 2 mg/m² IV	x	x	x	x	x		x		x			x			x			x					
Prednisone 40 mg/m² orally	Daily				Taper				5d			5d			5d			5d					
L-asparaginase 6,000 U/m² IM (max > 10,000 U)			5 doses																				
Methotrexate 12 mg IT			x		5 doses																		
Whole brain XRT					2,400 rad in 12 fractions																		
6-Mercaptopurine 75 mg/m² orally																					daily		
Methotrexate 30 mg/m² orally																					weekly		

Coleman *et al.* 1986; [6] Picozzi and Coleman 1990 [5]

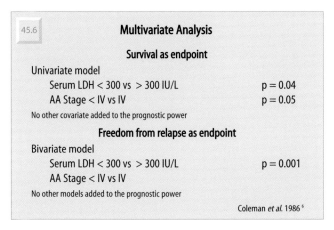

45.6

Multivariate Analysis

Survival as endpoint

Univariate model
  Serum LDH < 300 vs > 300 IU/L   p = 0.04
  AA Stage < IV vs IV   p = 0.05
No other covariate added to the prognostic power

Freedom from relapse as endpoint

Bivariate model
  Serum LDH < 300 vs > 300 IU/L   p = 0.001
  AA Stage < IV vs IV
No other models added to the prognostic power

Coleman *et al.* 1986 [6]

One of the unfortunate points in relation to lymphoblastic lymphoma therapy is that an attempt by the NCI to put together a nation-wide lymphoblastic lymphoma study group never came to fruition. Because of this, many patients today get treated with acute lymphoblastic leukemia protocols without any attempt to study this rare disease in the concerted way that co-operative groups can achieve.

Studies from France have analyzed clinical prognostic factors [45.9].[8] Most patients had a mediastinal mass, and a fair number were leukemic and many were of T cell type. They were treated with either CHOP or intensive acute lymphoblastic leukemia-like regimens. There was a high complete remission at about 80%, and the duration of remission was good for those who achieved it. Overall survival was about 50%.

The influence of prognostic factors was similar to that seen in the NCOG Stanford population [45.10]. Elevated LDH was associated with a poorer complete remission rate and survival, as was advanced stage and multiple site disease. It thus emerged that, as the lymphoma progressed into a leukemia, patients needed more leukemia-like therapies.

Some of the better studies come from pediatric experience. In a study comparing LSA_2-L_2 versus ADCOMP [45.11], the event-free survival for localized

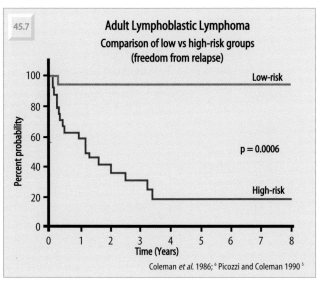

45.7

Adult Lymphoblastic Lymphoma

Comparison of low vs high-risk groups (freedom from relapse)

p = 0.0006

Low-risk

High-risk

Percent probability / Time (Years)

Coleman *et al.* 1986; [6] Picozzi and Coleman 1990 [5]

45.8 LBL Schema for High-risk Patients

Agent	Induction 1	2	3	4	5	CNS prophylaxis 6	7	8	9	Consolidation 10	11	12	13	14	15-26	Maintenance 27-104
Cyclophosphamide 400 mg/m² x 3 d IV	x		x									x				
Doxorubicin 50 mg/m² IV	x		x									x				
Vincristine 1.5 mg/m² IV (max 2 mg)	x	x	x	x	x	x						x	x			
Prednisone 60 mg/m² D PO	Daily	Taper														
L-asparaginase 6,000 U/m² IM (max > 10,000 U)	MWF xxx	MWF xxx	MWF xxx	MWF xxx		MW xx						MWF xxx	MW xx			
Methotrexate 12 mg IT	x			x	x	x	x	x							Repeat weeks x 2 9-14	
Whole brain XRT						2,400 rad in 12 fractions										
Cytarabine 300 mg/m² IV						MWF xxx										
VM-26, 165 mg/m² IV						xxx	F									
Methotrexate 200 mg/m² IV										x						
Leucovorin 10 mg/m² PO q6h x 6 doses										x						
Trimethoprimsulfamethoxazole 1DS bid		––														
Ketoconazole 200 mg PO qd																
Methotrexate 30 mg/m² PO																weekly
6-Mercaptopurine 75 mg/m² PO																daily

Picozzi and Coleman 1990 [5]

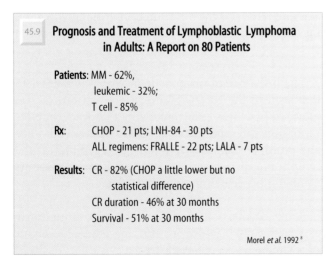

45.9 Prognosis and Treatment of Lymphoblastic Lymphoma in Adults: A Report on 80 Patients

Patients: MM - 62%,
leukemic - 32%;
T cell - 85%

Rx: CHOP - 21 pts; LNH-84 - 30 pts
ALL regimens: FRALLE - 22 pts; LALA - 7 pts

Results: CR - 82% (CHOP a little lower but no
statistical difference)
CR duration - 46% at 30 months
Survival - 51% at 30 months

Morel et al. 1992 [8]

45.10 Prognosis and Treatment of Lymphoblastic Lymphoma in Adults: A Report on 80 Patients

Characteristic	CR rate%	CR duration % at 2 years	Survival
Age < 40	94*	51*	68
≥ 40	55	30	35
LDH ≤ 2 x Normal	92	NA	73
> 2 x Normal	57		40
AA Stage I-III	92	45	73
Stage IV	78	48	54
No. of E sites 0-1	92	50	68
2 or more	72	44	51

Prognostic factors (* denotes p < 0.050)

Morel et al. 1992 [8]

disease was about 84%, but for disseminated disease it was about 67%.[9] Since the majority of patients were in the latter group, about 70% of these patients seemed to be curable. This is consistent with the literature, where we find fairly high overall response rates and overall survivals of about 50-60%.

first complete remission had a 70% overall survival and progression-free survival [45.14]. Bone marrow transplantation clearly seems to be necessary for patients who relapse, but the question is whether current intensive therapy regimens would give similar results. This question is still unanswered.

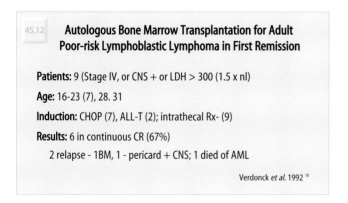

Summary of Results
Pediatrics, LBL: randomized trial: LSA$_2$-L$_2$ vs ADCOMP

RFS at 5 years

Localized (10% of patients) - 84%
Disseminated - 67%
BM neg. - 70%
BM pos. - 46%

Regimen	Evaluable patients	Complete response	Frequency of relapse	Overall survival rate
L2 or L10 or L10M or L17 or L17M	51	40 (78%)	25%	45% (5 year)
CHOP + L-asparaginase + methotrexate	44	42 (95%)	44%	56% (5 year)
Variable	34	28 (74%)	60%	22% (5 year)
CHOP	25	11 (44%)	-	30% (3 year)
APO	21	20 (95%)	42%	-
Mod. LSA$_2$-L$_2$	15	11 (73%)	36%	42% (4 year)
(CHOP 8 or CVP) + XRT	15	7 (47%)	-	-
(Bone marrow - negative) COOP/6-MP/Methotrexate	13	8 (62%)	-	-

Tubergen et al. 1995 [9]

The question which then arises concerns the role of bone marrow transplantation, and in the author's opinion this it still unanswered. Some of the first reports showed that in high risk patients in first remission about two thirds could achieve a sustained continuous complete remission, which was better than historic data [45.12].[10]

Autologous Bone Marrow Transplantation for Adult Poor-risk Lymphoblastic Lymphoma in First Remission

Patients: 9 (Stage IV, or CNS + or LDH > 300 (1.5 x nl)

Age: 16-23 (7), 28. 31

Induction: CHOP (7), ALL-T (2); intrathecal Rx- (9)

Results: 6 in continuous CR (67%)

2 relapse - 1BM, 1 - pericard + CNS; 1 died of AML

Verdonck et al. 1992 [10]

The European Transplant Group has reported on a very similar population treated with standard induction therapies, analyzing the benefit of bone marrow transplantation [45.13].[11] Patients transplanted during

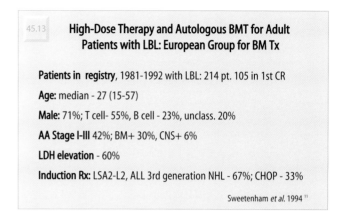

High-Dose Therapy and Autologous BMT for Adult Patients with LBL: European Group for BM Tx

Patients in registry, 1981-1992 with LBL: 214 pt. 105 in 1st CR

Age: median - 27 (15-57)

Male: 71%; T cell- 55%, B cell - 23%, unclass. 20%

AA Stage I-III 42%; BM+ 30%, CNS+ 6%

LDH elevation - 60%

Induction Rx: LSA2-L2, ALL 3rd generation NHL - 67%; CHOP - 33%

Sweetenham et al. 1994 [11]

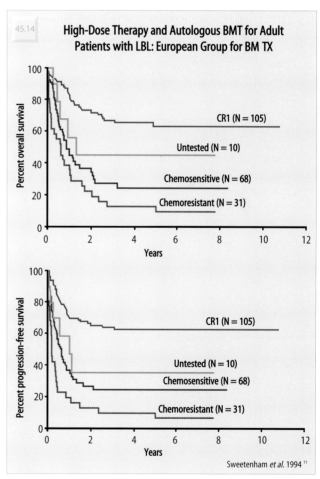

High-Dose Therapy and Autologous BMT for Adult Patients with LBL: European Group for BM TX

Sweetenham et al. 1994 [11]

The important prognostic factors are therefore age, bulk of disease, and advanced stage of disease, and these prompt the use of aggressive leukemia-like regimens [45.15]. Early data suggest that regimens using cyclophosphamide may give better results than those without this agent. Whether or not one should use a less intensive regimen for patients who have a true lymphoma, i.e. who are not leukemic, is unanswered. However, it is suggested that one may not need to use the very intensive treatment required for acute lymphoblastic leukemia. The role of bone marrow transplant during first complete remission is also unknown. The results that have been published are certainly better than those obtained with the old regimens, but more data are needed from very intensive induction chemotherapy regimens.

Bone marrow transplant is necessary in relapse, because conventional chemotherapy does not yield good results. CNS prophylaxis is used for all patients, but again it may be that more favorable risk patients need less of this treatment, and it is difficult to obtain good data on this because of the small patient numbers. Some groups have used involved field radiotherapy in slow responders to bring them into remission, but this is probably not useful, or at least not as a routine part of treatment.

Finally, what recent progress can we identify in this field [45.16]? The term "lymphoblastic lymphoma" has now progressed to "precursor T or B neoplasms". The treatment has progressed from lymphoma-like pulsed treatment to leukemia-like treatment. However, no single regimen is clearly superior. And the role of bone marrow transplantation in first complete remission, like the lymphocytes, remains "convoluted"!

45.15 **Treatment of Lymphoblastic Lymphoma in Adults**

Prognostic factors:

Advanced age, bulky disease, elevated LDH (> 1.5 - 2 x nl),

Advanced stage (BM, CNS), multiple E sites

Treatment:

- Aggressive anti-leukemia regimens,
    cyclophosphamide may be important

- More intensive for advanced disease (adverse Px factors)

- Role of BMT in CR 1 unknown

- BMT necessary for relapse

- CNS prophylaxis - unknown for "favorable" patients

- IF RT - possible for consolidation of slow responders
    not necessary as a routine except if used with CNS
    prophylaxis

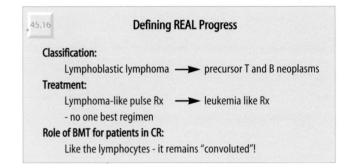

45.16 **Defining REAL Progress**

Classification:

Lymphoblastic lymphoma ➝ precursor T and B neoplasms

Treatment:

Lymphoma-like pulse Rx ➝ leukemia like Rx
- no one best regimen

Role of BMT for patients in CR:

Like the lymphocytes - it remains "convoluted"!

ACKNOWLEDGEMENTS

The following figures are reproduced by copyright permission of W.B. Saunders:
[45.3], [45.5], [45.6], [45.7] - reproduced from the *J Clin Oncol* 1986; **4**: 1628-37.
[45.4] - reproduced from *Blood* 1981; **57**: 679-684.
[45.8] - reproduced from *Semin Oncol* 1990; **17**: 96-103.
[45.9] and [45.10] - reproduced from *J Clin Oncol* 1992; **10**: 1078-85.
[45.13] and [45.14] - reproduced from *J Clin Oncol* 1994; **12**: 1358-65.

REFERENCES

1. Barcos MP, Lukes RJ. Malignant lymphoma of convoluted lymphocytes: a new entity of possible T-cell type. In: Sinks LF, Godden JO (eds). *Conflicts in childhood cancer: an evaluation of current management.* New York: Liss, 1975: 147-78.

2. Nathwani BN, Kim H, Rappaport H. Malignant lymphoma, lymphoblastic. *Cancer* 1976; **38**: 964-83.

3. Nathwani BN, Diamond LW, Winberg CD *et al.* Lymphoblastic lymphoma: a clinicopathologic study of 95 patients. *Cancer* 1981; **48**: 2347-57.

4. Rosen PJ, Feinstein DI, Pattengale PK *et al.* Convoluted lymphocytic lymphoma in adults: a clinicopathologic entity. *Ann Intern Med* 1978; **89**: 319-24.

5. Picozzi VJ Jr, Coleman CN. Lymphoblastic lymphoma. *Semin Oncol* 1990; **17**: 96-103.

6. Coleman CN, Picozzi VJ Jr, Cox RS *et al.* Treatment of lymphoblastic lymphoma in adults. *J Clin Oncol* 1986; **4**: 1628-37.

7. Coleman CN, Cohen JR, Burke JS, Rosenberg SA. Lymphoblastic lymphoma in adults: results of a pilot protocol. *Blood* 1981; **57**: 679-84.

8. Morel P, Lepage E, Brice P *et al.* Prognosis and treatment of lymphoblastic lymphoma in adults: a report on 80 patients. *J Clin Oncol* 1992; **10**: 1078-85.

9. Tubergen DG, Krailo MD, Meadows AT *et al.* Comparison of treatment regimens for pediatric lymphoblastic non-Hodgkin's lymphoma: a Childrens Cancer Group study. *J Clin Oncol* 1995; **13**: 1368-76.

10. Verdonck LF, Dekker AW, de Gast GC, Lokhorst HM, Nieuwenhuis HK. Autologous bone marrow transplantation for adult poor-risk lymphoblastic lymphoma in first remission. *J Clin Oncol* 1992; **10**: 644-6.

11. Sweetenham JW, Liberti G, Pearce R, Taghipour G, Santini G, Goldstone AH. High-dose therapy and autologous bone marrow transplantation for adult patients with lymphoblastic lymphoma: results of the European Group for Bone Marrow Transplantation. *J Clin Oncol* 1994; **12**: 1358-65.

Morphologic, immunologic and genetic features of lymphocyte predominance Hodgkin's disease

P M Banks

The main features of lymphocyte predominance Hodgkin's disease [46.1] are now well recognized. However, although most pathologists have a clear idea of the nature of Hodgkin's disease, it is a difficult concept to communicate to a non-medically qualified person. The only simple definition is the rather vague one that it is a grouping of malignant lymphomas which share distinctive common clinical and histologic features. It tends to arise in lymph nodes, at least in immunocompetent patients, and it progresses in a steady, predictable fashion, affecting contiguous lymph nodes.

46.1	Lymphocyte Predominance Hodgkin's Disease	
Definition:	In contrast to "classical " Hodgkin's disease, the tumor cells of LP type are microscopically more delicate and phenotypically B cell.	
Morphology:	At least focal, faint nodular concentration of delicate "L & H" or "popcorn" tumor giant cells. Background cells are almost exclusively lymphocytes and epithelioid histiocytes, without neutrophils, eosinophils, or plasma cells.	
Immunophenotype:	Tumor cells show a complete or nearly complete B cell phenotype and are surrounded by a collarette of T cells that express CD57.	
Genetic features:	Monoclonal versus polyclonal B cells.	
Differential diagnosis:	Progressive transformation of GC, follicle center, or mantle cell lymphomas, "T cell-rich B cell lymphoma".	

We categorize lymphocyte predominance Hodgkin's disease as a form of Hodgkin's disease because it shows a hiatus between the tumor giant cells and a benign background of inflammatory cells. In lymphocyte predominance disease, the acute inflammatory response seen in other Hodgkin's disease categories is absent [46.2]. Lymphocyte predominance disease lacks neutrophils and eosinophils in the background, having only lymphocytes and/or histiocytes, in particular epithelioid histiocytes.

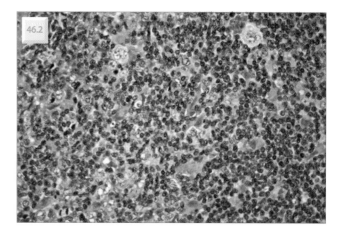

The pathologist initially reviewing a lymph node involved by this variant of Hodgkin's disease usually includes benign lymphoid hyperplasia in the differential diagnosis, as well as low grade non-Hodgkin's lymphoma, particularly follicle center lymphoma and mantle cell lymphoma.

This is because a very faint but distinct nodularity is often seen [46.3]. However, at intermediate and higher powers, one becomes aware of scattered large cells [46.4]. Shown in [46.5] are rather delicate cells, known as "L & H" cells or "popcorn" cells, and also at least one large benign epithelioid histiocyte. The typical background of lymphocytes, without eosinophils or neutrophils, is also seen.

When this disease was "rediscovered" by Dr. Poppema, working with the Kiel group, he recognized the common association of lymphocyte predominance Hodgkin's disease with so-called "progressively transformed" germinal centers [46.6]. These are large germinal centers with an irregular border and an expanded surrounding mantle zone [46.7 - left], and it is tempting to assume some histogenetic relationship between these peculiar germinal centers and the neoplasm [46.7 - right].

The Kiel group suggested that this disease is a B cell proliferation lymphocyte predominance Hodgkin's, differing in phenotype from other forms of Hodgkin's disease, and this proposal has been confirmed by many subsequent studies. With available paraffin-reactive antibodies, it is easy to demonstrate that the tumor cells stain strongly for B cell markers (CD20, CDw75 and CD79a). Compared in [46.8] are

a progressively transformed germinal center on the right with a nodular area involved by typical lymphocyte predominance Hodgkin's disease on the left. The pattern of B cell staining in the progressively transformed germinal center resembles a reactive follicle, with many cells, including the small lymphocytes in the background, staining as B cells.

The tumor cells characteristically stand out when stained with an anti-B cell antibody because they are surrounded by a collar or "rosette" of non-staining T cells, and this is a useful diagnostic aid. Dr. Poppema has reported that these T cells differ from those seen

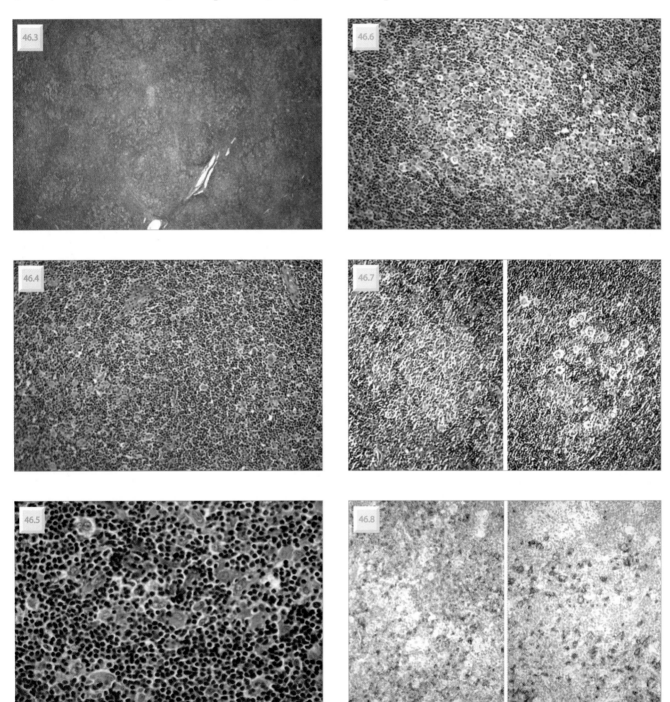

in classical Hodgkin's disease being CD57 (Leu-7)-positive T-helper cells (which resemble the T cells normally found in germinal centers), and this sometimes provides an additional diagnostic clue [46.9].

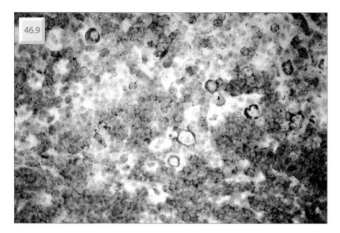

The case illustrated above is typical in that it shows at least faint nodularity. However, one occasionally encounters cases in which the growth pattern, in at least H and E stained sections is diffuse [46.10]. In these cases there is usually a higher proportion of L & H cells than in cases with nodular growth pattern [46.11]. However, immunostaining for B cells usually shows convincing nodularity of the tumor cell distribution [46.12]. The question has therefore been raised as to whether true diffuse lymphocyte predominance Hodgkin's disease even exists.

Lymphocyte predominance Hodgkin's disease has a favorable clinical course, but it has a risk, albeit low, of progressing or transforming to a histologically higher grade disease. This can be a straightforward diffuse large B cell lymphoma, as seen on the left [46.13]; or it can progress to the appearance, illustrated on the right, in which there is an ever-increasing number of recognizable "L & H" type cells. Dr. Jaffe and her colleagues have described this variant of lymphocyte predominance Hodgkin's disease.

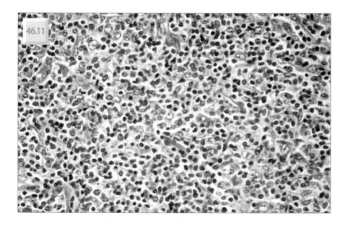

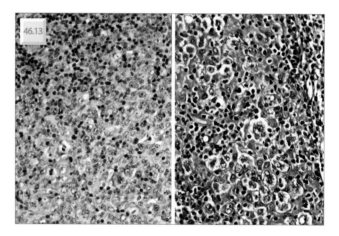

The nature of the disease is still not clear, despite much active work on the nature of the L & H cell. Elegant studies have been carried out using high resolution molecular biologic methods, and [46.14] is a photograph from a paper published by workers in the University of Nebraska.[1] Dr. Delabie and others have micropipetted individual L & H cells from tissue sections and then carried out PCR analysis for immunoglobulin heavy chain gene rearrangement. Variable results have emerged from such studies. Some groups, such as that of Hansmann in Cologne,[2] have found uniform clonal rearrangement among the L & H cells within an individual case, fulfilling expectations that this is indeed a clonal B cell neoplasm. Other groups, such as the workers at the University of Nebraska, have found variation from cell to cell within the same case, raising the question of whether this is truly a neoplasm, or whether it should be considered a preneoplastic polyclonal or oligoclonal process.

However, the most recent study,[3] representing an enormous amassed effort of single cells extracted by micromanipulation studies on a number of cases, indicate the process to be a clonal proliferation of highly mutated germinal center B cells.

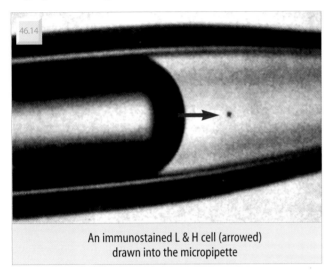

An immunostained L & H cell (arrowed) drawn into the micropipette

Finally, the nomenclature of this disease is of interest. Lukes, Butler and Hicks, in their original 1966 magnum opus on the classification of Hodgkin's disease,[4] categorized lymphocyte predominance Hodgkin's disease largely in the "nodular L & H" group, and emphasized its extremely favorable clinical behavior [46.15]. Lymphocyte predominance Hodgkin's disease represents the main area of change in the nomenclature of Hodgkin's disease over the last two decades. The Rye Conference took place almost immediately after the appearance of the classic proposal by Lukes, Butler and Hicks that Hodgkin's disease could be classified into six separate groups. It was agreed at the Rye meeting to simplify the system, and "lymphocytic/histiocytic" disease disappeared into a single category of lymphocyte predominance. Poppema and his colleagues at Kiel used the term which Mohri and Lennert had coined earlier, "para-granuloma, nodular and diffuse". However, in the REAL classification, the simple term "lymphocyte predominance" is used again, but now with the specific connotation that it is a B cell process, which differs in phenotype from classical Hodgkin's disease and has a particularly favorable prognosis [46.16].

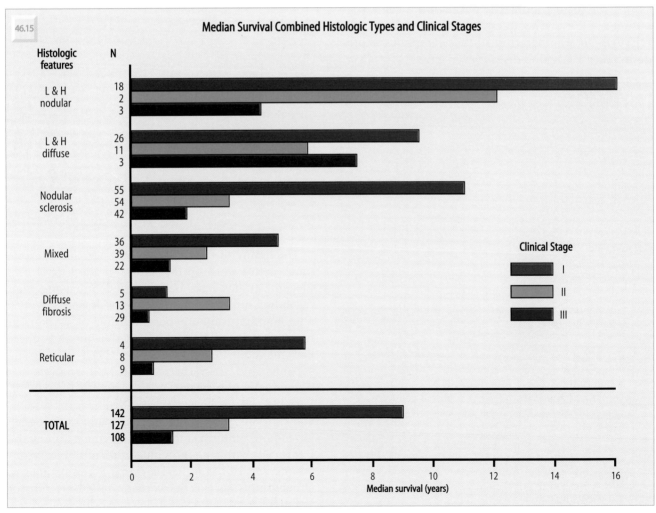

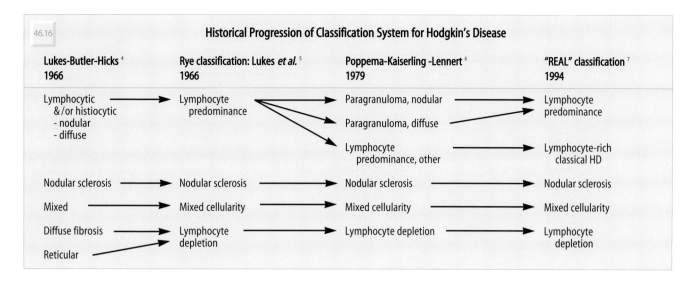

46.16 Historical Progression of Classification System for Hodgkin's Disease

Lukes-Butler-Hicks [4] 1966	Rye classification: Lukes *et al.* [5] 1966	Poppema-Kaiserling -Lennert [6] 1979	"REAL" classification [7] 1994
Lymphocytic &/or histiocytic - nodular - diffuse	Lymphocyte predominance	Paragranuloma, nodular / Paragranuloma, diffuse / Lymphocyte predominance, other	Lymphocyte predominance / Lymphocyte-rich classical HD
Nodular sclerosis	Nodular sclerosis	Nodular sclerosis	Nodular sclerosis
Mixed	Mixed cellularity	Mixed cellularity	Mixed cellularity
Diffuse fibrosis / Reticular	Lymphocyte depletion	Lymphocyte depletion	Lymphocyte depletion

REFERENCES

1. Delabie J, Tierens A, Wu G, Weisenburger DD, Chan WC. Lymphocyte predominance Hodgkin's disease: lineage and clonality determination using a single-cell assay. *Blood* 1994; **84**: 3291-8.

2. Küppers R, Rajewsky K, Zhao M *et al.* Hodgkin disease: Hodgkin and Reed-Sternberg cells picked from histological sections show clonal immunoglobulin gene rearrangements and appear to be derived from B cells at various stages of development. *Proc Natl Acad Sci U S A* 1994; **91**: 10962-6.

3. Marafioti T, Hummel M, Anagnostopoulos I *et al.* Origin of nodular lymphocyte-predominant Hodgkin's disease from a clonal expansion of highly mutated germinal-center B cells. *N Engl J Med* 1997; **337**: 453-8.

4. Lukes RJ, Butler JJ, Hicks EB. Natural history of Hodgkin's disease as related to its pathologic picture. *Cancer* 1966; **19**: 317-44.

5. Lukes RJ, Craver RF, Hall TC, *et al.* Report of the nomenclature committee. *Cancer* 1966; **26**: 1311.

6. Poppema S, Kaiserling E, Lennert K. Nodular paragranuloma and progressively transformed germinal centers. Ultrastructural and immunohistologic findings. *Virchows Arch B Cell Pathol Incl Mol Pathol* 1979; **31**: 211-25.

7. Harris NL, Jaffe ES, Stein H *et al.* A revised European-American classification of lymphoid neoplasms: a proposal from the International Lymphoma Study Group. *Blood* 1994; **84**: 1361-92.

Should lymphocyte predominance Hodgkin's disease be treated like classical Hodgkin's disease?

P M Mauch

Lymphocyte predominance Hodgkin's disease differs from nodular sclerosis and mixed cellularity disease both clinically and histopathologically [47.1]. This chapter is concerned with the patterns of presentation, stage, median time to recurrence, pattern of late recurrences, the risk of secondary non-Hodgkin's lymphomas, and the low mortality of this entity.

47.1	Differences from Nodular Sclerosing and Mixed Cellularity Hodgkin's Disease
	Histopathology
	Patterns of presentation
	Early stage distribution
	Late median time to recurrence
	Continuous late recurrences?
	High secondary NHL incidence?
	Low mortality from Hodgkin's disease

Summarized in [47.2] are seven studies from literature which cover a total of 426 patients from Boston University, Stanford University, the Christie Hospital in Manchester, the Mayo Clinic, and Melbourne, Australia, St. Bartholomew's Hospital in London, together with 71 of our own patients reviewed at the Joint Center for Radiation Therapy.[1-7]

47.2	Literature Studies (426 patients)
	Trudel *et al.* 1987 (Boston U, N = 35)[1]
	Regula *et al.* 1988 (Stanford U, N = 73)[2]
	Borg-Grech *et al.* 1989 (Christie Hosp, N = 101)[3]
	Tefferi *et al.* 1990 (Mayo Clinic, N = 32)[4]
	Crennan *et al.* 1995 (Melbourne, N = 64)[5]
	Pappa *et al.* 1995 (St. Bart's, N = 50)[6]
	Bodis *et al.* 1997 (N = 71)[7]

Illustrations [47.3], [47.4] and [47.5] relate to gender, age and site of disease, and come from a study, published in *Cancer* in 1993,[8] of 800 patients who had undergone a staging laparotomy at the Harvard Medical School Longwood Area Hospitals. When histology was correlated with sites of involvement, it was evident that patients with lymphocyte predominance pathology rarely had mediastinal involvement, whereas mediastinal disease was present in about 75% of patients with nodular sclerosis and in about half the patients with mixed cellularity disease [47.3]. In addition, the hilum was rarely involved, and the upper neck was much more commonly involved by lymphocyte predominance disease — 14% of the time versus 4% for the other categories. Another peripheral site, epitrochlear nodes, are also much more frequently involved in lymphocyte predominance disease, although overall this site is relatively rare.

47.3	Prevalence of Sites of Involvement Above the Diaphragm by Histologic Subtype			
Site	NS (433)	MC/LD (223)	LP (63)	p-value
Mediastinum	73%	46%	8%	< 0.0001
Left neck	62%	53%	41%	0.03
Right neck	55%	60%	46%	NS
Left axilla	15%	14%	14%	NS
Right axilla	11%	16%	13%	NS
Left hilum	15%	8%	5%	0.006
Right hilum	14%	9%	3%	0.005
Upper neck	4%	4%	14%	0.05
Epitrochlear	1%	1%	6%	0.12

Within the abdomen [47.4], upper abdominal nodes and the spleen are much less frequently involved in lymphocyte predominance disease, whereas peripheral sites, such as the inguinal nodes, are much more commonly involved.

There are also differences in age distribution, despite the fact that this was a laparotomy based series from which patients over 60 were excluded [47.5]. Almost 80% of patients with nodular sclerosis disease were between 16 and 39; only 10% were age 15 or under; and 11% were 40 or over. In contrast, 33% of patients with lymphocyte predominance disease were age 15 or under, 26% were age 40 or over, and only 41% were in the intermediate age interval. There was also a clear preponderance of male patients with lymphocyte predominance disease. In this study, three quarters of patients were male: other studies have reported an incidence of 80 or 85%.

47.4	Prevalence of Sites of Involvement Below the Diaphragm by Histologic Subtype			
Site	NS (433)	MC /LD (223)	LP (63)	p-value
Spleen	24%	35%	17%	0.006
Upper abdomen	13%	18%	5%	0.008
Lower abdomen	8%	17%	8%	0.008
Right inguinal	1%	3%	10%	0.03
Left inguinal	1%	3%	10%	0.02

47.5	Histology versus Age and Sex			
Co-variate	LP (63)	NS (433)	MC /LD (223)	p-value
Age < 15	33%	10%	11%	
Age 16-39	41%	79%	68%	< 0.0001
Age ≥ 40	26%	11%	21%	
Male	75%	51%	63%	0.0001
Female	25%	49%	37%	

Laparotomy staging data are available from 66 patients in our series and from about 25 to 30 patients in the Boston University study [47.6]. Patients underwent laparotomy in the other studies, but the number that were "upstaged" was not reported. The striking finding is that lymphocyte predominance patients who were clinically Stage IA were rarely reassigned to Stages III or IV after laparotomy. This occurred in the combined Harvard and Boston University series in only two out of 42 patients. Since this is largely a male population, about 15-20% of patients with nodular sclerosis or mixed cellularity histology initially categorized as Stage IA would normally be upstaged, so the figure is significantly lower for lymphocyte predominance disease. For patients with Stage IIA disease, 21% were upstaged, similar to other histologies. The other finding of note is the very low percentage of patients with lymphocyte predominance histology who presented with B symptoms or with Stage III or IV disease.

Information about median times to recurrence can be gleaned from the Stanford study, from Tefferi's series and from our own investigation [47.7]. The total number of relapses was 38, and the median time to relapse was nearly four years. If patients with Stage III or IV disease are excluded, the median time to recurrence exceeds five years. To put that in perspective, patients with early stage mixed cellularity or nodular sclerosis Hodgkin's disease have a median time to recurrence of about two and a half years, and for patients with large mediastinal disease the figure is about a year and a half.

47.6	Results of Staging Laparotomy (Trudel /JCRT)				
	Pathology Stage				
Clinical stage	1A	11A	III-IVA	IB-IIB	III-IVB
IA (42)	40		2 /0		
IIA (33)		26	6 /1		
IIIA (10)	4	3	3 /0		
IB-IIB (3)				2	1
III-IVB (1)					1

47.7	Median Time to Recurrence		
Report	N relapsed	Median	
Trudel [1]	—	—	
Regula [2]	15 /73	3.75 years	
Borg-Grech [3]	—	—	
Tefferi [4]	10 /32	4 years	
Crennan [5]	—	—	
Pappa [6]	—	—	
Bodis [7]	13 /71	4 years	
— not available			

The issue of continuing late recurrences (CLR) is also of interest [47.8]. It is worth pointing out, however, that whether one interprets one or two late recurrences as indicating that the survival curve has yet to plateau is a matter of interpretation. This Table also lists the number of nodular and diffuse cases in each study. In our series, even minimal nodularity was enough to classify the histology as nodular. In the St. Bartholomew's series there were no diffuse cases. In other studies, such as the Stanford 1988 series, more patients had diffuse than nodular disease.

47.8	Continuing Late Recurrences Nodular vs Diffuse		
Report	N nod /dif	Difference	CLR > 10 year
Trudel [1]	—	—	—
Regula [2]	32 /41	Yes	Yes
Borg-Grech [3]	59 /32	No	Yes
Tefferi [4]	13 /19	No	No
Crennan [5]	31 /33	No	+/-
Pappa [6]	50 /0	—	No
Bodis [7]	52 /17	No	No
— not available			

Also shown in [47.8] is whether there was a difference in disease-free survival between nodular and diffuse disease. Only one study, the *New England Journal of Medicine* paper from Stanford,[2] argues that the nodular cases have a continuing risk of late recurrences and a poorer disease-free survival than the diffuse cases. The other four studies showed superimposable curves, and provided no evidence for differences between nodular and diffuse subtypes.

Shown in [47.9] are the 1988 Stanford survival curves, the only study that found clear differences for freedom from recurrence between the nodular and the diffuse subgroups. It is difficult, however, to tell whether the disease recurs late but then reaches a true plateau or not, and there are certainly not enough patients after twelve or thirteen years to make this clear.

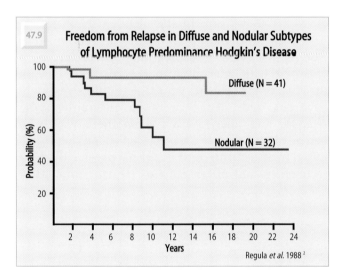

The survival curves in [47.10] from the Christie Hospital group in Manchester show no differences, in terms of relapse-free survival, between the diffuse and the nodular subtypes of lymphocyte predominance Hodgkin's disease.[3] This Figure also shows the very favorable prognosis of this group of Hodgkin's patients. The ten year survival is about 80%, which is good considering that there were some advanced stage patients in the study.

The St. Bartholomew's group is shown in [47.11]; all cases were of nodular type.[6] The two curves compare the remission duration of lymphocyte predominance Hodgkin's disease with other types of Hodgkin's disease (nodular sclerosis and mixed cellularity). In this group one could argue that, although there are late recurrences, some after ten or twelve years, there is a point beyond which no further recurrences are seen. In contrast, if this were a low grade lymphoma, one would expect to see continuing recurrences.

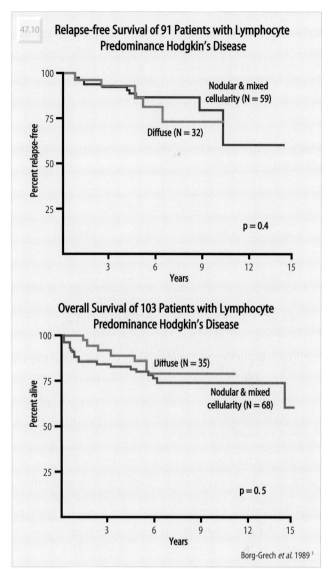

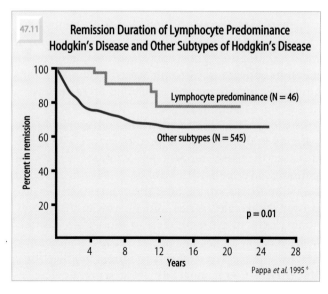

Shown in [47.12] is the incidence of second malignancy, and specifically of non-Hodgkin's lymphoma in patients with lymphocyte predominance Hodgkin's disease. All of these series have a relatively long follow up and one would expect to see second tumors if they are going to arise. These are not actuarial numbers, but crude figures, and normally one would expect an actuarial risk for second tumors of about 15% after 15 years. The frequencies here are close to that figure, and thus there does not appear to be an increased risk of second malignancy in lymphocyte predominance Hodgkin's disease patients compared to nodular sclerosis or mixed cellularity patients.

47.12	2nd Malig /NHL after HD		
Report	N 2nd malig	N NHL	Histology
Trudel [1]	5/35 (14%)	2/35 (6%)	DLCL (2)
Regula [2]	9/73 (12%)	2/73 (3%)	DLCL (2)
Borg-Grech [3]	—	—	—
Tefferi [4]	8/32 (25%)	1/32 (3%)	—
Crennan [5]	3/64 (5%)	1/64 (2%)	DLCL
Pappa [6]	6/50 (12%)	2/50 (4%)	HG-B-NHL (2)
Bodis [7]	7/71 (10%)	0/71 (0%)	
TOTAL	**38/325 (12%)**	**8/325 (2.5%)**	

In terms of non-Hodgkin's lymphoma, the striking finding is that only eight out of the 325 patients (2.5%) analyzed in these six studies developed secondary non-Hodgkin's lymphomas. Furthermore, all of them are intermediate or high grade lymphomas, the type of neoplasm one sees typically following Hodgkin's disease. This frequency is perhaps slightly higher than one would normally find in a group of patients with nodular sclerosis or mixed cellularity disease. Some investigators have argued that lymphocyte predominance Hodgkin's disease is associated with a high risk of secondary non-Hodgkin's lymphoma. One explanation is that in some reports the initial histopathologic diagnosis may have been in error. In all of the above studies, some cases of secondary non-Hodgkin's lymphoma were excluded on re-review.

Shown in [47.13] are the causes of mortality for patients with lymphocyte predominance Hodgkin's disease. In these reports an average of 22% of patients have died, with a range of 14% to 31%. In the Stanford series, the St. Bartholomew's series, the Boston University series and our own series, only about 1-4% of patients died of Hodgkin's disease, compared to about 8% due to second malignancy, and a similar percentage due to other complications. In all six studies, mortality from lymphocyte predominance Hodgkin's disease was only 6.5%, compared to an overall mortality of 22%; thus deaths due to the neoplasm itself are rare. This may be partly due to the early stage distribution; for example, in our series of about 400 patients with early stage Hodgkin's

disease, only fifteen deaths (about 3%) have been due to the disease. Thus, when dealing with aggressively treated patients with favorable early stage disease, there may be more deaths from other causes than from Hodgkin's disease.

47.13	Cause of Mortality				
Report	N deaths	HD	2nd malig	Cardiac	Other
Trudel [1]	8/35 (23%)	3%	9%	3%	9%
Regula [2]	17/73 (23%)	4%	10%	6%	4%
Borg-Grech [3]	25/110 (23%)	14%	5%	3%	2%
Tefferi [4]	10/32 (31%)	9%	6%	—	16%
Crennan [5]	—	—	—	—	—
Pappa [6]	12/50 (24%)	2%	8%	8%	6%
Bodis [7]	10/71 (14%)	1%	7%	4%	1%
TOTAL	**82/371 (22%)**	**6.5%**	**7.0%**	**4.0%**	**4.6%**

[47.14] shows very limited data on the effectiveness of chemotherapy for lymphocyte predominance Hodgkin's disease. Disappointing results have been obtained with adriamycin-based chemotherapy in that five of six patients who received this treatment have relapsed. These were patients either who relapsed and then received chemotherapy, or who had advanced disease and received chemotherapy as initial treatment. In contrast, we have seen only three recurrences out of ten patients treated with MOPP chemotherapy.

47.14	Recurrences After Chemotherapy Alone		
Report	Relapses	MOPP-like	ABVD-like
Trudel [1]	—	—	—
Regula [2]	—	—	—
Borg-Grech [3]	—	—	—
Tefferi [4]	—	—	—
Crennan [5]	—	—	—
Pappa [6]	—	—	—
Bodis [7]	8/16	3/10	5/6
— not available			

To summarize, the clinical presentation of lymphocyte predominance Hodgkin's disease is distinct from other subtypes. There is a strong predominance of males, and it is more common in children and adolescents than in young adults. The majority of patients are at Stage I or II. The disease at presentation involves peripheral nodal sites, involvement of mediastinal nodes and central abdominal nodes being rare.

When lymphocyte predominance Hodgkin's disease is treated like classical Hodgkin's disease, the prognosis is very favorable. Deaths from other causes are more common than from Hodgkin's disease, the time of recurrence is longer, and there are more late recurrences. Development of non-Hodgkin's lymphoma is unusual, and the evidence for continuing late recurrences is questioned.

Finally, should lymphocyte predominance Hodgkin's disease be treated like classical Hodgkin's disease? The author's view is that it should be, but with some modifications [47.14]. Because of the very favorable prognosis, one can eliminate surgical staging for the early stage patient, and consider smaller radiation fields and lower doses, although the details of this reduced treatment remain to be established, and the number of patients is small. However, there certainly appear to be more deaths from causes other than Hodgkin's disease itself, suggesting that currently some of these patients may be overtreated.

SELECTED REFERENCES

1. Trudel MA, Krikorian JG, Neiman RS. Lymphocyte predominance Hodgkin's disease. A clinicopathologic reassessment. *Cancer* 1987; **59**: 99-106.

2. Regula DP Jr., Hoppe RT, Weiss LM. Nodular and diffuse types of lymphocyte-predominance Hodgkin's disease. *N Engl J Med* 1988; **318**: 214-9.

3. Borg-Grech A, Radford JA, Crowther D, Swindell R, Harris M. A comparative study of the nodular and diffuse variants of lymphocyte predominant Hodgkin's disease. *J Clin Oncol* 1989; **7**: 1303-9.

4. Tefferi A, Zellers RA, Banks PM, Therneau TM, Colgan JP. Clinical correlates of distinct immunophenotypic and histologic subcategories of lymphocyte-predominance Hodgkin's disease. *J Clin Oncol* 1990; **8**: 1959-65.

5. Crennan E, D'Costa I, Liew KH *et al.* Lymphocyte predominant Hodgkin's disease: a clinicopathologic comparative study of histologic and immunophenotypic subtypes. *Int J Radiat Oncol Biol Phys* 1995; **31**: 333-7.

6. Pappa VI, Norton AJ, Gupta RK, Wilson AM, Rohatiner AZ, Lister TA. Nodular type of lymphocyte predominant Hodgkin's disease. A clinical study of 50 cases. *Ann Oncol* 1995; **6**: 559-65.

7. Bodis S, Kraus MD, Pinkus G *et al.* Clinical presentation and outcome in lymphocyte-predominant Hodgkin's disease. *J Clin Oncol* 1997; **15**: 3060-6.

8. Mauch PM, Kalish LA, Kadin M *et al.* Pattern of presentation of Hodgkin's disease. Implications for etiology and pathogenesis. *Cancer* 1993; **71**: 2062-71.

FURTHER READING

Pinkus GS, Said JW. Hodgkin's disease, lymphocyte predominance type, nodular — a distinct entity? Unique staining profile for L&H variants of Reed-Sternberg cells defined by monoclonal antibodies to leukocyte common antigen, granulocyte-specific antigen, and B-cell-specific antigen. *Am J Pathol* 1985; **118**: 1-6.

Should lymphocyte predominance Hodgkin's disease be treated as a low grade lymphoma?

S J Horning

This chapter updates the Stanford series of lymphocyte predominance Hodgkin's patients, and also considers how the morphologic pattern relates to prognosis.

Lymphocyte predominance Hodgkin's disease is a distinctive histologic subtype with characteristic morphologic and immunophenotypic features [48.1]. There is a striking male predominance and, at least in the Stanford series, it is usually a disease of adults. The great majority of cases, as amply confirmed in the literature, present asymptomatically with limited Stage I or II disease involving peripheral sites, particularly the cervical, axillary and inguinal nodes. Mediastinal presentations are unusual, in contrast to nodular sclerosing disease, as is bulky mediastinal involvement.

48.1	Lymphocyte Predominance Hodgkin's Disease A Distinctive Histologic Subtype
	- Characteristic morphology, immunophenotype
	- Clinical features: male predominance, adults, limited stage, peripheral sites
	- Association with diffuse aggressive B cell lymphoma
	- ? Unique pattern of relapse

It is commonly thought that there is an association with diffuse aggressive B cell lymphoma, but that may need to be re-evaluated since many assumptions about this complication have been based on individual case reports or on small series in the literature. However, a large retrospective analysis has been performed by the BNLI,[1] in which the incidence of secondary non-Hodgkin's lymphoma in lymphocyte predominance cases was found to be 3-4%, which is greater than the figures for nodular sclerosing disease (0.8%).

Does one see a unique pattern of relapse in lymphocyte predominance Hodgkin's disease and should it be considered a form of low grade B cell lymphoma?

Our 1988 paper [2] has now been updated, based on a patient population which has expanded to 101 [48.2]. One interesting point is that diffuse lymphocyte predominance Hodgkin's disease is now very rarely diagnosed, so that only about five cases have been added to this group, whereas more than twenty cases have been added to the nodular category. These data have been compiled by two radiation oncologists at Stanford, Drs. Tate and Hoppe. The paper by Regula *et al.* was authored by a pathologist, and changing views on the nature of lymphocyte predominance Hodgkin's disease mean that it might be appropriate to review these cases again.

48.2	Lymphocyte Predominance Hodgkin's Disease Characteristics of 101 Stanford Patients	
Nodular:diffuse		55:46
Median age		29 years
M:F		82:19
Laparotomy		61
Stage	IA:IIA	42:37
	IIB	6
	IIIA	16
Treatment	IFRT	29
	EFRT	42
	CM	30

Despite the additional patients, the median age of the patient population is unchanged at 29 years, and a striking male predominance is again seen. Sixty one of the 101 patients underwent staging laparotomy, which is a low percentage but reflects usual staging practice for patients with clinical Stage I and IIA. Few patients were symptomatic, and only sixteen had advanced stage disease.

When considering classical Hodgkin's disease, it is customary to focus on treatment, whereas with lymphocyte predominance disease the treatment often receives less attention than the pathology. However, it is noteworthy that at Stanford many more patients have been treated with only involved field radiotherapy, whereas this limited therapy ceased to be used in laparotomy staged patients in about 1970 because the relapse rate was well over 50%.

With that background, [48.3] shows actuarial freedom from progression in the 101 patients related to the pattern (diffuse versus nodular). At first glance these curves appear different, but the p value indicates that there is about a one in eleven probability that this occurred by chance alone. There were two late relapses in the diffuse group, and one occurred very late, after more than twelve years. There appears to be a plateau in the freedom from progression curve for patients with the nodular pattern of disease, but time will tell if this is the case.

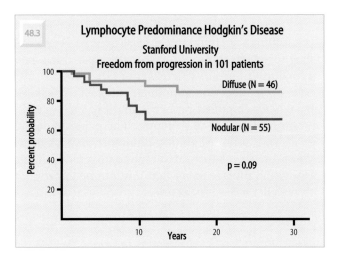

Patients who relapse with lymphocyte predominance Hodgkin's disease can of course be successfully treated secondarily, and the overall survival results are, as expected, excellent [48.4].

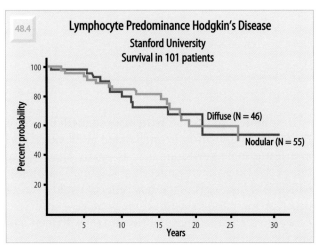

It is of interest to compare these patients with cases of nodular sclerosing disease of similar stage - Stages I and IIA. Kaplan-Meier plots of freedom from progression [48.5] compare a large group of nodular sclerosing patients with the subsets of lymphocyte predominance Hodgkin's disease. The results at ten, fifteen and more years are similar, but at earlier stages there is a clear difference, in that lymphocyte predominance Hodgkin's disease is more indolent in its relapse pattern. With regard to overall survival [48.6], the data are very similar when patients of comparable stage are evaluated, despite the difference in numbers.

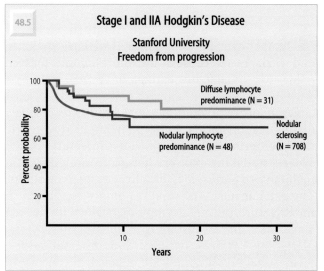

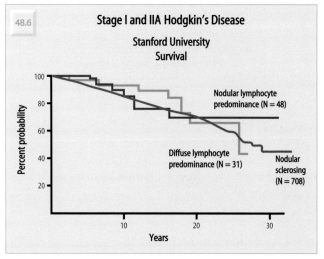

Another question of interest concerns the freedom from progression of patients with lymphocyte predominance Hodgkin's disease, particularly of nodular pattern [48.7]. When early stage asymptomatic patients were reviewed, there was no difference between those who received limited radiation and those treated with extended fields. Among patients who had an extended field of radiation, there was a single relapse, occurring beyond five years.

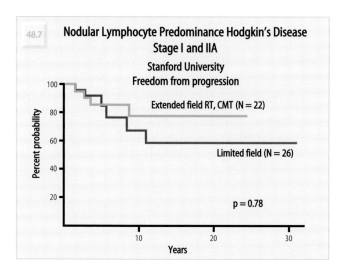

48.7 Nodular Lymphocyte Predominance Hodgkin's Disease Stage I and IIA. Stanford University. Freedom from progression. Extended field RT, CMT (N = 22). Limited field (N = 26). p = 0.78

A total of 24 patients died in this series of 101 cases [48.8]. The major cause of death was cardiac disease - this was usually myocardial infarction, although there were cases of congestive heart failure and radiation carditis. Four patients developed non-Hodgkin's lymphoma (all diffuse large B cell lymphomas), four developed solid cancers and only three died of Hodgkin's disease. Two patients developed acute myeloid leukemia, both of whom had received alkylating agents. Two deaths were due to infection and one was due to radiation hepatitis.

48.8	Lymphocyte Predominance Hodgkin's Disease Late Causes of Death in 24 Patients	
	Cardiac disease	8
	Non-Hodgkin's lymphoma	4
	Solid cancers	4
	Hodgkin's disease	3
	Acute myeloid leukemia	2
	Infection	2
	Radiation hepatitis	1

It is of interest to compare other series with the Stanford data. A group of 64 patients was analyzed retrospectively at the Peter MacCallum Cancer Institute [48.9].[3] They are similar in terms of the proportions with nodular versus diffuse disease. The median age was the same as in the Stanford group. There was a male predominance as expected, and patients frequently had early stage disease. The majority appear to have received extended field radiotherapy, although it is not clear in all cases what this meant in practice. Most of the patients who relapsed did so at sites distant from those of presentation, which is similar to the experience at Stanford.

The Manchester group [48.10] assigned cases not only into nodular and diffuse groups, but also into a "mixed" category.[4] They also reviewed cytologic features, and 56 of the 104 patients showed what was

considered to be characteristic L & H histology. The median age was approximately ten years greater than in other series. Again there was a male predominance, and a marked propensity for limited asymptomatic disease, although there were more patients with either symptomatic or advanced disease. Treatment varied according to the particular protocols being used.

48.9	Lymphocyte Predominance Hodgkin's Disease Characteristics of 64 Peter MacCallum Patients		
	Nodular:diffuse		31:33
	Median age		29 years
	M:F		52:12
	Stage	I:IIA	33:17
		IIIA:IIIB	8:3
		IV	1
	Treatment	EFRT	52
		Other	12

Crennan *et al.* 1995 [3]

48.10	Lymphocyte Predominance Hodgkin's Disease Characteristics of 104 Manchester Patients		
	Nodular (mixed):diffuse		69:35
	L + H histology		56
	Median age		38 years
	M:F		81:22
	Stage	I:IIA	61:10
		IIB:IIIA:IIIB	1:17:5
		IV	9
	Treatment	RT	61
		CT	15
		CM	28

Borg-Grech *et al.* 1989 [4]

Shown in [48.11] are the results at ten years from the MacCallum Cancer Institute, from Manchester and from Stanford, in terms of freedom from relapse and overall survival. The MacCallum review also considered the impact of immunophenotype, and cases are divided into B cell and non-B cell types. It is striking that the data show greater similarities than differences, and the morphologic pattern has no clear influence on either freedom from relapse or overall survival.

48.11	Lymphocyte Predominance Hodgkin's Disease Comparative Results of Treatment at 10 Years		
		FFR%	OS%
Peter MacCallum			
	Nodular (31)	72	83
	Diffuse (33)	76	87
	B cell (19)	68	77
	Non-B cell (17)	77	82
Manchester			
	Nodular/mixed (69)	73	78
	Diffuse (35)	77	74
Stanford University			
	Nodular (55)	69	78
	Diffuse (46)	93	82

Is lymphocyte predominance Hodgkin's disease a low grade B cell lymphoma and should it be treated accordingly [48.12]? It is clear that lymphocyte predominance Hodgkin's disease has distinctive clinical features, and in general these clinical features, particularly at presentation, if not throughout the natural history of the disease, do not vary with the morphologic pattern. Lymphocyte predominance Hodgkin's disease is clearly different from the low grade B cell lymphomas, at least as they are currently recognized in the Working Formulation. There is a marked male predominance, which is unusual, and patients tend to be younger and to present with limited asymptomatic disease. It is rare for pathologic staging, based on CT scanning or bone marrow biopsy, to "upstage" cases of lymphocyte predominance Hodgkin's disease. It is also relevant that lymphocyte predominance Hodgkin's disease does not express BCL-2, nor has the (14;18) translocation been seen. However, expression of the CD20 B cell surface marker and J chain does indicate that the L & H cells are of B cell lineage.

Further studies of the correlation between immunophenotype, morphology, extent of treatment and clinical outcomes are clearly needed in lymphocyte predominance Hodgkin's disease, particularly in view of pathologists' current thinking in relation to morphologic features.

Should lymphocyte predominance Hodgkin's disease be treated like low grade lymphoma? The answer is yes if by that one means involved field radiotherapy. In effect, the same treatment is used, without laparotomy staging, in lymphocyte predominance disease.

48.12 Should LPHD Be Treated Like Low Grade Lymphoma?

LPHD has distinctive clinical features that do not vary with morphologic pattern

Pathologic staging less frequently upstages LPHD

Further correlation of immunophenotype, morphology, extent of treatment and clinical outcomes is needed in LPHD

Intercurrent deaths constitute the major adverse outcome after a diagnosis of either limited stage low grade lymphoma or LPHD

Finally, it should be recognized that intercurrent death constitutes the major adverse outcome after diagnosis in both limited stage low grade lymphoma and lymphocyte predominance Hodgkin's disease. This provides an interesting opportunity to look at causes of death, at observed versus expected outcomes, and perhaps to provide an insight into the underlying biology and whether the patients are predisposed to secondary malignancy or whether this is related to treatment. And in lymphocyte predominance Hodgkin's disease, as in all other types of Hodgkin's disease, clinicians need to continue the search for effective but less toxic means of therapy.

REFERENCES

1. Bennett MH, MacLennan KA, Vaughan Hudson G, Vaughan Hudson B. Non-Hodgkin's lymphoma arising in patients treated for Hodgkin's disease in the BNLI: a 20-year experience. British National Lymphoma Investigation. *Ann Oncol* 1991; **2** (Suppl 2): 83-92.

2. Regula DP Jr, Hoppe RT, Weiss LM. Nodular and diffuse types of lymphocyte predominance Hodgkin's disease. *N Engl J Med* 1988; **318**: 214-9.

3. Crennan E, D'Costa I, Liew KH, Thompson J, Laidlaw C, Cooper I, Quong G. Lymphocyte predominant Hodgkin's disease: a clinicopathologic comparative study of histologic and immunophenotypic subtypes. *Int J Radiat Oncol Biol Phys* 1995; **31**: 333-7.

4. Borg-Grech A, Radford JA, Crowther D, Swindell R, Harris M. A comparative study of the nodular and diffuse variants of lymphocyte-predominant Hodgkin's disease. *J Clin Oncol* 1989; **7**: 1303-9

Morphologic, immunologic and genetic features of "Classical" Hodgkin's disease

P M Banks

	"Classical" Hodgkin's Disease
Definition:	Microscopic - striking microscopic hiatus between tumor giant cells and background inflammatory cellularity.
	Clinical - bimodal age incidence affects lymph nodes or thymus, spreads slowly and predictably.
Morphology	Diagnostically large bizarre Reed-Sternberg cells
	Types - lymphocyte-rich (provisional); mixed cellularity; lymphocyte depletion; nodular sclerosis.
Immunophenotype	In paraffin section CD45RB-, CD30+, CD15+/-.
Genetic features	Clonal hyperdiploid abnormalities.
Differential diagnosis	Lymphocyte-rich versus lymphocyte predominance; mixed cellularity versus peripheral T cell lymphoma or T cell rich B cell lymphoma; lymphocyte depletion versus ALCL.
Postulated normal counterpart	B or ?T cell of unknown type

49.1

The histologic hallmark of classical Hodgkin's disease is the hiatus between the bizarre Reed-Sternberg cells (and their mononuclear variants) and the background infiltrate, which features a diversity of cellular elements [49.1] and [49.2]. This chapter considers types of Hodgkin's disease other than "lymphocyte predominance" [49.3] starting with the lymphocyte-rich subgroup. This is not an entirely satisfactory term but it was adopted in the REAL classification to make a distinction from lymphocyte predominance disease.

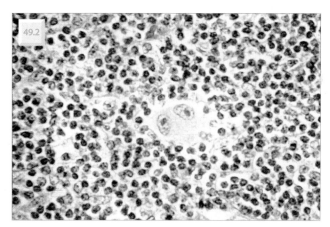

49.2

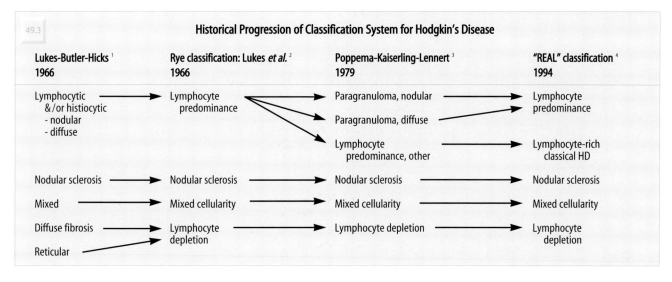

Historical Progression of Classification System for Hodgkin's Disease

49.3

Lukes-Butler-Hicks [1] 1966	Rye classification: Lukes *et al.* [2] 1966	Poppema-Kaiserling-Lennert [3] 1979	"REAL" classification [4] 1994
Lymphocytic &/or histiocytic - nodular - diffuse	Lymphocyte predominance	Paragranuloma, nodular	Lymphocyte predominance
		Paragranuloma, diffuse	
		Lymphocyte predominance, other	Lymphocyte-rich classical HD
Nodular sclerosis	Nodular sclerosis	Nodular sclerosis	Nodular sclerosis
Mixed	Mixed cellularity	Mixed cellularity	Mixed cellularity
Diffuse fibrosis	Lymphocyte depletion	Lymphocyte depletion	Lymphocyte depletion
Reticular			

Immunophenotyping is sometimes needed to distinguish lymphocyte predominance Hodgkin's disease from diffuse lymphocyte-rich classical disease. With paraffin-reactive antibodies this is now simple, and the staining pattern of R-S cells in classical Hodgkin's disease is well established, the cells being positive for CD30 and negative for B cell markers, such as CD20, CDw75 or CD79a [49.4].

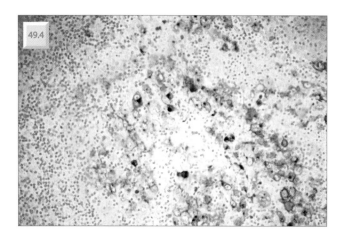

The term "lymphocyte-rich" implies a very low ratio of neoplastic tumor cells to reactive cells [49.5]. If even occasional eosinophils are seen in the background, the diagnosis is unlikely to be lymphocyte predominance type disease. It is important to use the term lymphocyte-rich classical Hodgkin's disease sparingly, and one should not make this diagnosis if there is only limited focal involvement of the lymph node [49.6]. This is in contradistinction to so-called "interfollicular" Hodgkin's disease, which represents limited early focal involvement [49.7]. The Stanford group[5] coined the term "interfollicular" to indicate a situation in which one cannot reliably distinguish between nodular sclerosis and mixed cellularity disease. Thus involvement of the lymph node has to be advanced and extensive if one is to classify the process confidently as lymphocyte-rich classical Hodgkin's disease.

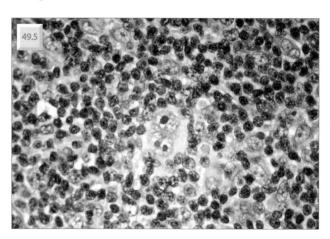

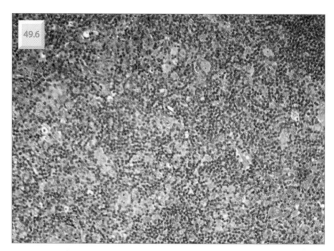

The mixed cellularity subtype is in many ways the prototype of Hodgkin's disease. One often sees large expanses of partial nodal involvement, notably in the paracortex [49.8], and, by definition, neoplastic cells are relatively abundant [49.9]. In practice one does not necessarily have to see numerous classical Reed-Sternberg cells, provided that a few are present. However, a relatively high proportion of presumably neoplastic mononuclear variants are needed to classify the process as mixed cellularity disease, and a sclerosing nodular stromal reaction excludes the diagnosis.

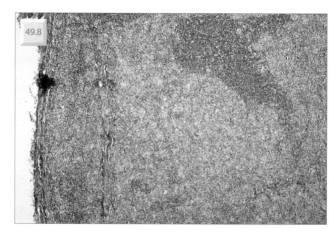

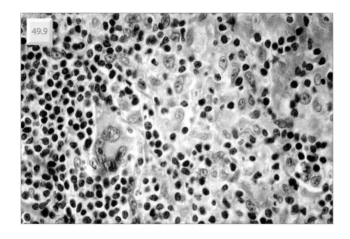

The differential diagnosis in cases of mixed cellularity disease includes "T cell-rich B cell lymphoma" and the occasional pleomorphic peripheral T cell lymphoma.

There are two variant forms of lymphocyte depletion Hodgkin's disease. These were first delineated by Lukes and Butler in their 1966 classification.[6] The non-controversial category is the "diffuse fibrosis" variant [49.10] in which one sees effacement of the nodal architecture by a peculiarly hypocellular process featuring abundant pre-collagenous matrix material and relatively scant cellularity [49.11]. Paradoxically, one often sees in these cases relatively few neoplastic Hodgkin's cells, but an even smaller number of reactive background cells is present.

It can occasionally be difficult to recognize this variant of Hodgkin's disease, and immunostains are sometimes useful in highlighting the neoplastic cells. They often have a dark and crushed appearance, rather than the classical aspect of Reed-Sternberg cells. This variant is often seen in the setting of relapsed Hodgkin's disease, or when there is diminished host immunity, but it can also occur as a primary manifestation of Hodgkin's disease.

The controversial category of "lymphocyte depletion" Hodgkin's disease is the subtype described by Lukes, Butler and Hicks, as the "reticular" variant [49.12].[1] In the earlier Jackson and Parker system,[7] it was described as "Hodgkin's sarcoma". It is controversial because of differing usage of the term in the United States and Europe. However, many American pathologists reserve a space in their classification concepts for the most aggressive type of Hodgkin's disease in which there is a striking predominance of neoplastic cells. In support of this interpretation, they will point to borderline areas in which there is minimal residual inflammatory cellularity, and perhaps even some hyaline fibrosis, and will suggest that this is the most aggressive extreme of nodular sclerosis Hodgkin's disease [49.13]. However, many of these cases are interpreted by European pathologists as "Hodgkin's-like anaplastic large cell lymphoma". This explains why the latter category is included (as a provisional category) in the REAL classification.

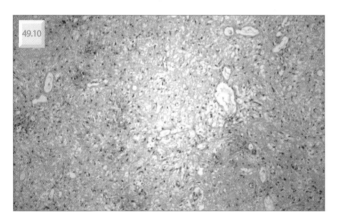

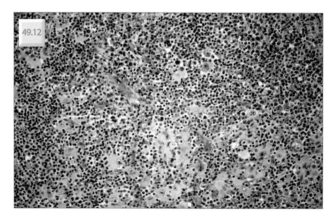

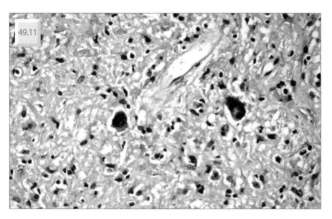

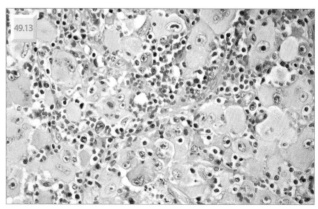

The differential diagnosis for this disease (whether one calls it Hodgkin's sarcoma, the reticular variant of lymphocyte depleted Hodgkin's, or Hodgkin's-like anaplastic large cell lymphoma) is quite different from that other forms of Hodgkin's disease. The pathologist has to consider diverse possibilities, including metastatic carcinoma or even malignant melanoma. True histiocytic malignancy (if there is such an entity) also has to be considered [49.14].

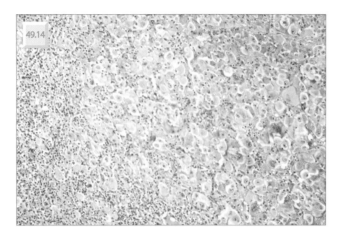

One way to minimize the difference between European and American interpretations is to take the view that there are a number of Hodgkin's like lesions, including lymphomatoid papulosis and anaplastic large cell lymphomas, and that, even if they are different from Hodgkin's disease, there is nevertheless great overlap, at least morphologically and immunophenotypically and possibly in the genetic features of the neoplastic cells [49.15].

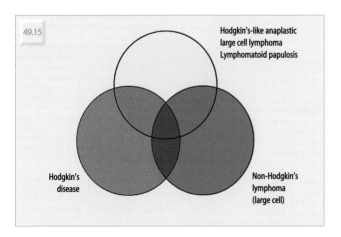

Nodular sclerosis is the commonest histologic type of Hodgkin's disease in developed countries, and pathologists have little difficulty in making this diagnosis [49.16]. When the classic proliferative fibroblastic transformation of the lymph node capsule and trabeculae encircling cellular nodules are seen [49.17], the neoplastic cells are often of the so called "lacunar" type, in which abundant clear cytoplasm

imparts a characteristic appearance in conventional formalin fixed tissue blocks [49.18]. These cells display delicate multilobated nuclear appearances, with nucleoli smaller than those of classic Reed-Sternberg cells.

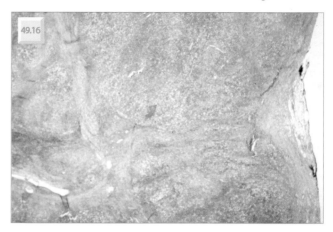

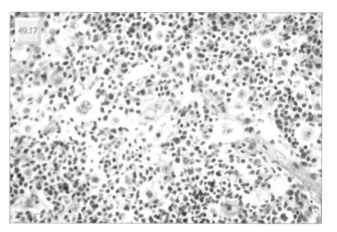

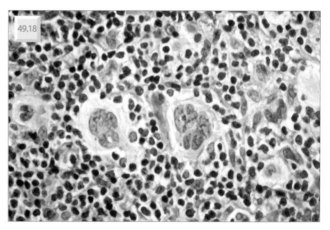

This "smiling" Reed-Sternberg cell [49.19] is a reminder that pathologists like Hodgkin's disease because they can recognize it in most cases by conventional microscopy alone. Pathologists are also now able to predict the likely progression of the disease, and oncologists have learned how to treat the majority of patients successfully. However, the nature of these cells, in particular their genetic features, is only now coming to light. This has been an elusive problem because it is difficult to isolate these rare cells and to study them in sufficient numbers, but elegant and powerful molecular techniques have been applied in recent years to individual tumor cells. There is still no universal agreement over the nature of the Reed-Sternberg cell, but most evidence today suggests that they are B lymphoid cells, perhaps in a very abnormal activated form.[8] We also know that they are neoplastic cells. It was suggested at one point that the cell was an end-stage, possibly degenerating, cell, and perhaps not even neoplastic. However, there is now no doubt about their neoplastic nature. The relatively few karyotypic studies that have been done all show a very abnormal, usually hyperdiploid, pattern. Thus the secrets of this mysterious cell, with its enigmatic Mona Lisa smile, are finally being revealed.

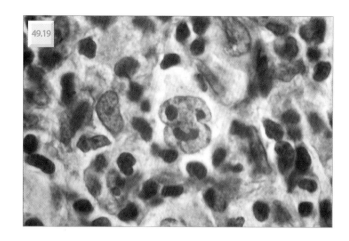

REFERENCES

1. Lukes RJ, Butler JJ, Hicks EB. Natural history of Hodgkin's disease as related to its pathologic picture. *Cancer* 1966; **19**: 317-344.

2. Lukes RJ, Craver RF, Hall TC, *et al*. Report of the nomenclature committee. *Cancer* 1966; **26**: 1311.

3. Poppema S, Kaiserling E, Lennert K. Nodular paragranuloma and progressively transformed germinal centers. Ultrastructural and immunohistologic findings. *Virchows Arch B Cell Pathol Incl Mol Pathol* 1979; **31**: 211-25.

4. Harris NL, Jaffe ES, Stein H *et al*. A revised European-American classification of lymphoid neoplasms: a proposal from the International Lymphoma Study Group. *Blood* 1994; **84**: 1361-92.

5. Doggett RS, Colby TV, Dorfman RF. Interfollicular Hodgkin's disease. *Am J Surg Pathol* 1983; **7**: 145-9.

6. Lukes RJ, Butler JJ. The pathology and nomenclature of Hodgkin's disease. *Cancer Res* 1966; **26**: 1063-83.

7. Jackson H. and Parker H. *Hodgkin's Disease and Allied Disorders*. New York: Oxford University Press 1947; 28-33.

8. Küppers R, Rajewsky K, Zhao M *et al*. Hodgkin disease: Hodgkin and Reed-Sternberg cells picked from histological sections show clonal immunoglobulin gene rearrangements and appear to be derived from B cells at various stages of development. *Proc Natl Acad Sci U S A* 1994; **91**: 10962-6.

Butler JJ. The histologic diagnosis of Hodgkin's disease. *Semi Diag Pathol* 1992; **9**: 252-6.

Gulley ML, Eagan PA, Quintanilla-Martinez L *et al*. Epstein-Barr virus DNA is abundant and monoclonal in the Reed-Sternberg cells of Hodgkin's disease: Associated with mixed cellularity subtype and Hispanic American ethnicity. *Blood* 1994; **83**: 1595-602.

Hummel M, Ziemann K, Lammert H, Pileri S, Sabattini E, Stein H. Hodgkin's disease with monoclonal and polyclonal populations of Reed-Sternberg cells. *N Engl J Med* 1995; **333**: 901-6.

Kamel OW, Chang PP, Hsu FJ *et al*. Clonal VDJ recombination of the immunoglobulin heavy chain gene by PCR in Classical Hodgkin's disease. *Am J Clin Pathol* 1995; **104**: 419-23.

McBride JA, Rodriguez J, Luthra R, Ordóñez, Cabanillas F, Pugh WC. T-cell-rich B large-cell lymphoma simulating lymphocyte-rich Hodgkin's disease. *Am J Surg Pathol* 1996; **20**: 193-201.

MacLennan KA, Bennett MH, Tu A *et al*. Relationship of histopathologic features to survival and relapse in nodular sclerosing Hodgkin's disease. A study of 1659 patients. *Cancer* 1989; **64**: 1686-93.

Patsouris E, Noël H, Lennert K. Cytohistologic and immunohistochemical findings in Hodgkin's disease, mixed cellularity type, with a high content of epithelioid cells. *Am J Surg Pathol* 1982; **13**: 1014-22.

Weber-Matthiesen K, Deerberg J, Poetsch M, Grote W, Schlegelberger B. Numerical chromosome aberrations are present within the CD30+ Hodgkin and Reed-Sternberg cells in 100% of analyzed cases of Hodgkin's disease. *Blood* 1995; **86**:1464-8.

FURTHER READING

Banks PM. The pathology of Hodgkin's disease. *Sem Oncol* 1990; **17**: 683-95.

Weiss LM, Lopategui JR, Sun L-H, Kamel OW, Koo CH, Glackin C. Absence of the t(2;5) in Hodgkin's disease. *Blood* 1995; **85**: 2845-7.

Treatment of early-stage Hodgkin's lymphoma

C N Coleman

This chapter considers some of the controversial questions concerning the treatment of Hodgkin's disease. Before doing that, it may be commented that, although there is a general acceptance of the inclusion of Hodgkin's disease with other lymphomas in the REAL classification, there are a few voices who question whether this is justified. Apparently, Thomas Hodgkin was asked recently for his opinion, but his only response was a Rye smile! [50.1]

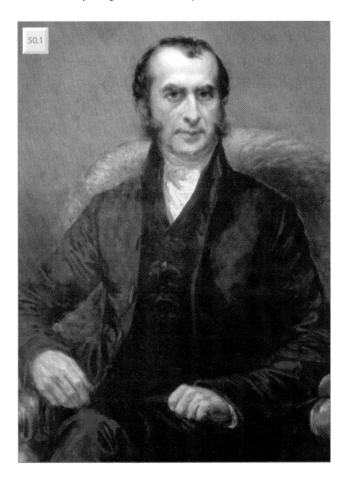

The problem posed by Hodgkin's disease is a problem of success. If patients who have been treated with early stage disease, Stages IA and IIA, are reviewed,[1]

about 80% are alive after 25 years, and most are relapse-free [50.2]. This has been achieved using very effective intensive therapies. The question is therefore — can we now reduce our efforts in staging and can we also reduce the treatment we give?

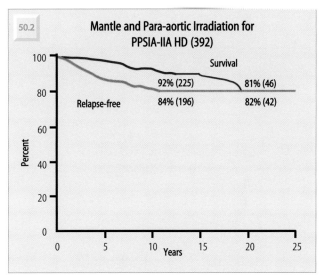

What is the necessity of staging and the possibility of using prognostic factors to replace surgical staging? It should be emphasized that many of the good results achieved in treating this disease were based on careful staging — essentially the more is known about the patient, the better equipped the oncologist is to devise a tailor-made treatment. However, it is now clear that in some patients the judicious use of prognostic factors can avoid the need for laparotomy.

Work from Stanford[2] [50.3] showed that clinical Stage I patients, if they were female or had only mediastinal involvement, or had lymphocyte predominance disease, very rarely had evidence of widespread disease at laparotomy. These patients could therefore be treated on the basis of clinical prognostic factors alone. For other patients, males in particular, there were no prognostic factors with an upstaging rate of less than 15%, and for all these other characteristics, there was an upstaging rate of about 25-30%. Similarly, with clinical Stage II young female patients, assessment of the number of involved sites identifies a low risk population [50.4]. All other Stage II patients have a significant risk of microscopic abdominal disease.

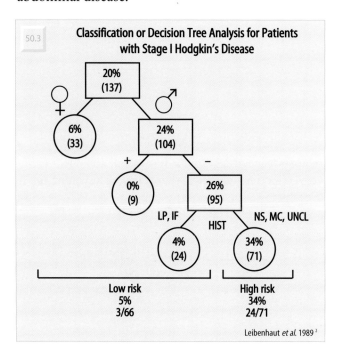

Classification or Decision Tree Analysis for Patients with Stage I Hodgkin's Disease

Leibenhaut *et al.* 1989 [2]

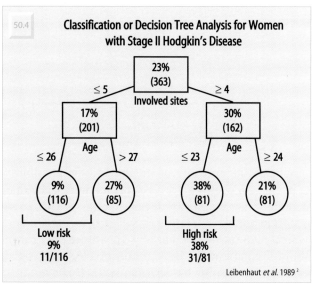

Classification or Decision Tree Analysis for Women with Stage II Hodgkin's Disease

Leibenhaut *et al.* 1989 [2]

In a multivariate analysis [50.5] Dr. Mauch[3] of the Joint Center found various factors that together give lower risks of upstaging — being female, having no B symptoms, having few sites of involvement, being young and having favorable histology. It is therefore clear that a subset of patients can be identified who have a very low risk of upstaging following laparotomy. These patients can be treated without laparotomy, and indeed many centers now treat all patients without laparotomy.

50.5	CS I-II Upstaging by Clinical Factors (552)	
Male vs female	29% vs 18%	0.003
Symptoms vs none	34% vs 21%	0.027
≥ 2 sites vs none	27% vs 17%	0.003
Age ≥ 40 vs ≤ 39	30% vs 23%	0.081
NS/LP vs MC/LD	27% vs 23%	NS

Mauch *et al.* 1988 [3]

Is it better to understage and overtreat — or to overstage and undertreat? If minimal staging and less toxic therapy is given (which is becoming the trend), can patients given these relatively less aggressive early treatments be salvaged when they relapse? The question is — does reducing initial therapy compromise the success rate?

If one adopts a general policy of doing very little clinical staging, and giving limited radiotherapy, one gets very poor freedom from relapse. A classic paper from Stanford many years ago [50.6] showed that at least half of the patients would relapse if treated with limited radiotherapy alone. It is true that in early stage Hodgkin's disease, even if one chooses the wrong treatment initially, salvage therapy is so effective that survival differences are very rarely related to the choice of initial therapy. But clearly it is undesirable for the patient's initial treatment to have a high failure rate. In that sense radiotherapy alone, without staging, is not an acceptable choice, except in a highly selected group of patients.

50.6	Wide-field RT (STLI/TLI) Versus Limited-field RT		
Study	**Stage**	**Design (N patients)**	**FFR (year)**
Stanford U (15) [4]	PS IA-IIA	STLI/TLI (35) vs IF (28)	80% vs 32%
COLL CLIN Trial (10) [5]	PS I-II	STLI(84) vs II (81)	66% vs 52%
BNLI (12) [6,7]	PS IA-IIA	Reg (181) vs IF (147)	48% vs 50%
COLLAB CLIN Trial [5]	CS I-II	STLI (98) vs IF (88)	59% vs 32%
BNLI [6,7]	CS IA-IIA	Reg (95) vs IF (114)	43% vs 40%

Mauch *et al.* 1994 [1]

Dr. Mauch[8] [50.7] has conducted a study of mantle radiotherapy alone, and there has been a similar study from the Princess Margaret Hospital. This was a prospective one arm trial for selected pathologically staged patients of Stage IA and IIA. The entry criteria were quite strict and included nodular sclerosis or lymphocyte predominance histology, no B symptoms, negative laparotomy, and disease limited to sites above the carina. Patients were carefully staged with CT and gallium scans, so that the number of sites and their location were well established.

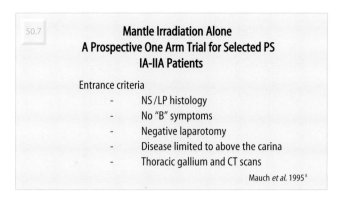

**Mantle Irradiation Alone
A Prospective One Arm Trial for Selected PS
IA-IIA Patients**

Entrance criteria
- NS/LP histology
- No "B" symptoms
- Negative laparotomy
- Disease limited to above the carina
- Thoracic gallium and CT scans

Mauch *et al.* 1995 [8]

The 20 year relapse-free survival for 79 carefully staged patients was about 75%, and survival was also high, at 80-90% [50.8]. Hence, with laparotomy staging and careful selection, one can identify a group of patients who require limited amounts of radiation and enjoy excellent long-term results.

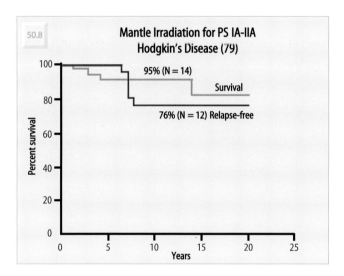

Mantle Irradiation for PS IA-IIA Hodgkin's Disease (79)

95% (N = 14) Survival
76% (N = 12) Relapse-free

The other approach, reported by the EORTC [50.9] in their H6 trial[9] (and also by a number of other groups), is to base treatment on clinical staging. In the H6 trial patients were randomized between clinical and laparotomy staging, and entry criteria were again very selective. Patients all had clinical Stage I or very limited Stage II disease with only two sites of involvement, no large mediastinal masses, no markers of advanced disease (B symptoms or a high ESR). The histology was mostly nodular sclerosis or lymphocyte predominance.

About 30% of patients were up-staged, all of whom received combined modality therapy. The patients were laparotomy staged: if they were Stage I they were given mantle treatment; and if they had more extensive disease they received subtotal nodal radiotherapy.

When staging laparotomy was compared with clinical staging, there was a slight difference in progression-free survival but this was not significant

[50.10]. The difference between the two survival curves was also not significant. Consequently, it is equally acceptable to treat early stage Hodgkin's disease with either laparotomy staging and tailor-made treatment, or with clinical staging and combined modality therapy.

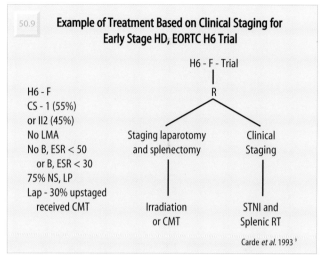

Example of Treatment Based on Clinical Staging for Early Stage HD, EORTC H6 Trial

Carde *et al.* 1993 [9]

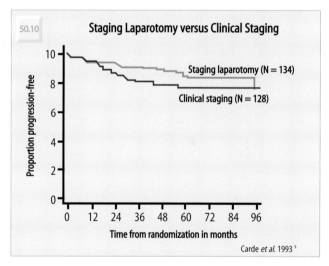

Staging Laparotomy versus Clinical Staging

Carde *et al.* 1993 [9]

Many studies have been performed with the aim of avoiding the need for pathologic staging. A classic one was from Stanford [50.11].[10] These studies investigated whether what one may call "chemo-lite" regimes with limited radiotherapy is as good as more extensive radiotherapy. At least half a dozen such randomized studies have been carried out around the world, but long-term follow-up is needed to see if the good preliminary results are substantiated over time.

The next question is whether the dose and volume can be limited when patients are treated with radiotherapy (either as part of combined modality therapy or as the sole treatment). The main reasons to reduce radiation are to reduce the risk of second tumors and also to limit other organ toxicity. Volume is probably much more important than dose — once one gives

20 Gy or 30 Gy to treat Hodgkin's disease, one is in the carcinogenic risk range, and it is clearly preferable to reduce the tissues exposed to radiation. Furthermore, there are some specific subgroups who require special consideration — for example young females, who have a high risk of breast cancer.

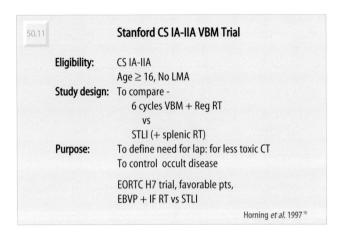

50.11	**Stanford CS IA-IIA VBM Trial**	
Eligibility:	CS IA-IIA	
	Age ≥ 16, No LMA	
Study design:	To compare -	
	6 cycles VBM + Reg RT	
	vs	
	STLI (+ splenic RT)	
Purpose:	To define need for lap: for less toxic CT	
	To control occult disease	
	EORTC H7 trial, favorable pts,	
	EBVP + IF RT vs STLI	
		Horning et al. 1997[10]

For these reasons in our current studies of chemotherapy and radiation, we use mantles which exclude the axillary fields (if axillary nodes were not involved), and we try to avoid irradiating breast tissue. These issues have not been adequately addressed yet in the literature, but the risk of secondary tumors means that volume is more of a problem than dose.

When is combined modality treatment required [50.12]? There are a number of clinical features (of which the classic one is a large mediastinal mass) which suggest that radiotherapy alone is unlikely to be successful, and that a staging laparotomy is not needed.[1] The other indication for chemotherapy is probably the presence of multiple B symptoms, particularly weight loss and fever. In the Stanford analysis that group fared very poorly, and such patients require upfront chemotherapy.

50.12	**When Is Combined Modality Treatment Required?**
	Are there high-risk subgroups that are "bad actors" that need very aggressive treatment?
	Is "chemo-lite" plus involved field radiation the optimal approach for favorable patients?

Some of the classic data for large mediastinal masses are shown in [50.13] where combined modality therapy is compared to radiotherapy alone. The relapse rate after radiotherapy alone is relatively high — about 50%. But again these patients can be salvaged with chemotherapy. However, an important issue is the location of the mass and what it is overlying,

and not necessarily its size. Some large masses can be treated with radiotherapy alone, whereas some narrow elongated masses that run down to the diaphragm require combined modality therapy. It may therefore not be appropriate simply to measure the ratio of the mass to the chest width, and to follow the rule that if it is greater than a third it requires combined modality therapy. It is necessary to know, for example, whether one can give high dose radiotherapy without compromising the heart or lung. If this is possible, radiotherapy alone may be reasonable, but if not, combined modality therapy is appropriate. If radiotherapy alone is reasonable, laparotomy may or may not be required, depending on other presenting factors.

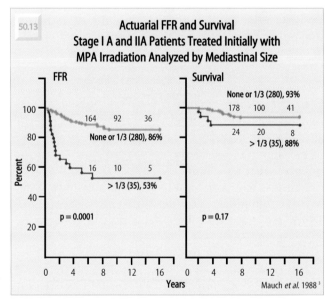

50.13	**Actuarial FFR and Survival** **Stage I A and IIA Patients Treated Initially with** **MPA Irradiation Analyzed by Mediastinal Size**

Mauch et al. 1988[3]

The last question is — what is the role of chemotherapy alone? One current issue, now that less toxic regimens are being proposed, is whether there is a risk of developing drug resistance and thereby compromising survival? It is evident today from Hodgkin's survival curves that late relapses occur, so that it is important to know whether "chemo-lite" regimes will induce a drug resistant phenotype in some patients, making it difficult to salvage them later?

There have been two major studies on the use of chemotherapy alone, one by medical oncologists[11] and one by radiation oncologists[12] [50.14]. These data can be analyzed in a variety of ways — for example, one can include cases with large mediastinal masses or take out poor prognosis Stage II patients. These different ways of studying the data obviously influence the final conclusions. In the NCI study, when very favorable prognosis patients were excluded and some high risk patients were included, the radiotherapy group fared worse. The reason was that some patients with large mediastinal masses were initially included, and some Stage I patients with limited peripheral disease, all of whom were cured, were not included. If they had been included in the radiotherapy group, the survival curves would have been improved. Nevertheless, optimal chemotherapy, as used in the NCI study — in other words aggressive treatment with MOPP (or likely other regimens) — in good hands is an effective treatment.

50.14	CT Alone versus Wide-field RT (STLI /TLI)	
	NAT Cancer Inst. [11]	Ital PROS RAND S [12]
N patients	82	89
Stage	PS IB, IIA, IIB	PS IA - IIA
Design	MOPP vs STLI	MOPP vs STLI
FFR (8 year)	82% vs 74%	64% vs 76%
Survival (8 year)	90% vs 85%	56% vs 93%
		Mauch et al. 1994 [1]

In the Italian randomized study freedom from relapse was worse with chemotherapy alone, and survival was worse because there was great difficulty in salvaging the chemotherapy relapses. In consequence, treating all patients with chemotherapy is not necessarily appropriate. If that strategy starts to be adopted with the less intensive "chemo-lite" regimens, there may be difficulty in the future in salvaging patients.

Hodgkin's disease is a lesson in long-term follow-up and a lesson in complications. Of the patients who die over the long-term, many still die of Hodgkin's disease [50.15].[13] As we reduce our therapies, and give less aggressive treatment, we run the risk of having patients fail. It would obviously be undesirable to see an increase in Hodgkin's deaths as a result of giving less aggressive treatment.

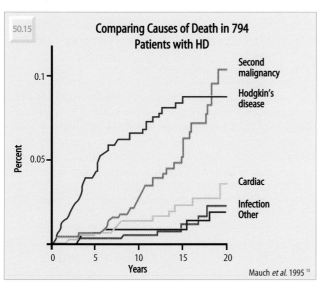

50.15 Comparing Causes of Death in 794 Patients with HD

Mauch et al. 1995 [13]

An aspect which emerges over time is that of second malignancies or late organ dysfunction, and we are faced with the issue of how to balance a maximal cure rate with a minimum of complications. To evaluate this, long-term follow-up, of fifteen or twenty years, is needed since there are no good surrogate endpoints earlier in the disease course.

The approach to the treatment of Hodgkin's disease that is currently used at the Joint Center for Radiation Therapy is shown in [50.16] to [50.18]. For favorable presentations, such as Stage IA lymphocyte predominance cases and some Stage IA nodular sclerosis female patients, mantle radiotherapy alone may be appropriate. For Stage IA nodular sclerosis cases and Stage IIA patients, with disease that is subcarinal but high up in the chest, staging by laparotomy is still performed. In effect, a strategy which could be described as overstaging and undertreating is adopted, using mantle irradiation alone or some modifications of this [50.16].

50.16	Recommendations 1995 Favorable Prognosis CS I-II
Presentation	CS IA LP HD
Treatment	Mantle RT alone
Presentation	CS IA NS/MC, CS IIA NS/LP, No subcarinal or hilar disease, no LMA
Staging	Negative laparotomy
Treatment	Mantle RT alone, or MPA RT

For patients with a more intermediate prognosis, who have a 25-30% chance of being upstaged, laparotomy staging and radiotherapy alone can be used [50.17]. Alternatively, one of the many current chemotherapy approaches can be adopted, such as EBVP, or a few cycles of MOPP or ABVD or a related regimen, together with involved field radiotherapy.

50.17	Recommendations 1995 Intermediate Prognosis CS I-II
Presentation (1)	CS IIA with subcarinal or hilar disease CS IIA MC, CS IB-IIB with night sweats
Staging	Negative laparotomy
Treatment	MPA RT
Presentation (2)	CS IIA with subcarinal or hilar disease, CS IIA MC, CS IB-IIB with night sweats
Treatment	ABVD x6, and IF or MANTLE RT: Clinical trials of RT and CT

To summarize, the current challenge in early stage Hodgkin's disease is how to minimize treatment toxicity while maintaining a high cure rate. Staging and treating patients by pre-treatment prognostic factors is now popular. IIowever, it is not always valid to use prospective factors derived retrospectively from a prior clinical trial. Does this approach require more treatment, using chemotherapy for more patients as part of the primary treatment, or is there a risk of a higher relapse rate from the less intensive treatments? Are less toxic chemotherapeutic regimens as effective and can relapses be salvaged? Careful long-term follow-up is essential [50.18].

Finally, the advice of Dr. Glatstein, one of the author's mentors, is worth quoting:

"there are three or four right ways of treating early stage Hodgkin's disease, and three or four wrong ways — just make sure you don't pick one of the wrong ones!"

> **50.18** **Summary - Early Stage HD**
>
> Current issues are how to deal with successful treatment
> -   minimizing toxicity while maintaining high cure rate
>
> Staging and treating by pre-treatment prognostic factors
> -   do retrospectively derived factors hold when used prospectively?
> -   does this approach ultimately require more treatment by using chemotherapy as part of primary treatment or for relapse?
>
> Less toxic chemotherapeutic regimens
> -   are these as effective and can relapses be salvaged?
>
> Careful, long-term follow-up is essential

ACKNOWLEDGEMENTS

Figure [50.1] is a reproduction of the portrait of Thomas Hodgkin, which hangs in the Gordon Museum, KCL (Guy's Campus), and is reproduced here by permission of the Curator.

The following figures are reproduced with copyright permission of W.B. Saunders:
[50.3] and [50.4] - reproduced from *J Clin Oncol* 1989; **7**: 81-91.
[50.5] and [50.13] - reproduced from *J Clin Oncol* 1988; **6**: 1576-83.
[50.6] and [50.14] - reproduced from *Blood* 1994; **83**: 318-329.
[50.7] - reproduced from *J Clin Oncol* 1995; **13**: 947-52
[50.9] - reproduced from *J Clin Oncol* 1993; **11**: 2258-72.
[50.11] - reproduced from *J Clin Oncol* 1997; **15**: 1736-1744.

Figure [50.15] is reproduced from *Cancer J Sci Am* 1995; **1**: 33-42 with copyright permission of Scientific American, Inc.

REFERENCES

1. Mauch PM. Controversies in the management of early stage Hodgkin's disease. *Blood* 1994; **83**: 318-29.

2. Leibenhaut MH, Hoppe RT, Efron B, Halpern J, Nelsen T, Rosenberg SA. Prognostic indicators of laparotomy findings in clinical stage I-II supradiaphragmatic Hodgkin's disease. *J Clin Oncol* 1989; **7**: 81-91.

3. Mauch P, Tarbell N, Weinstein H *et al.* Stage IA and IIA Supradiaphragmatic Hodgkin's disease: Prognostic factors in surgically staged patients treated with mantle and paraortic irradiation. *J Clin Oncol* 1988; **6**: 1576-83.

4. Rosenberg SA, Kaplan HS. The evolution and summary results of the Stanford randomized clinical trials of the management of Hodgkin's disease: 1962-1984. *Int J Radiat Oncol Biol Phys* 1985; **11**: 5-22.

5. Fuller LM, Hutchison GB. Collaborative clinical trial for stage I and II Hodgkin's disease: significance of mediastinal and nonmediastinal disease in laparotomy- and non-laparotomy-staged patients. *Cancer Treat Rep* 1982; **66**: 775-87.

6. Haybittle JL, Hayhoe FG, Easterling MJ *et al.* Review of British National Lymphoma Investigation studies of Hodgkin's disease and development of prognostic index. *Lancet* 1985;**1**: 967-72.

7. Hope-Stone HF. The place of radiotherapy in the management of localised Hodgkin's disease (Report no 11). *Clin Radiol* 1981; **32**: 519-22.

8. Mauch PM, Canellos GP, Shulman LN *et al.* Mantle irradiation alone for selected patients with laparotomy-staged IA to IIA Hodgkin's disease: preliminary results of a prospective trial. *J Clin Oncol* 1995; **13**: 947-52.

9. Carde P, Hagenbeek A, Hayat M *et al.* Clinical staging versus laparotomy and combined modality with MOPP versus ABVD in early-stage Hodgkin's disease: the H6 twin randomized trials from the European Organization for Research and Treatment of Cancer Lymphoma Cooperative Group. *J Clin Oncol* 1993; **11**: 2258-72.

10. Horning SJ, Hoppe RT, Mason J *et al.* Stanford-Kaiser Permanente G1 study for clinical stage I to IIA Hodgkin's disease: subtotal lymphoid irradiation versus vinblastine, methotrexate, and bleomycin chemotherapy and regional irradiation. *J Clin Oncol* 1997; **15**: 1736-44.

11. Longo DL, Glatstein E, Duffey PL *et al.* Radiation therapy versus combination chemotherapy in the treatment of early-stage Hodgkin's disease: seven-year results of a prospective randomized trial. *J Clin Oncol* 1991; **9**: 906-17.

12. Biti GP, Cimino G, Cartoni C *et al.* Extended-field radiotherapy is superior to MOPP chemotherapy for the treatment of pathologic stage I-IIA Hodgkin's disease: eight-year update of an Italian prospective randomized study. *J Clin Oncol* 1992; **10**: 378-82.

13. Mauch PM, Kalish LA, Marcus KC *et al.* Long-term survival in Hodgkin's disease. *Cancer J Sci Am* 1995; **1**: 33-42.

Treatment of advanced Hodgkin's disease

G P Canellos

Question: Is alternating combination chemotherapy superior to a single combination?

The principles of chemotherapy and the drugs used, and the general problems of toxicity associated with chemotherapy regimens, are now well known. However, several unresolved issues have emerged over the years in relation to the treatment of Hodgkin's disease.

The MOPP regimen was the standard chemotherapy treatment for this disease in the United States from about 1970 to 1985, but in the early 1980s interest developed in regimens in which MOPP was alternated with some other drug combinations. The Golde-Coleman hypothesis, based on data from Vancouver, argued that the capacity of tumor cells to become resistant to chemotherapy would be reduced if alternating chemotherapy were to be given in successive cycles. This idea had a certain theoretical appeal and some experimental support from animal work. Some early clinical studies therefore compared alternating combination chemotherapy with single regimen treatment. They aimed to establish whether the better therapeutic result outweighed the increased toxicity due to the additive effect of all the drugs.

Outlined in [51.1] are most of these randomized trials that have been performed, and shows the drug combinations compared in different series.[1-7] The conclusion is that these alternating regimens proved superior to MOPP in terms of progression-free survival and also, in many circumstances, of overall survival. The possible exceptions are one EORTC trial and the first Bethesda/NCI series, in which OPP alternated with CABS regimen. In most series, MOPP was alternated with ABVD or an ABVD-like regime. Consequently, the clear message was that alternating chemotherapy was better than MOPP alone in the treatment of advanced Hodgkin's disease.

51.1 Randomized Trials Comparing Alternating Combination Chemotherapy Regimens to MOPP or a Variant

	CR rate	RFS	PFS	Survival
Milan [1]				
MOPP	74%	46%	37%	58%
MOPP/ABVD	89%	68%	61%	69%
p value	NS	0.002	0.005	NS at 10 years
CALGB [2]				
MOPP	67%	48%	50%	64%
ABVD	82%	64%	62%	72%
MOPP/ABVD	83%	64%	65%	75%
p value	0.006	—	0.02	NS
ECOG [3]				
BCVPP	73%	56%	49%	68%
MOPP/ABVD	80%	61%	61%	75%
p value	NS	NS	NS	NS
EORTC [4]				
MOPP	57%	61%	43%	57%
MOPP/ABVD	59%	69%	60%	65%
p value	NS	NA	0.013	NS
UK/BNLI [5]				
LOPP	57%	52%	32%	66%
LOPP/EVAP	64%	72%	47%	75%
p value	NS	< 0.001	—	< 0.05
NCI/Bethesda [6]				
MOPP	91%	65%	68%	80%
MOPP/CABS	92%	72%	54%	72%
p value	NS	NS	NS	NS
Manchester/Bart's [7]				
MVPP	55%	—	66%	71%
ChlVPP/EVA	68%	—	80%	80%
p value	—	—	NS	NS

Alternating chemotherapy was not, however, easy to administer, since it required, at least in the early Milan experience, twelve months of alternation. The Vancouver group therefore created a hybrid regime based on combining the MOPP and ABVD regimens.

This raised the question of whether this hybrid program, involving a multiplicity of agents, was superior to alternating chemotherapy, and at least three randomized trials suggested it was not [51.2].[8] There is one unpublished study from the ECOG, which used more of a sequential than an alternating regime, that did show an advantage, but to the best of the author's knowledge most of the studies of "hybridization" of chemotherapy agents have shown, perhaps not surprisingly, no advantage over alternating regimes.

51.2	Trials in Which Hybrid Regimens of MOPP / ABVD Were Randomized Against Alternating or Sequential Therapy			
	CR rate	RFS	PFS	Survival
Milan				
MOPP / ABVD Hybrid	89%	78%	71%	75% (8 years)
MOPP / ABVD Alternating	91%	76%	69%	74%
p value	NS	NS	NS	NS
ECOG				
MOPP / ABV	81%	70%	80%	90% (30 months)
Sequential MOPP x 6-8, ABVD x 3	76%	56%	67%	85%
p value	NS	0.04	0.007	0.04
NCI / Canada				
MOPP / ABV	85%	---	75%	84% (5 years)
MOPP / ABVD Alternating	82%	---	70%	84%
p value	---	---	NS	NS
				Duggan et al. 1997 [8]

This Table does not include the current intergroup trial, in which the hybrid regimen was compared to ABVD alone. That intergroup trial was closed with 856 patients. The toxicity of the hybrid arm was excessive without any advantage over ABVD at three years of follow-up.[8]

When the Dana-Farber Center joined the CALGB in 1982, a study was organized which compared alternating chemotherapy with classical MOPP and classical ABVD [51.3]. At that time there was great concern over MOPP, because it was apparent that at least 3% of the patients, and probably more, developed myelodysplasia or acute leukemia. Practically all males are sterilized by it, as were probably all females above the age of 25 or 30. It was a difficult regimen to give, being associated with considerable toxicity, poor patient tolerance, the need for great dose modification, and marrow intolerance. The ABVD regimen, which was pioneered in Milan, was claimed not to induce secondary leukemia, nor to cause sterilization, and to produce only minimal cardiotoxicity, with modest pulmonary toxicity. In consequence, about 400 patients were prospectively randomized, and a "crossover" was incorporated, i.e. patients who failed to respond to one regime were switched to the other.

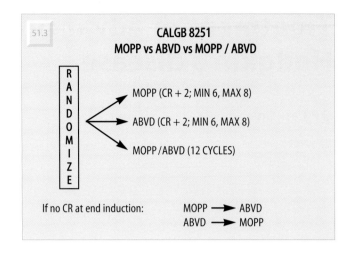

Data were published in the *New England Journal of Medicine* [51.4], and have been updated to cover the following two years. The progressionfree and treatment failure curves show the poorest results for the MOPP group. The curves for the alternating regimen and ABVD alone are similar. This again suggests that it is not necessary to give twelve months of chemotherapy to achieve a good result in Stage III or IV disease, and that both of these regimes are clearly superior to MOPP.[2]

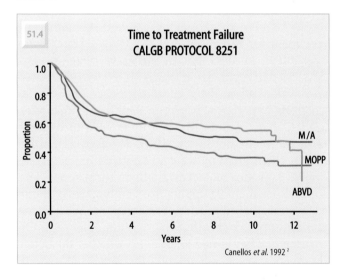

The long survival currently achieved for Hodgkin's disease [51.5] reflects our ability to salvage patients who relapse, and also the relatively indolent nature of the disease, even in relapse. The survival curves for different regimens are essentially the same, although some statisticians predict that, with the passage of time, significant differences will emerge. The important lesson is that it is not necessary to use MOPP, and this has led to a "counter-revolution" in the use of alkylating agent regimens. ABVD has become the most commonly used regimen, at least in this country. It may be noted, however, that, despite all of its advantages, it does have some side effects, including bleomycin induced pulmonary toxicity.

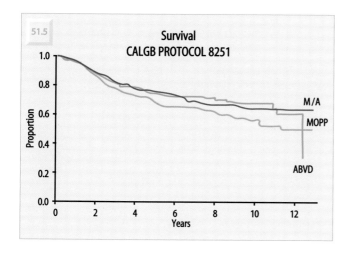

Survival
CALGB PROTOCOL 8251

One of the other interesting spinoffs of the trial was that when patients "crossed over", because of incomplete remission, there was a difference in survival related to their first regime. Survival was poorer for patients changing from MOPP to ABVD, although it should be noted that this is no longer statistically significant [51.6]. This suggests, however, that there may be less cross-resistance if a patient starts on a regimen which does not contain an alkylating agent and crosses over to one that does.

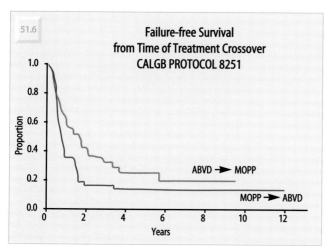

Failure-free Survival
from Time of Treatment Crossover
CALGB PROTOCOL 8251

Such studies have led to the development of a large number of non-alkylating agent regimens, not all of which have been tested in advanced disease. The regimes summarized here all avoid alkylating agents, and use etoposide, anthrocyclines and vinca drugs, with or without prednisolone [51.7].

In the author's view, the popularity of some of these regimes stems from their avoidance of the unpredictable pulmonary toxicity that one occasionally sees with bleomycin, with or without radiation, which can still be fatal in 1-2% of patients. However, whether these regimens would prove equivalent to ABVD if compared directly has never been demonstrated.

Non-alkylating Chemotherapy Regimens	Mg/m²	Days
ABVD		
Doxorubicin	25 IV	1, 15
Bleomycin	10 units	1, 15
Vinblastine	6	1, 15
Dacarbazine	375	1, 15
EVA		
Etoposide	100	1, 2, 3
Vinblastine	6	1
Doxorubicin	50	1 q. 28 days
EVAP		
Etoposide	150 p.o.(200)	1-3
Vinblastine	6 (10)	1, 8
Doxorubicin	25	1, 8
Prednisone	25	1, 8
VEEP		
Vincristine	1.4 (2.0)	1, 8
Epirubicin	50	1 q. 21 days
Etoposide	100	1-4
Prednisolone	100 p.o.	1-8
NOVP		
Mitoxantrone	10	1
Vincristine	1.4	8 q. 21 days
Vinblastine	6	1
Prednisone	100 p.o.	1-5

Another issue is how bulky a tumor must be in advanced disease to require complementary radiation therapy. Does this influence survival? There have been several randomized trials - for example, in one from the South West Oncology Group, patients with masses bigger than 6 cms were given radiation therapy. A study, published in the *Annals of Internal Medicine*, showed no survival advantage for complementary radiation therapy in advanced stage disease.[9]

The issue is probably accentuated by the fact that most patients have a residual mass, detectable either radiographically or by CT scan. [51.8] is from a study published by our group some years ago of patients with residual masses.[10] Patients were separated into those with large versus minimal masses, and their progress and that of the mass itself were analyzed. The relapse rate was not significantly related to the size of residual mass, and it was evident that residual abnormalities can persist for a long time.

Gallium scans have made it possible to assess these residual masses. Pilot data from the Duke group [51.9] show that patients with residual positive gallium scans have strikingly different likelihoods of relapse and overall survival compared to patients with negative scans, and this may possibly offer a means of assessing residual masses and targeting positive patients for complementary radiotherapy. It is generally accepted that large mediastinal masses are candidates for complementary radiotherapy, but it is the smaller ones that pose a problem.   It has never been clearly established how big a mass should be to justify radiotherapy.

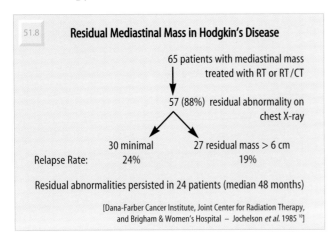

Is there a role for complementary radiotherapy in Stage III and IV patients? A randomized trial from Germany, in which 2,000 rads was compared with continuation of chemotherapy in patients who achieved a clinical remission, showed no difference.[11] The author's own bias is that there is no value in radiating lesser masses once a good partial or complete remission (as assessed radiographically and from a negative gallium scan) has been achieved. The only exceptions are patients with very large mediastinal masses who remain at Stage III or IV.

Chemotherapy can be given over twelve weeks, as was shown for the British regimen VAPEC-B and for the Stanford V protocol [51.10].[12,13] This has the advantage that treatment is complete in twelve weeks, but it does involve the patient in weekly chemotherapy. Some of the side effects of these agents are probably avoidable, but it is an interesting way of giving chemotherapy based on the MACOP-B principle of the Vancouver group.

The next issue to consider is that of salvage therapy for patients who fail chemotherapy. Several studies (from Stanford, the NCI and Vancouver) have assessed risk factors [51.11].[13] These are relevant because of the current enthusiasm for using high dose therapy, sometimes without taking into account its intrinsic toxicity, morbidity, and mortality. It may be possible in some cases to achieve similar results with less intensive therapy.

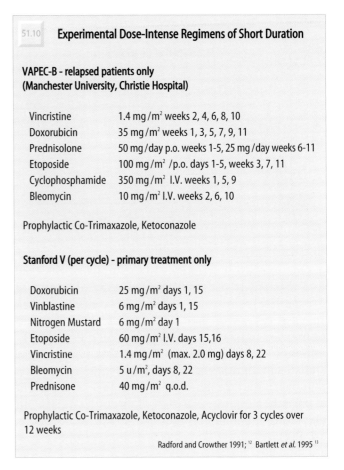

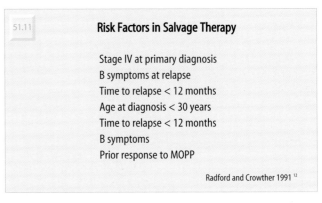

The Vancouver series [51.12], published some years ago, showed that patients who do not have adverse prognostic features respond very well to second line treatment, whatever regime is used.[14] In contrast, patients with poor prognostic characteristics do extremely poorly.

The NCI/Bethesda data [51.13] on patients who received further treatment with MOPP after having relapsed on this protocol showed a clear difference in relapse-free survival between patients whose first remission was greater than twelve months and those whose remission lasted less than twelve months.[15] Clearly, patients who relapse within twelve months have a poor prognosis, with a survival of only 10-20%.

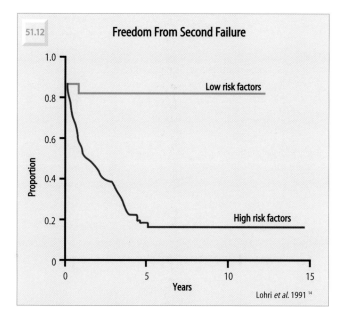

Freedom From Second Failure

Lohri et al. 1991 [14]

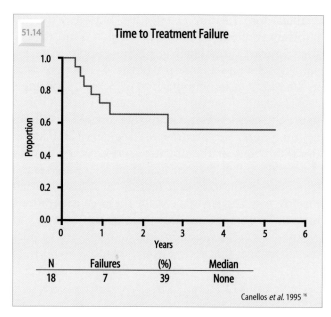

Time to Treatment Failure

N	Failures	(%)	Median
18	7	39	None

Canellos et al. 1995 [16]

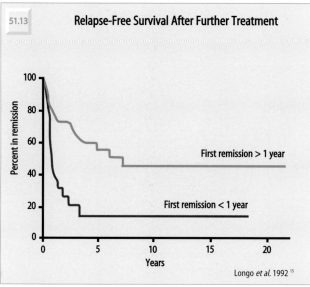

Relapse-Free Survival After Further Treatment

Longo et al. 1992 [15]

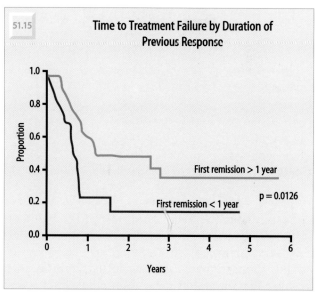

Time to Treatment Failure by Duration of Previous Response

p = 0.0126

Shown in [51.14] is the time to relapse from complete remission for those 18 who achieved a CR following EVA used as a salvage regimen for MOPP failures. When the data is analyzed in terms of the length of the first remission, the results are almost the same as those reviewed above.

The duration of first remission is therefore significant. Shown in [51.15] is what can be achieved with second line therapy if the initial remission lasts more than a year.

These criteria can be applied not only in the context of conventional dose chemotherapy, but also to high dose chemotherapy. Many multivariate analyses have identified risk factors, as shown in [51.16], such as the amount of prior therapy, the patient's condition, duration of first remission, performance status, and bulky disease.

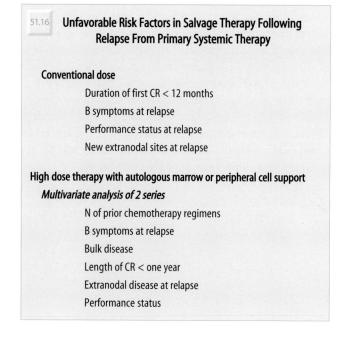

51.16 Unfavorable Risk Factors in Salvage Therapy Following Relapse From Primary Systemic Therapy

Conventional dose

    Duration of first CR < 12 months

    B symptoms at relapse

    Performance status at relapse

    New extranodal sites at relapse

High dose therapy with autologous marrow or peripheral cell support

  Multivariate analysis of 2 series

    N of prior chemotherapy regimens

    B symptoms at relapse

    Bulk disease

    Length of CR < one year

    Extranodal disease at relapse

    Performance status

High dose therapy is effective, but there is still uncertainty about the setting in which it is most effective. However, it is likely to be most appropriate for patients who have a poor prognosis. Series published in the recent years, summarized in [51.17], show high responsiveness and variable progression-free survival figures.[17-22] Generally speaking, the longer the follow-up, the poorer the progression-free survival, making the point that in therapeutic studies of Hodgkin's disease the full pattern only emerges after many years. One other point to note is that the death rate due to toxicity was about 10%. All of these considerations have to be brought into the equation, and one has to balance a 1015% morbidity/mortality figure against the advantages that accrue from high dose therapy.

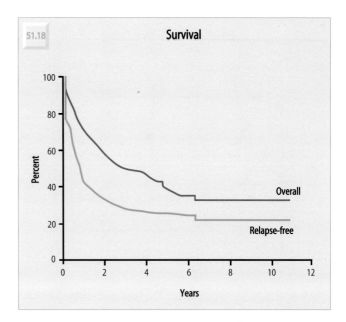

51.18   **Survival**

| 51.17 | **Overall Results of ABMT in Hodgkin's Disease (1993-95)** |

Series date	Total patients	Progression-free survival (time)	Median follow-up (months)	Toxic deaths
City of Hope, 1995 [17]	85	52% (3 years)	28	11
Vancouver, 1994 [18]	58	64% (4 years)	27	3
Toronto, 1993 [19]	73	38.6% (4 years	30	7
Nebraska, 1993 [20]	128	25% (4 years)	77	11
Rochester, 1993 [21]	47	49% (3 years)	24	8
UCH/London, 1993 [22]	155	50% (5 years)	36	20
TOTAL	**546**			**60**

Results from the Nebraska series [51.18], based on long follow-ups, show overall survival and relapse-free survival which are less than 30% at 5 years.[20] When these figures are re-plotted, taking into account the amount of prior chemotherapy (i.e. one regimen, two regimens or more), the results resemble those achieved with second line regular dose chemotherapy [51.19]. There is a benefit of 10%, or at the most 20%, from using intensification. Very few studies, if any, have compared regular chemotherapy directly with transplantation in the salvage setting, and there is some scepticism about the advantages of transplantation, especially when the patient selection involved is taken into account. However, transplantation may offer a clear-cut benefit for a minority of patients who have been heavily pretreated.

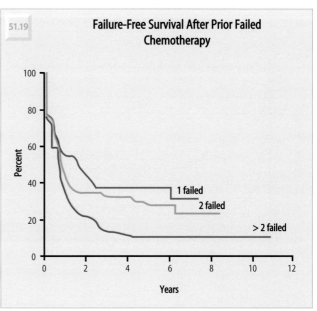

51.19   **Failure-Free Survival After Prior Failed Chemotherapy**

Finally, is there a role for dose intensification as part of initial therapy? This is an important question, but there is no scientific answer. However, a prognostic factor analysis has been performed in Hodgkin's disease, and thus far this shows no group which has such a poor prognosis that high dose therapy is justified as initial treatment, given its side effects. It was not possible to identify a substantial subgroup with an outcome worse than 50%.

REFERENCES

1. Bonadonna G, Valagussa P, Santoro A. Alternating non-cross-resistant combination chemotherapy or MOPP in stage IV Hodgkin's disease. A report of 8-year results. *Ann Intern Med* 1986; **104**: 739-46.

2. Canellos GP, Anderson JR, Propert KJ *et al.* Chemotherapy of advanced Hodgkin's disease with MOPP, ABVD, or MOPP alternating with ABVD. *N Engl J Med* 1992; **327**: 1478-84.

3. Glick J, Tsiatis A, Schilsky R *et al.* A randomized Phase III trial of MOPP/ABV hybrid versus sequential MOPP-ABVD for advanced Hodgkin's disease: preliminary results of the intergroup trial [abstract #1074]. *Proc ASCO* 1991; **10**: 271.

4. Somers R, Carde P, Henry-Amar M *et al.* A randomized study in Stage IIIB and IV Hodgkin's disease comparing eight courses of MOPP versus an alternation of MOPP with ABVD: a European Organization for Research and Treatment of Cancer Lymphoma Cooperative Group and Groupe Pierre-et-Marie-Curie controlled clinical trial. *J Clin Oncol* 1994; **12**: 279-87.

5. Hancock BW, Vaughan Hudson G, Vaughan Hudson B *et al.* LOPP alternating with EVAP is superior to LOPP alone in the initial treatment of advanced Hodgkin's disease: results of a British National Lymphoma Investigation trial. *J Clin Oncol* 1992; **10**: 1252-8.

6. Longo DL, Duffey PL, De Vita VT Jr *et al.* Treatment of advanced-stage Hodgkin's disease: alternating non-crossresistant MOPP / CABS is not superior to MOPP. *J Clin Oncol* 1991; **9**: 1409-20.

7. Radford JA, Crowther D, Rohatiner AZ *et al.* Results of a randomized trial comparing MVPP chemotherapy with a hybrid regimen, ChlVPP/EVA, in the initial treatment of Hodgkin's disease. *J Clin Oncol* 1995; **13**: 2379-85.

8. Duggan D, Petroni G, Johnson J *et al.* MOPP/ABV vs. ABVD for advanced Hodgkin's disease - a preliminary report of CALGB 8952 (with SWOG, ECOG, NCIC). *Proc ASCO* 1997; **15**: 12a.

9. Fabian CJ, Mansfield CM, Dahlberg S *et al.* Low-dose involved field radiation after chemotherapy in advanced Hodgkin disease. A Southwest Oncology Group randomized study. *Ann Intern Med* 1994; **120**: 903-12.

10. Jochelson M, Mauch P, Balikian J, Rosenthal D, Canellos G. The significance of the residual mediastinal mass in treated Hodgkin's disease. *J Clin Oncol* 1985; **3**: 637-40.

11. Diehl V, Loeffler M, Pfreundschuh M *et al.* Further chemotherapy versus low-dose involved-field radiotherapy as consolidation of complete remission after six cycles of alternating chemotherapy in patients with advance Hodgkin's disease. German Hodgkins' Study Group (GHSG). *Ann Oncol* 1995; **6**: 901-10.

12. Radford JA, Crowther D. Treatment of relapsed Hodgkin's disease using a weekly chemotherapy of short duration: results of a pilot study in 20 patients. *Ann Oncol* 1991; **2**: 505-9.

13. Bartlett NL, Rosenberg SA, Hoppe RT, Hancock SL, Horning SJ. Brief chemotherapy, Stanford V, and adjuvant radiotherapy for bulky or advanced-stage Hodgkin's disease: a preliminary report. *J Clin Oncol* 1995; **13**: 1080-8.

14. Lohri A, Barnett M, Fairey RN *et al.* Outcome of treatment of first relapse of Hodgkin's disease after primary chemotherapy: identification of risk factors from the British Columbia experience 1970 to 1988. *Blood* 1991; **77**: 2292-8.

15. Longo DL, Duffey PL, Young RC *et al.* Conventional-dose salvage combination chemotherapy in patients relapsing with Hodgkin's disease after combination chemotherapy: the low probability for cure. *J Clin Oncol* 1992; **10**: 210-8.

16. Canellos GP, Petroni GR, Barcos M, Duggan DB, Peterson BA. Etoposide, vinblastine, and doxorubicin: an active regimen for the treatment of Hodgkin's disease in relapse following MOPP. Cancer and Leukemia Group B. *J Clin Oncol* 1995; **13**: 2005-11.

17. Nademanee A, O'Donnell MR, Snyder DS *et al.* High-dose chemotherapy with or without total body irradiation followed by autologous bone marrow and/or peripheral blood stem cell transplantation for patients with relapsed and refractory Hodgkin's disease: results in 85 patients with analysis of prognostic factors. *Blood* 1995; **85**: 1381-90.

18. Reece DE, Connors JM, Spinelli JJ *et al.* Intensive therapy with cyclophosphamide, carmustine, etoposide +/- cisplatin, and autologous bone marrow transplantation for Hodgkin's disease in first relapse after combination chemotherapy. *Blood* 1994; **83**: 1193-9.

19. Crump M, Smith AM, Brandwein J *et al.* High-dose etoposide and melphalan, and autologous bone marrow transplantation for patients with advanced Hodgkin's disease: importance of disease status at transplant. *J Clin Oncol* 1993; **11**: 704-11.

20. Bierman PJ, Bagin RG, Jagannath S *et al.* High dose chemotherapy followed by autologous hematopoietic rescue in Hodgkin's disease: long-term follow-up in 128 patients. *Ann Oncol* 1993; **4**: 767-73.

21. Rapoport AP, Rowe JM, Kouides PA *et al.* One hundred autotransplants for relapsed or refractory Hodgkin's disease and lymphoma: value of pretransplant disease status for predicting outcome. *J Clin Oncol* 1993; **11**: 2351-61.

22. Chopra R, McMillan AK, Linch DC *et al.* The place of high-dose BEAM therapy and autologous bone marrow transplantation in poor-risk Hodgkin's disease. A single-center eight-year study of 155 patients. *Blood* 1993; **81**: 1137-45.

Diagnosis of Hodgkin's disease, Hodgkin's-like anaplastic large cell lymphoma, and T cell/histiocyte-rich B cell lymphoma

H Stein

Although Hodgkin's disease is relatively well defined, there are borderline cases in which this disease overlaps with non-Hodgkin's lymphoma. Fortunately, there are only two such areas: lymphocyte predominance Hodgkin's disease (LPHD) versus T-cell-rich B cell lymphoma (TCRBCL); and classical Hodgkin's disease versus anaplastic large cell lymphoma (ALCL) [52.1]. Before dealing with these overlaps in detail, we should consider why it is necessary to be concerned about the distinction between these diseases. The answer lies in their different clinical behavior. TCRBCL is an aggressive disorder – as reflected in the fact that patients suffering from this disease are usually at Stage III and IV – whereas LPHD is indolent, and usually presents at Stage I or II. Bone marrow involvement is frequent in TCRBCL but rarely in LPHD. There are also hints that ALCL progresses more rapidly than classical Hodgkin's disease, and that patients with ALCL benefit more from aggressive treatment than do classical Hodgkin's disease patients [52.2].

as concrete as possible, participants were asked to submit atypical cases of Hodgkin's disease and related disorders. The cases were carefully reviewed by the expert panel of hematopathologists before the Workshop and a list of possible diagnostic criteria was drawn up. These and other criteria were discussed at the Workshop along with the cases presented.

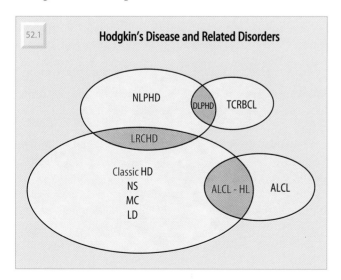

52.1 **Hodgkin's Disease and Related Disorders**

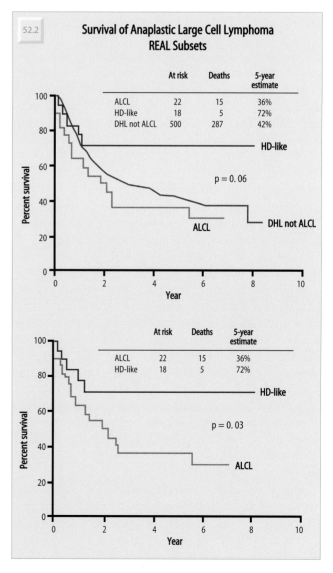

52.2 **Survival of Anaplastic Large Cell Lymphoma REAL Subsets**

Because of their clinical relevance, these borderline problems were discussed extensively at a Workshop in Toledo in 1994. To make the discussions

As far as the distinction between TCRBCL and LPHD is concerned, the expert panel felt, and this was agreed by the majority of the participants, that the most important criterion for the differential diagnosis is the architectural pattern. In LPHD there is always some degree of nodularity, due to accumulations of B cells. This may be difficult to recognize in H and E stained sections, but is easily revealed by staining for a pan-B cell marker, such as CD20. At the Workshop it was confirmed that B cell staining in LPHD will reveal in all instances some degree of nodularity and if this is completely missing the diagnosis should be TCRBCL.

The distribution of the neoplastic cells was also considered to be of importance, since they are found in a nodular distribution in LPHD, whereas in TCRBCL they are more diffusely scattered in the cellular background. A "popcorn" appearance of the neoplastic cells was seen more frequently in LPHD. Immunologic markers on the other hand proved to be of little help because the tumor cells in both neoplasms exhibit the same antigen profile (i.e. positivity for CD20 and J chain and often for EMA).

Concerning the reactive cellular component, the general opinion was that the infiltrating T cells found in TCRBCL are more irregular in their nuclear shape than those occurring in LPHD. Finally, there was agreement that meshworks of follicular dendritic cells are seen in nearly all cases of LPHD, but not in TCRBCL.

Although the Toledo Workshop was informative, the criteria which it considered did not resolve the diagnostic problems. The author therefore subsequently organized, in collaboration with Dr. Diehl and on behalf of the European Lymphoma Task Force, a new Workshop on LPHD. Oncology centers throughout the world were asked to submit typical and atypical cases. Paraffin blocks and clinical data were submitted on 550 cases by 16 centers. This material is under evaluation, but it is already clear that the real problem is not the differential diagnosis between LPHD and TCRBCL, but between LPHD and classical Hodgkin's disease, at least if one tackles the issue from the starting point of a diagnosis of LPHD. Around a third of the cases submitted with the diagnosis of LPHD proved in reality to be classical Hodgkin's disease.

The other area of overlap – between ALCL and classical Hodgkin's disease – was first addressed at a Workshop on ALCL and its possible subtypes in Berlin in 1987. It was agreed that cases can be found that appear to show features of both classical Hodgkin's disease and ALCL, and the term "ALCL-Hodgkin's related" was proposed for these borderline cases. The International Lymphoma Study Group adopted this concept but changed the term to "ALCL-Hodgkin's-like".[1]

If one considers the criteria which emerged from the Toledo Workshop for distinguishing between classical Hodgkin's disease and ALCL-Hodgkin's-like, it is evident that the neoplastic component is more cohesive in ALCL-Hodgkin's-like than in classical Hodgkin's disease. Cells with the typical morphology of Hodgkin's and Reed-Sternberg cells are constantly present in Hodgkin's disease, but are absent or rare in ALCL-Hodgkin's-like. Intrasinusoidal spread of the tumor cells was regarded as a very important criterion in favor of ALCL-Hodgkin's-like or true ALCL.

In terms of markers, it was agreed that there is a tendency for ALCL-Hodgkin's-like to be CD45-positive, whereas this molecule is usually absent in classical Hodgkin's disease. Furthermore, EMA is frequently expressed by ALCL cells, but rarely by Reed-Sternberg cells in classical Hodgkin's disease, whereas the reverse is true for CD15. The p53 molecule was found less frequently in ALCL than in Hodgkin's disease, and the same appeared to be true for EBER. Follicular dendritic cells are frequently present in Hodgkin's disease, but are usually absent in ALCL. A typical feature of Hodgkin's disease is the presence of T cell rosettes around Hodgkin and Reed-Sternberg cells. These rosettes are missing or infrequent in ALCL-Hodgkin's-like.

The application of criteria listed in [52.3] to the cases submitted for the Toledo Workshop revealed that none of the criteria discussed are really suitable for a reliable distinction between "classical Hodgkin's disease", "ALCL-Hodgkin's-like" and true ALCL.

This disappointing outcome of the Toledo Workshop prompted one of the participants, Andrew Norton, to make this drawing [52.4].

One year after the Toledo meeting, a paper in the Lancet by Orscheschek et al.[2] described the presence of the (2;5) translocation in the majority of cases of classical Hodgkin's disease, implying that this disease is closely related to ALCL and that they may represent variants of the same neoplastic disease. This very provocative finding prompted many groups to attempt to reproduce these results. Eight groups investigated a total of 250 cases of Hodgkin's disease for the (2;5) translocation, using RT-PCR, but in none of these cases was there any evidence for the translocation. The author's own group[3] has investigated

85 Hodgkin's disease cases for the presence of the (2;5) translocation by looking for ALK gene transcripts or protein products in tissue sections, using *in situ* hybridization and immunohistology. In none of the cases was there evidence for expression of the ALK gene, confirming the absence of the (2;5) translocation in Hodgkin and Reed-Sternberg cells at the single cell level. In contrast a significant proportion of ALCL cases were positive.

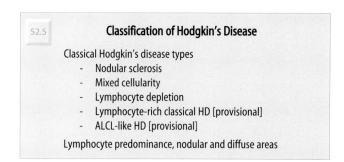

52.5 Classification of Hodgkin's Disease

Classical Hodgkin's disease types
- Nodular sclerosis
- Mixed cellularity
- Lymphocyte depletion
- Lymphocyte-rich classical HD [provisional]
- ALCL-like HD [provisional]

Lymphocyte predominance, nodular and diffuse areas

In conclusion, it may be noted that it can be of clinical interest to measure soluble CD30 (sCD30) in the sera of patients with primary systemic ALCL. Recent data have shown that levels of sCD30 are greatly increased in nearly all instances [52.6].[4] After treatment there is a fall to normal levels when complete remission is attained, and at relapse the levels increase again [52.7]. Thus, sCD30 may provide a valuable means for monitoring the response of ALCL to treatment. It remains to be seen whether this is also true for cases of ALCL-Hodgkin's-like.

52.3 Criteria for Distinction between ALCL-Hodgkin's-like and Hodgkin's Disease as Formulated at the EAHP Workshop in Toledo 1994

	ALCL-HL	Hodgkin's disease
Morphologic features		
Neoplastic component	Usually cohesive	Usually separated
Reactive component	Often minor	Usually major
Reed-Sternberg cells	May be present	Always present
Intrasinusoidal spread	Characteristic	The exception
Phenotypic features		
CD30 (Ber H2)	+*	+
CD45	+/−	−
CD15 (C3D1)	−/+	+/−
EMA (E29)	+/−	−/+
CBF.78	+ (80-90%)	−/+ (few cells) ?
BNH-9	+ (60%)**	− (5%)**?
CD3	−/+***	−/+ (heterogeneous in the same case)
CD43	+/−	−
CD20 (L26)	−/+****	−/+ (heterogeneous in the same case)
CD79a (JCB117)	−/+****	−/+
p53	−/+	+
EBER	−/+	+
FDC (CD21/1F8)	Usually absent	Often present (tumor cells within FDC meshwork)
T cell rosetting	−	+/−

Used by the panel: * positive staining; ** results can vary according to fixation; *** membrane positive and/or dot-like positivity in the Golgi area; **** positive in anaplastic variants of diffuse large B cell lymphoma

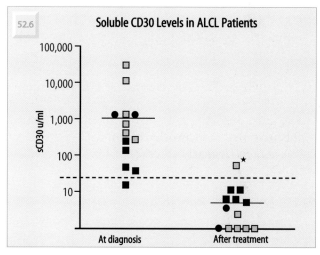

52.6 Soluble CD30 Levels in ALCL Patients

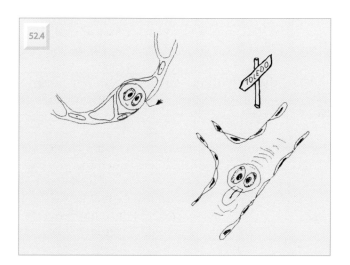

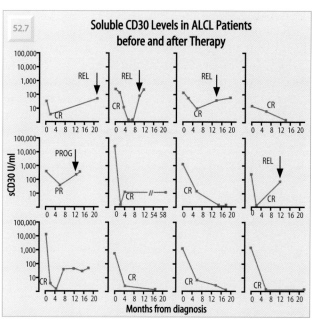

52.7 Soluble CD30 Levels in ALCL Patients before and after Therapy

In the light of all these data, ALCL-Hodgkin's-like seems very likely to be more closely related to Hodgkin's disease than to ALCL, but this requires confirmation by additional studies [52.5].

REFERENCES

1. Harris NL, Jaffe ES, Stein H *et al.* A revised European-American classification of lymphoid neoplasms: a proposal from the International Lymphoma Study Group. *Blood* 1994; **84**: 1361-92.

2. Orscheschek K, Merz H, Hell J, Binder T, Bartels H, Feller AC. Large-cell anaplastic lymphoma-specific translocation (t[2;5] [p23;q35]) in Hodgkin's disease: indication of a common pathogenesis? *Lancet* 1995; **345**: 87-90.

3. Herbst H, Anagnostopoulos J, Heinze B, Durkop H, Hummel M, Stein H. ALK gene products in anaplastic large cell lymphomas and Hodgkin's disease. *Blood* 1995; **86**: 1694-1700.

4. Nadali G, Vinante F, Stein H *et al.* Serum levels of the soluble form of CD30 molecule as a tumor marker in CD30+ anaplastic large-cell lymphoma. *J Clin Oncol* 1995; **13**: 1355-60.

Clinical relevance of Hodgkin's-like anaplastic large cell lymphoma

F Cabanillas

There are still instances in which it is difficult to define Hodgkin's disease precisely. Although in many instances the pathologist can give a confident diagnosis of Hodgkin's disease or anaplastic large cell lymphoma, a small number of cases show morphologic and/or immunophenotypic overlap [53.1].

53.1 Anaplastic Large Cell Lymphoma and Hodgkin's Disease Project Background

- Most cases of Hodgkin's disease and anaplastic large cell lymphoma (ALCL) are readily distinguished but occasionally morphologic and immunophenotypic features overlap

- Nodular Sclerosis Hodgkin's can be divided into two types:
    - Grade I (classical HDNS)
    - Grade II ("syncytial variant")

- Primary ALCL can be divided into two major types:
    - ALCL classic type (ALCL-CT)
    - ALCL Hodgkin's-like (ALCL-HL)

- Well defined morphologic and immunophenotypic criteria are not available but most ALCL-HL are reputedly CD15-, EMA+.

- Question: is ALCL-HL clinically different from classical HDNS and from ALCL-CT?

It is also known, from the work of the BNLI group, that nodular sclerosis Hodgkin's disease can be divided into two grades. Grade I corresponds to classical nodular sclerosis Hodgkin's, whereas Grade II is what in the United States is called the syncytial variant of the disease. It is important to mention that the Grade II form is not synonymous with Hodgkin's-like anaplastic large cell lymphoma, since some oncologists have assumed that the two disorders are equivalent.

It has been suggested that there are two major types of primary anaplastic large cell lymphoma - classic or common type, and the Hodgkin's-like group. Prof. Stein feels that the latter group is more closely related to anaplastic large cell lymphoma, but some data are presented in this chapter that may

contradict that view. These result from a study in which we attempted to see how Hodgkin's-like anaplastic large cell lymphoma differed clinically from Hodgkin's disease on the one hand, and from anaplastic large cell lymphoma on the other. Although there are no absolute morphological or immunotypic criteria, most Hodgkin's-like anaplastic large cell lymphomas are supposed to be CD15-negative and EMA-positive. However, this cannot be used as the sole deciding factor, and morphology remains the most important aspect in attempting to define this entity.

To provide a background, [53.2] shows data from the Pileri series which showed that the complete response rate in 28 cases of so-called Hodgkin's-like anaplastic large cell lymphoma was identical to that of classical anaplastic large cell lymphoma.[1] The relapse rate was a little lower than in classical anaplastic large cell lymphoma but not significantly so, and the mortality rates were the same. They thus concluded that the two diseases are clinically similar, but the question that was not addressed in that study was whether there was any difference in outcome when compared to classical Hodgkin's disease. One can only make that kind of comparison if patients are treated similarly. This poses a problem: if these Hodgkin's-like anaplastic large cell lymphoma patients are treated with large cell lymphoma chemotherapy regime (as was the case in Pileri's study) it may appear that the outcome is similar to that of common type anaplastic large cell lymphoma. But what if they had been treated with therapy designed for Hodgkin's disease? Would the outcome then have been different?

If one wants to find cases of Hodgkin's-like anaplastic large cell lymphoma, how can they be identified [53.3]? Some of them might be found among cases diagnosed as nodular sclerosis Hodgkin's disease. Others might be found among cases of lymphocyte-depleted Hodgkin's disease. However, the latter is something of a vanishing diagnosis, because most of these patients are now diagnosed as classical anaplastic large cell lymphoma. In consequence, we did not look at cases in this group, because we did not have any to look at! The other source comprises patients who have been diagnosed as having anaplastic large cell lymphoma. These are divided into the common-type and the Hodgkin's-like type, with two additional rare variants.

53.2	**Treatment Outcome of ALCL-Hodgkin's-like vs ALCL-Classic Type** *Pileri Series*		
Feature		**ALCL-HD** (N = 28)	**ALCL-CT** (N = 41)
CR rate		68%	68%
Relapse from CR		21%	32%
NED		54%	46%
Dead		32%	34%

Conclusions: No major difference in outcome between ALCL-HD-like and ALCL common type
Question: Any difference in outcome from classic Hodgkin's?

Pileri *et al.* 1994 [1]

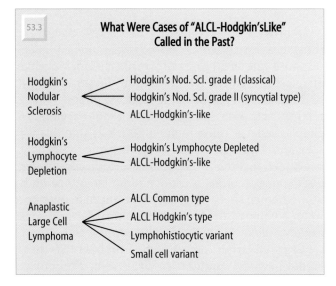

| 53.3 | **What Were Cases of "ALCL-Hodgkin'sLike" Called in the Past?** |

Hodgkin's-like anaplastic large cell lymphoma is not a diagnosis that we made previously in our institution, although we do constantly see patients in whom there is difficulty in distinguishing between Hodgkin's disease and large cell lymphoma. However, at the suggestion of Dr. Pugh in our hematopathology section, we have reviewed all cases of nodular sclerosis Hodgkin's disease registered in our studies – so that we would have a uniformly treated group of patients – and reviewed the anaplastic large cell lymphoma cases that have been entered in our clinical trials since 1988 [53.4].

| 53.4 | **Anaplastic Large Cell Lymphoma and Hodgkin's Disease Project Methodology** |

- Review of all cases of Hodgkin's nodular sclerosis stage I-III and anaplastic large cell lymphoma entered on clinical trials since 1988
- Reclassify cases using consensus diagnosis rendered by two expert blinded hematopathologists.
- Cases reclassified using morphologic criteria and immunophetype into:
    - Hodgkin's nodular sclerosis grade I
    - Hodgkin's nodular sclerosis grade II
    - Anaplastic large cell lymphoma-Hodgkin's-like (ALCL-HL)
    - Anaplastic large cell lymphoma, classic type (ALCL-CT)

Dr. Pugh reclassified those cases, based on a consensus between himself and Dr. McBride after blind review, and classified the cases into four categories: Grade I nodular sclerosis; Grade II nodular sclerosis; Hodgkin's-like anaplastic large cell lymphoma; and classic anaplastic large cell lymphoma. We attempted to put every patient into one of these four categories and did not have a group of borderline cases. We used phenotyping to support the morphological findings.

The defining criteria that were used are shown in [53.5]. It is well known how classic-type anaplastic large cell lymphoma is defined, but the Hodgkin's-like type of anaplastic large cell lymphoma was more difficult to define. When Dr. Pugh attempted to put his criteria in writing, he had to work on it overnight! The definition he came up with the following morning is that of a large cell lymphoma with certain histologic features of Hodgkin's disease including lacunar cells or Reed-Sternberg cell variants and collagenous bands. This definition does not include immunophenotypic features, because of the uncertainty about how they should be interpreted.

| 53.5 | **Definitions Used for ALCL-HD MD Anderson Project** |

- **HDNS Grade I:** Collagenous bands producing nodules of lacunar cells, classic RS cells, and variable inflammatory background.

- **HDNS Grade II:** Histologic features of HDNS with either lympho cyte depletion, increased numbers of anaplastic RS cells and variants of a prominent fibrohistiocytic pattern

- **ALCL classic type:** A large cell lymphoma composed of anaplastic cells with a cohesive growth pattern, often with prominent sinusoidal involvement.

- **ALCL Hodgkin's-like:** Large cell lymphoma with certain histologic features of Hodgkin's disease (lacunar cells, Reed-Sternberg variants and collagenous bands).

Of our initial total of 170 cases [53.6], suitable slides or blocks were not available for 50 cases (since many of our patients are referred from elsewhere). In consequence, we identified 21 that had been previously diagnosed by the M D Anderson hematopathologist as anaplastic large cell lymphoma, and 99 which had been diagnosed as Hodgkin's disease. When these cases were reviewed and reclassified, 18 of the 21 retained the original diagnosis, but two were changed to nodular sclerosis Hodgkin's disease, and one of them turned out to be the rare entity we were looking for, Hodgkin's-like anaplastic large cell lymphoma.

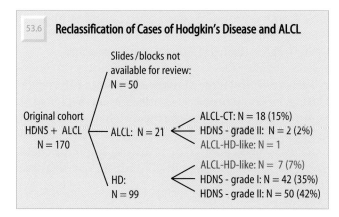

When the Hodgkin's cases were reviewed, seven were reclassified as Hodgkin's-like anaplastic large cell lymphoma, and 92 were still called nodular sclerosis disease, with 42 and 50 respectively in the Grades I and II groups. Thus only 7% of all these cases ended up as Hodgkin's-like anaplastic large cell lymphoma.

Some of the interesting clinical features which emerged are shown in [53.7]. Firstly there was some difference in mediastinal involvement. A mediastinal mass was clearly seen on chest X-ray in 74% of the cases of Grade I Hodgkin's disease, whereas this was seen in 94% of the Grade II cases. This was statistically significant. The size of the mediastinal mass was even more striking. 50% of Grade II patients had a mass larger than 7.5 cm, compared to only 30% for Grade I patients.

53.7	Comparison of Mediastinal Involvement and Size of Mediastinal Mass According to Histology		
Histology	N	Mediastinum involvement	Mediast. mass ≥ 7.5 cm
HDNS Grade I	42	74%	30%
HDNS Grade II	52	94% $p = 0.06$	50% $p = 0.03$
ALCL-HL	8	63%	50%
ALCL-CT	18	33%	0

Among the Hodgkin's-like anaplastic large cell lymphoma cases, 63% had a mediastinal mass, and in 50% it was bulky, being more than 7.5 cm in size. However, none of the patients with the classic type of anaplastic large cell lymphoma had a large mediastinal mass.

When LDH, β2-microglobulin, constitutional symptoms, clinical stage, and median age were assessed [53.8], Grade II Hodgkin's tended to present more frequently with elevated LDH than did Grade I Hodgkin's. These patients also had higher β2-microglobulin although this was not quite statistically significant. Constitutional symptoms were also more than twice as frequent in Grade II than in Grade I patients. The median age was not significantly different.

53.8	Comparison of Clinical Features According to Histology					
Histology	N	High LDH	High β-2M	B Sx	Stage III-IV	Median age
HDNS Grade I	42	15% $p < 0.05$	17%	10% $p < 0.05$	14%	30
HDNS Grade II	52	38%	30%	25%	14%	27 $p < 0.05$
ALCL-HL	8	25%	38%	38%	38%	30
ALCL-CT	18	38%	43%	50%	44%	30

B Sx = fever, night sweats or weight loss ≥ 10%

Hodgkin's-like anaplastic large cell lymphoma tended to present with less favorable features. 25% had high LDH levels, 38% had high β2-microglobulin and constitutional symptoms, 38% were Stage III and IV. The median age was slightly higher than for the Grade II cases, and this was statistically significant, but it is not a very striking difference because these were mostly young patients. The classic type of ALCL also presented with more advanced features, or worse prognostic factors than the others.

When the failure-free survival was assessed according to the diagnosis before pathologic reclassification, the nodular sclerosis Hodgkin's cases achieved a failure free survival of almost 80%, with only one late relapse [53.9]. The failure-free survival curve for classic type anaplastic large cell lymphoma showed a rapid fall off and then a plateau, as has been noted before. These cases were not subdivided before reclassification according to Grade, so cases of nodular sclerosis Hodgkin's disease of both Grade I and II are shown.

When failure-free survival according to diagnosis following reclassification was assessed, common type anaplastic large cell lymphoma had a very good outcome, and Grade I nodular sclerosis Hodgkin's also had a good prognosis [53.10]. The Grade II cases were not clearly different, although there is a hint that they might fare slightly worse, and this is not surprising because they had more adverse prognostic factors. The BNLI have also found that Grade II cases fare worse, but we cannot say that we have found a statistically significant difference at this point.

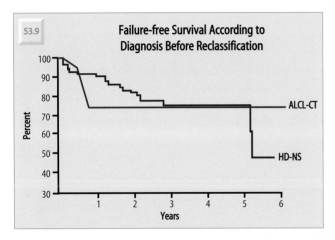

A striking aspect was the rapid initial mortality for Hodgkin's-like anaplastic large cell lymphoma patients, with a survival curve which fell to a plateau

of approximately 30%. This may seem a very poor result, but these patients were diagnosed and treated as Hodgkin's disease with the NOVP regimen plus radiation. Had they been treated with a large cell lymphoma-like regime, the outcome might have been very different. The important message is that they may represent a subset of patients who should be treated as if they had large cell lymphoma.

In conclusion [53.11], cases of Hodgkin's-like anaplastic large cell lymphoma usually present with more advanced disease, more constitutional symptoms, older age and larger mediastinal masses than Grade I nodular sclerosis Hodgkin's. Furthermore, they may have a worse prognosis than Grade I and II nodular sclerosis Hodgkin's, but this is in the context of their being treated like Hodgkin's disease patients.

Patients with Grade II disease present with higher LDH levels and more frequent mediastinal involvement than Grade I cases, as well as with larger mediastinal masses. There is no significant difference in outcome between Grade I and Grade II disease, although there is perhaps a suggestion that Grade II has a worse prognosis.

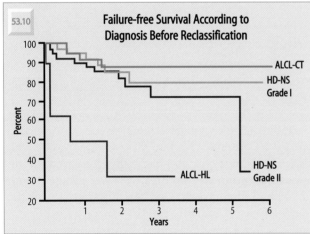

53.11

**ALCL-Hodgkin's Like
Conclusions**

- In comparison with HDNS, patients with ALCL-HL usually present with:
    – more advanced disease
    – constitutional symptoms
    – older age
    – larger mediastinal masses than HDNS grade I

- ALCL -HL has a worse prognosis than HDNS grade I / II

- In comparison with HDNS grade I, HDNS-grade II presents with higher LDH, more frequent mediastinal involvement and larger mediastinal masses.

- No significant difference in outcome between HDNS grade I and grade II.

REFERENCES

1. Pileri S, Bocchia M, Baroni CD *et al.* Anaplastic large cell lymphoma (CD30 +/Ki-1+): results of a prospective clinico-pathological study of 69 cases. *Br J Haematol* 1994; **86**: 513-23.

Is it necessary to make clinical groupings of lymphoid neoplasms?

J O Armitage

The issue addressed in this chapter can be phrased as a question. Is it desirable to incorporate clinical information into a histopathologically based system for classifying lymphomas?

It is evident, if one considers previous classification systems for lymphomas, that the first of these made little attempt to incorporate clinical features. Nodularity was said to have clinical implications in the Rappaport classification, and the Lukes-Collins classification made a distinction between T and B cell lymphomas, and indicated that this had some clinical implications [54.1]. In contrast, the Kiel scheme and the Working Formulation both incorporated clinical features.

54.1	"Clinical" Groupings	
Classification		**Basis**
Rappaport		Nodularity
Lukes		T vs B
Kiel		Grade x 2
Working Formulation		Grade x 3

For clinicians, the greatest difference between the Rappaport and the Lukes-Collins schemes on the one hand and the Kiel scheme and the Working Formulation on the other lies in this aspect [54.2]. One can take the view that this is a trivial observation - that it is of little importance if we distinguish, as these schemes did, between high and low grade lymphomas. However, we should appreciate that participants in specialist courses on lymphoma are not representative of most clinicians. Most clinicians do not think that lymphomas are the most important thing in the world, nor do they spend all their waking hours thinking about them! They are physicians who, on average, see one case of Hodgkin's disease and four or five cases of non-Hodgkin's lymphoma a year. For them a simplistic approach which says "this is a good one, and this is a bad one" is important.

54.2	The biggest difference to clinicians between Kiel and Rappaport / Lukes is the addition of clinical groupings

This is certainly a major reason for the popularity of those schemes. The reason why the Kiel classification was never supplanted in Europe, and why the Working Formulation did supplant other schemes among the physicians in the United States is that they gave clinicians simple practical information. In consequence, these schemes had a huge impact because they told clinicians what they wanted to hear.

The next four figures [54.3 - 54.6], from Dr. Lister, relate to cases of non-Hodgkin's lymphoma seen at St. Bartholomew's Hospital over almost three decades. Shown in [54.3] is the survival curve of more than 1,400 cases. These are subdivided in various ways. In [54.4] they are divided on the basis of histology into high and low grade lymphomas, using the Kiel classification. These curves have the features one would anticipate - the low grade tumors continue to fall away steadily, whereas the high grade tumors fall and then tend to plateau.

There are of course other clinically related features that can be used. There is a clear distinction between groups separated on the basis of age [54.5], and [54.6] shows separation on the basis of Stage for all non-Hodgkin's lymphomas. The curves are clearly very different.

There are thus a variety of clinically relevant ways in which one can divide up non-Hodgkin's lymphomas, and it is desirable to unite histopathologic observations with clinical ones [54.7]. Any classification which keeps them separate will never become popular with clinicians.

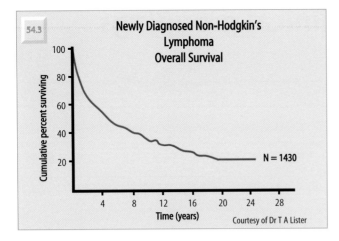

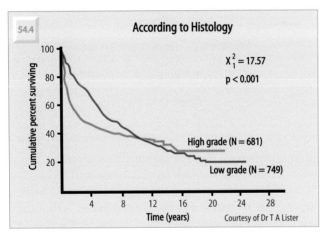

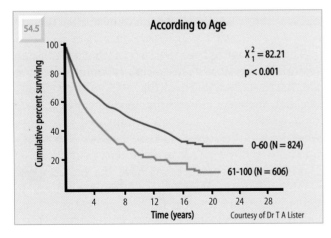

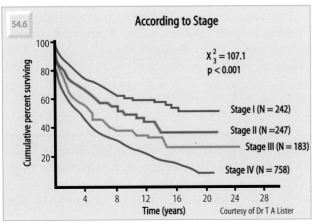

One other point is of importance for anybody interested in lymphomas. There is a tendency sometimes to take criticisms of our ideas as "personal and not business". It is wise to remember that we are not, when we try to name and separate out these diseases, aiming for the truth [54.8]. We are trying to formulate guidelines which allow us to take better care of our patients. That is of course a clinician's viewpoint, but it would be desirable if that viewpoint provided the background against which we advanced our common cause.

54.8   We are not aiming for "Truth" - merely a plan that

allows us to use clinically our understanding of solid

tumours of the immune system

The way a clinician now approaches a lymphoma patient is that he or she expects to be told by the pathologist what kind of disorder it is [54.9]. What the clinician then does, whether or not it is a formal process, is to use that diagnosis to put the patient into a clinical group, which provides some indication of outcome, suitable therapy, the chances of involving certain parts of the body, etc. With that information one plans staging and then, with that combined information, one treats the patient.

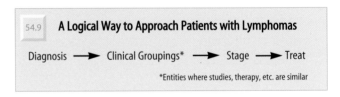

54.9   A Logical Way to Approach Patients with Lymphomas

Diagnosis ⟶ Clinical Groupings* ⟶ Stage ⟶ Treat

*Entities where studies, therapy, etc. are similar

Physicians will always tend to follow this procedure, whether or not a classification system provides explicit help with doing it. Most clinicians who manage lymphoma patients are not primarily lymphoma doctors, so that anything that helps them with this step of moving from diagnosis to clinical grouping is likely to prove popular.

The scheme shown in [54.10] shows how lymphomas can be divided up in this way into clinically relevant groups. Clinicians can then take other information and subdivide those groups.

54.10	A Proposal for Clinical Groups		
Disease extent	**Histologic groupings**		
	Indolent (Rarely curable)	**Aggressive** (Sometimes curable)	**Highly aggressive** (Urgent Rx, CNS, Rx)
Local / minimal	XRT vs chemo +/- XRT	Comb. chemo +/- XRT	Comb. chemo + CNX Rx
Extensive	Observation vs chemo	Comb. chemo	Comb. chemo+ NNS Rx

54.11	Sub-groups of NHL Possible Subdivisions	
Basic groups:	Small cell	
	Follicular	
	Mantle cell	
	Large cell	
	Very high grade	
Subcategories:	International Prognostic Index	
	Localized vs disseminated	
	Response to specific Rx	
	Unusual clinical course	
	Histology / genetics / immunology	

An important question is therefore: can pathologists provide information which will allow these disorders to be subdivided in a logical way by their clinical colleagues? [54.11] shows how this might be done. Today, when we receive a diagnosis of non-Hodgkin's lymphoma, these are the five broad groups that one immediately thinks about. Follicular lymphomas are distinctive, as are other lymphomas made up of small cells, with the exception of mantle cell lymphoma, which also seems to be a separate entity. Next there are the large cell lymphomas, that we know we can cure fairly regularly; and finally there are the unusual ones, that are more common in children and are often leukemic.

These are the five broad groups, and there are many ways in which they can now be further subdivided. One might divide them on the basis of prognostic index or anatomic distribution. Specific therapy is also relevant - for example, small cell lymphomas of the stomach need to be separated out because antibiotics may be effective but will not of course work for other kinds of lymphomas.

Some unusual clinical courses are recognized which also need to be taken into account when we subdivide these groups. For example lymphomas associated with HIV infection carry a special prognosis. We are also now particularly interested in whether or not histopathologic or genetic or immunologic observations allow us to subdivide any of these groups in a clinically useful way. A logical way to do this is to take these groups and see if, on the basis of available information, one can find useful ways to subdivide them clinically.

Any such scheme has to be simple - if a pocket calculator is needed to assign patients into subgroups, one might as well save one's time, because people won't use it. Successful systems should be simple and easy to remember. However, if we achieve this – if it is possible to take the concepts of the REAL classification and find a way of integrating in a similar fashion the insight gained by clinicians in treating lymphoproliferative disorders – this will become the most popular classification, at least in the eyes of clinicians.

POST-SCRIPT

The concepts involved in the REAL classification have been rapidly accepted by clinicians and pathologists. In the time since the meeting where this talk was given, it has become increasingly clear that lymphomas are better considered as specific clinical/pathologic entities and not grouped. Patients will receive the best care if the natural history and response to therapy of the specific entity (such as follicular lymphoma, diffuse large B cell lymphoma, mantle cell lymphoma, peripheral T cell lymphoma, small lymphocytic lymphoma, the MALT lymphomas, and others) are accurately diagnosed. The clinician then needs to know the common sites of involvement, typical pace of disease, and appropriate therapies for the specific lymphoma. Lumping two or more entities under the rubric of "intermediate grade" or "low grade" is more likely to lose important information than to facilitate management.

However, it is important to realize that the only change from Table [54.9] is that the "clinical groupings" now represent the major subtypes of lymphoma. The follicular lymphomas and the diffuse large B cell lymphomas certainly still represent a spectrum of conditions. However, lumping follicular lymphoma with MALT lymphoma is only likely to confuse the issue.

Can aggressive lymphomas be grouped for treatment?

M A Shipp

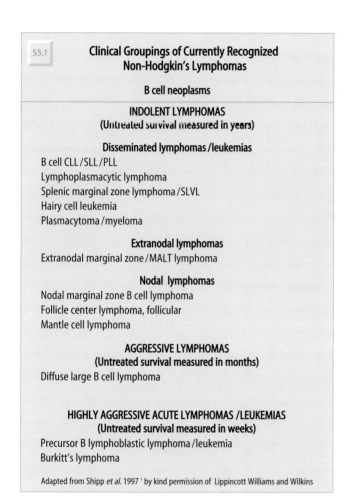

A classification of the entities described in the REAL formulation is shown in [55.1] and [55.2], but set out in a way that corresponds to how clinicians think about these disorders.

These entities are divided into three categories. First, there are the indolent lymphomas: untreated patients with these neoplasms typically have survivals that are measured in years. A second category comprises the aggressive lymphomas, for which the survival without treatment can be measured in months. Finally, there are the highly aggressive lymphomas and leukemias. Untreated patients with these diseases have survivals that are measured in weeks.

If the aggressive lymphomas in the Working Formulation and the REAL classification are compared, there are several obvious differences. Two Working Formulation entities are not found in the REAL classification: diffuse small cleaved cell lymphoma and the diffuse mixed small and large cell lymphoma. The reason is that today, with new information, we realise that these Working Formulation categories did not represent discrete entities.

To be more specific, if we list the diseases that make up the category of diffuse small cleaved cell lymphoma, one of the main entities previously classified as diffuse small cleaved cell lymphoma is now recognized as mantle cell lymphoma [55.3]. Mantle cell lymphoma is a unique entity that combines some of the least favorable characteristics of both indolent and aggressive non-Hodgkin's lymphomas.

55.3	Diffuse Small Cleaved Cell Lymphoma is Not a Discrete Entity	
Working Formulation	**REAL classification**	
	B cell neoplasms	**T cell neoplasms**
Intermediate grade		
E. Diffuse small	Mantle cell	T cell CLL/PLL
cleaved cell	Follicle center, diffuse	LGL
	small cell	ATL/L
	Marginal zone/MALT	Angioimmunoblastic
		Angiocentric

Adapted from Shipp *et al.* 1997 [1] by kind permission of Lippincott Williams and Wilkins

Patients with mantle cell lymphoma have significantly lower failure-free survival and overall survival than patients with other indolent lymphomas. Recent retrospective analyses from SWOG and EORTC [55.4] have shown that mantle cell lymphoma patients treated on indolent lymphoma protocols had rates of relapse that were similar to other low grade diseases, but had overall survivals that were only half those of other low grade patients, as defined in the Working Formulation. On the other hand, mantle cell lymphoma patients treated with aggressive lymphoma regimens had response rates that were similar to those of other Working Formulation immediate grade patients. However, none of the mantle cell lymphoma patients appeared to be curable.

55.4	Mantle Cell Lymphoma - Natural History

SWOG retrospective analysis

Patients with MCL had significantly lower failure-free survivals and overall survivals than patients with other "indolent" lymphomas (FFS 6% vs 25%, p = 0.0002 and OS 8% vs 35%, p = 0.0001).

Fisher *et al.* 1995 [2]

EORTC retrospective analysis

MCL patients treated with CHVm-VP or PROMACE-MOPP had response rates that were similar to those of WF intermediate grade patients. No curable subset. MCL patients treated with CVP+/- interferon had rates of relapse that were similar to those of patients with WF low grade disease. Overall survivals were only half that of WF low grade patients.

Teodorovic *et al.* 1995 [3]

An important point to remember is that mantle cell lymphoma is associated with a specific molecular abnormality, and, as we learn more about the basic biology of the disease, our therapeutic approaches may be very different.

The other Working Formulation entity that is no longer identified as a discrete aggressive lymphoma is diffuse mixed small and large cell lymphoma. The different entities that used to be included in this category are listed in [55.5]. One of the major entities in this category is T-cell-rich large B cell lymphoma. This disease is now considered to be simply a variant of large B cell lymphoma. The peripheral T cell neoplasms constitute the other major category which used to be in the diffuse mixed small and large cell lymphoma group.

55.5	Diffuse Mixed Small and Large Cell Lymphoma is Not a Discrete Entity	
Working Formulation	**REAL classification**	
	B cell neoplasms	**T cell neoplasms**
Intermediate grade		
F. Diffuse mixed small	Large B cell (T cell rich)	Peripheral T cell,
and large cell	Follicle center, diffuse	unspecified
	small cell	ATL/L
	Lymphoplasmacytoid	Angioimmunoblastic
	Marginal zone/MALT	Angiocentric
	Mantle cell	Intestinal T cell
		lymphoma

Adapted from Shipp *et al.* 1997 [1] by kind permission of Lippincott Williams and Wilkins

If we consider the remaining Working Formulation aggressive lymphomas, the diffuse large cell lymphomas correspond to diffuse large B cell and peripheral T cell lymphomas in the REAL classification [55.6]. There is an ongoing debate as to whether B cell immunoblastic lymphoma is a discrete entity.

55.6	Aggressive Lymphomas	
Working Formulation	**REAL classification**	
	B cell neoplasms	**T cell neoplasms**
Intermediate grade		
G. Diffuse large cell	Diffuse large B cell	Peripheral T cell
	lymphoma	
High grade		
H. Large cell	Diffuse large B cell	Peripheral T cell
immunoblastic	lymphoma	ATL/L
		Anaplastic large cell

Adapted from Shipp *et al.* 1997 [1] by kind permission of Lippincott Williams and Wilkins

In summary, the aggressive non-Hodgkin's lymphomas that remain in the REAL classification include diffuse large B cell, anaplastic large cell and peripheral T cell neoplasms [55.7].

> **55.7   Clinical Groupings of Currently Recognized Non-Hodgkin's Lymphomas**
>
> | B cell neoplasms | T/NK cell neoplasms |
> | --- | --- |
> | **AGGRESSIVE LYMPHOMAS** (Untreated survival measured in months) | |
> | Diffuse large B cell lymphoma | Anaplastic large cell lymphoma |
> | | Peripheral T cell lymphomas |
> | **HIGHLY AGGRESSIVE ACUTE LYMPHOMA / LEUKEMIA** (Untreated survival measured in weeks) | |
> | Precursor B lymphoblastic lymphoma / leukemia | Precursor T lymphoblastic lymphoma / leukemia |
> | Burkitt's lymphoma | Adult T cell lymphoma / leukemia (HTLV1+) |
>
> Adapted from Shipp et al. 1997 [1] by kind permission of Lippincott Williams and Wilkins

We usually treat aggressive B cell lymphomas on the basis of clinical prognostic factors, and think about subdividing these diseases according to their clinical presentation. There are now different approaches to the treatment of patients depending on whether they have low risk, low intermediate risk or high intermediate/high risk disease [55.8]. Again, as we learn more about the biologic heterogeneity of these diseases, our approaches to these different risk categories are likely to be refined and improved.

> **55.8   Treatment Strategies for Aggressive B Cell Lymphomas**
>
> Aggressive B cell lymphomas can be grouped for risk-related therapy:
>
> Low risk - standard therapy (combination chemotherapy +/- RT)
>
> Low intermediate risk - judgement call
>
> High intermediate / high risk - dose intensive experimental therapy

The other two entities in the aggressive non-Hodgkin's lymphoma category are anaplastic large cell lymphoma and peripheral T cell lymphoma [55.9]. There is now enough information on the distinctiveness of anaplastic large cell lymphoma to consider this a unique entity. It is a disease that is curable with combination chemotherapy. However, there is clearly clinical heterogeneity in this disease. Many of the prognostic factors that are clinically relevant for large B cell lymphoma are also relevant for anaplastic large cell lymphoma. For example, there is a striking difference in outcome in patients who present with localized versus advanced stage disease.

It is also important to remember that there is a primary cutaneous form of anaplastic large cell lymphoma which behaves in a more indolent manner than does systemic disease. There are now data to suggest that anaplastic large cell lymphoma patients who have the (2;5) translocation constitute a clinically

unique group. Patients with this anomaly who have T cell or null cell neoplasms tend to be younger and to have better five year disease-free survivals. This hallmark karyotypic abnormality may eventually provide insights into the basic biology of this disease.

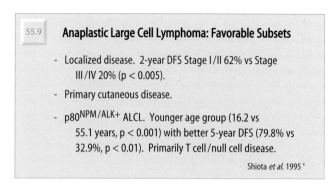

> **55.9   Anaplastic Large Cell Lymphoma: Favorable Subsets**
>
> - Localized disease. 2-year DFS Stage I/II 62% vs Stage III/IV 20% ($p < 0.005$).
> - Primary cutaneous disease.
> - p80[NPM/ALK+] ALCL. Younger age group (16.2 vs 55.1 years, $p < 0.001$) with better 5-year DFS (79.8% vs 32.9%, $p < 0.01$). Primarily T cell/null cell disease.
>
> Shiota et al. 1995 [4]

Finally, a brief comment should be made on peripheral T cell lymphomas [55.10], a category that requires further subclassification. One important point is that patients with peripheral T cell lymphoma have unique clinical characteristics: for example, they are more likely to present with advanced stage disease and B symptoms, and to have splenic and skin involvement. Patients with peripheral T cell lymphomas who achieve complete remission also have a higher risk of relapse. The data in [55.10] are from a GELA study comparing relapse rates between T cell and B cell aggressive lymphomas, which showed that 43% of T cell aggressive lymphoma patients are likely to relapse from CR compared with less then a third of B cell cases. It is therefore likely that information regarding the immunophenotype will begin to affect our decisions regarding treatment.

> **55.10   Peripheral T Cell Lymphoma (PTCLs)**
>
> - Require further subclassification: unspecified, ATL/L, angioimmunoblastic, angiocentric, intestinal T cell lymphomas.
> - More likely to present with advanced stage disease and B symptoms and to have splenic and skin involvement.
> - More likely to relapse from CR: T cell vs B cell relapse rates 43% vs 29%, $p < 0.001$.
>
> Coiffier et al. 1990 [5]

In summary [55.11], there are two aggressive non-Hodgkin's lymphoma entities from the Working Formulation that are not recognised in the REAL classification - diffuse small cleaved cell lymphoma and diffuse mixed cell lymphoma. Mantle cell lymphoma is a unique entity, with the least favorable characteristics of both indolent and aggressive lymphomas. The aggressive lymphomas that we now recognise are diffuse large B cell, anaplastic large cell and peripheral T cell lymphomas.

We can treat aggressive B cell lymphomas on the basis of clinical risk categories. Anaplastic large cell lymphoma includes certain favorable subsets that are important to distinguish. And finally, the peripheral T cell lymphomas require further subclassification, and are also more likely to relapse after achieving complete remission.

55.11   **Conclusions**

1. Working Formulation diffuse small cleaved cell lymphoma (E) and diffuse mixed small and large cell lymphoma (F) are not discrete entities.

2. Mantle cell lymphoma is a unique entity that shares some of the least favorable characteristics of both the indolent and the aggressive lymphomas.

3. Aggressive lymphomas include diffuse large B cell lymphoma, anaplastic large cell lymphoma and peripheral T cell lymphoma.

4. Aggressive B cell lymphomas can be grouped for risk-related therapy:
   Low risk - standard therapy
   Low intermediate risk - judgement call
   High intermediate / high risk - dose intensive experimental therapy

5. Anaplastic lymphoma includes favorable subsets:
   Primary cutaneous disease p80 [NPM/ALK+]
   (T cell / null cell) anaplastic lymphoma

6. Peripheral T cell lymphomas (PTCLs) require further subclassification. PTCLs are more likely to relapse from CR.

ACKNOWLEDGEMENT

Figures [55.1], [55.2], [55.3], [55.5], [55.6], and [55.7] are reproduced from DeVita VT, Hellman S, Rosenberg SA, eds. *Cancer Principles & Practice of Oncology.* Lippincott-Raven. 1997; Vol 2: 2165-2220, with copyright permission of Lippincott Williams and Wilkins.

REFERENCES

1. Shipp MA, Harris NL, Mauch PM. Non-Hodgkin's Lymphomas. In: DeVita VT, Hellman S, Rosenberg SA, eds. *Cancer Principles & Practice of Oncology.* Lippincot-Raven. 1997; Vol 2: 2165-2220.

2. Fisher RI, Dahlberg S, Nathwani BN, Banks PM, Miller TP, Grogan TM. A clinical analysis of two indolent lymphoma entities: mantle cell lymphoma and marginal zone lymphoma (including the mucosa-associated lymphoid tissue and monocytoid B-cell subcategories): a Southwest Oncology Group study. *Blood* 1995; **85**: 1075-82.

3. Teodorovic I, Pittaluga S, Kluin-Nelemans JC *et al.* Efficacy of four different regimens in 64 mantle-cell lymphoma cases: clinicopathologic comparison with 498 other non-Hodgkin's lymphoma subtypes. European Organization for the Research and Treatment of Cancer Lymphoma Cooperative Group. *J Clin Oncol* 1995; **13**: 2819-26.

4. Shiota M, Nakamura S, Ichinohasama R *et al.* Anaplastic large cell lymphomas expressing the novel chimeric protein p80NPM/ALK: a distinct clinicopathologic entity. *Blood* 1995; **86**: 1954-60.

5. Coiffier B, Brousse N, Peuchmaur M *et al.* Peripheral T-cell lymphomas have a worse prognosis than B-cell lymphomas: a prospective study of 361 immunophenotyped patients treated with the LNH-84 regimen. The GELA (Groupe d'Etude des Lymphomes Agressives). *Ann Oncol* 1990; **1**: 45-50.

FURTHER READING

Armitage JO, Greer JP, Levine AM *et al.* Peripheral T-cell lymphoma. *Cancer* 1989; **63**: 158-63.

Cheng AL, Chen YC, Wang CH *et al.* Direct comparisons of peripheral T cell lymphoma with diffuse B-cell lymphoma of comparable histological grades - should peripheral T-cell lymphoma be considered separately? *J Clin Oncol* 1989; **7**: 725-31.

Coiffier B, Berger F, Bryon PA, Magaud JP. T-cell lymphomas: immunologic, histologic, clinical, and therapeutic analysis of 63 cases. *J Clin Oncol* 1988; **6**: 1584-9.

Fisher RI, Gaynor ER, Dahlberg S *et al.* Comparison of a standard regimen (CHOP) with three intensive chemotherapy regimens for advanced non-Hodgkin's lymphoma. *N Engl J Med* 1993; **328**: 1002-6.

Gordon LI, Harrington D, Andersen J *et al.* Comparison of a second generation combination chemotherapy regimen (m-BACOD) with a standard regimen (CHOP) for advanced diffuse non-Hodgkin's lymphoma. *N Engl J Med* 1992; **327**: 1342-9.

Greer JP, Kinney MC, Collins RD *et al.* Clinical features of 31 patients with Ki-1 anaplastic large-cell lymphoma. *J Clin Oncol* 1991; **9**: 539-47.

Kwak LW, Wilson M, Weiss LM *et al.* Similar outcome of treatment of B-cell and T-cell diffuse large-cell lymphomas: the Stanford experience. *J Clin Oncol* 1991; **9**: 1426-31.

Nakamura S, Takagi N, Kojima M *et al.* Clinicopathologic study of large cell anaplastic lymphoma (Ki-1-positive large cell lymphoma) among the Japanese. *Cancer* 1991; **68**: 118-29.

Reiter A, Schrappe M, Tiemann M *et al.* Successful treatment strategy for Ki-1 anaplastic large-cell lymphoma of childhood: A prospective analysis of 62 patients enrolled in three consecutive Berlin-Frankfurt-Munster group studies. *J Clin Oncol* 1994; **12**: 899-908.

Shulman LN, Frisard B, Antin JH *et al.* Primary Ki-1 anaplastic large-cell lymphoma in adults: Clinical characteristics and therapeutic outcome. *J Clin Oncol* 1993; **11**: 937-42.

Index